Advances in Science, Technology & Innovation

IEREK Interdisciplinary Series for Sustainable Development

Advances in Science, Technology & Innovation (ASTI) is a series of peer-reviewed books based on important emerging research that redefines the current disciplinary boundaries in science, technology and innovation (STI) in order to develop integrated concepts for sustainable development. It not only discusses the progress made towards securing more resources, allocating smarter solutions, and rebalancing the relationship between nature and people, but also provides in-depth insights from comprehensive research that addresses the **17 sustainable development goals (SDGs)** as set out by the UN for 2030.

The series draws on the best research papers from various IEREK and other international conferences to promote the creation and development of viable solutions for a **sustainable future and a positive societal** transformation with the help of integrated and innovative science-based approaches. Including interdisciplinary contributions, it presents innovative approaches and highlights how they can best support both economic and sustainable development, through better use of data, more effective institutions, and global, local and individual action, for the welfare of all societies.

The series particularly features conceptual and empirical contributions from various interrelated fields of science, technology and innovation, with an emphasis on digital transformation, that focus on providing practical solutions to **ensure food, water and energy security to achieve the SDGs.** It also presents new case studies offering concrete examples of how to resolve sustainable urbanization and environmental issues in different regions of the world.

The series is intended for professionals in research and teaching, consultancies and industry, and government and international organizations. Published in collaboration with IEREK, the Springer ASTI series will acquaint readers with essential new studies in STI for sustainable development.

ASTI series has now been accepted for Scopus (September 2020). All content published in this series will start appearing on the Scopus site in early 2021.

More information about this series at http://www.springer.com/series/15883

Jihad Alja'am · Somaya Al-Maadeed ·
Osama Halabi

Editors

Emerging Technologies in Biomedical Engineering and Sustainable TeleMedicine

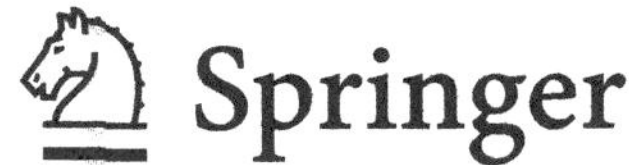 Springer

Editors
Jihad Alja'am
Department of Computer Science and Engineering
College of Engineering, Qatar University
Doha, Qatar

Somaya Al-Maadeed
Department of Computer Science and Engineering
College of Engineering, Qatar University
Doha, Qatar

Osama Halabi
Department of Computer Science and Engineering
College of Engineering, Qatar University
Doha, Qatar

ISSN 2522-8714   ISSN 2522-8722   (electronic)
Advances in Science, Technology & Innovation
IEREK Interdisciplinary Series for Sustainable Development
ISBN 978-3-030-14646-7   ISBN 978-3-030-14647-4   (eBook)
https://doi.org/10.1007/978-3-030-14647-4

Foreword

I am delighted to be given the opportunity to introduce this manuscript to a wider audience and impart its scientific value and benefits. One can pinpoint a plethora of publications, revolving around a specific thematic area, on diverse platforms and in various forms and presentation styles. However, it is seldom possible to put one's hand on a scientific asset that addresses a particular thematic area whilst putting the real-world applications right in the heart of its technical content and scientific coverage. This book pulls together the most recent research and innovation findings in bioinformatics and biomedical engineering achieved by a collection of experts from several international labs. The book consists of 12 very different but complementary chapters addressing novel enabling technologies in the field, highlighting their applicability to recently emerging global challenges.

Chapter "Internet of Medical Things (IoMT) Applications in E-Health Systems Context" displays a thorough coverage of the state of the art in Internet of Medical Things applications focussing on the underlying IoT technologies as well as fog and cloud infrastructures. Chapter "Artificial Intelligent and Machine Learning Methods in Bioinformatics and Medical Informatics" exhibits a comprehensive study of the use of artificial intelligence and machine learning methods in bioinformatics and medical informatics with particular emphasis on the use of learning processes, machine learning, text mining methods and their application to health informatics. Chapter "Human Facial Age Estimation: Handcrafted Features Versus Deep Features" presents a new method for age estimation using human facial feature extraction and analysis. The method consists of a pre-processing state and a subsequent linear regressor for handling the extracted features in such a way that can reliably estimate human age. Chapter "Multi-scale Multi-block Covariance Descriptor for a Compact Face Texture Representation: Application to Kinship Verification" presents a technique facial representation based on the pyramid multi-level scheme aiming particularly at kinship verification applications. The technique enables the encoding of the facial parts without having to detect the facial landmarks and contains a covariance descriptor that fuses several texture features for optimal identification/verification of human faces. Chapter "Continuous Wavelet Analysis and Extraction of ECG Features" proposes a wavelet-based algorithm that extracts and analyses the salient features of electrocardiogram records, whilst providing an overview of wavelet transforms and their properties. The effectiveness algorithm has been demonstrated in terms of sensitivity, positive predictivity and error rate, hence outlining its suitability for improving the processing capabilities of health systems. Chapter "e-Health Education Using Automatic Question Generation-Based Natural Language (Case Study: Respiratory Tract Infection)" addresses a particularly exciting application aiming at enhancing the reliability and validity of the myriad of information available about the coronavirus pandemic. This study presents an educational e-health platform with a particular focus on the upper respiratory tract infection, as a case study, providing critical answers that are purely based on valid information. The study harnesses a combination of enabling technologies including dynamic neural networks to create a virtual assistant that is capable of providing automatically generated bespoke answers about matters related to the infection of the upper respiratory tract with an accuracy higher than 70%. Chapter "A Novel Machine Learning Model for Adaptive Tracking and Real-Time Forecasting COVID-19 Dynamic Propagation" proposes a machine learning model for the adaptive tracking and real-time forecasting of COVID-19 outbreak. The model has been applied for the real-time forecasting of the propagation behaviour of COVID-19 in Brazil, with the simulation results and comparative analysis illustrating the efficiency and reliability of the model. Chapter "Heart Failure Occurrence: Mining Significant Patterns and 10 Days Early Prediction" outlines a study aiming at the early detection of heart failures using mining of significant patterns found in electronic health records. This study encompasses a bespoke algorithm aiming at detecting the specific patterns that come along with heart failure occurrences and then employs a recurrent neural network to predict the risk of a potential cardiac failure. Chapter "The Efficiency of the Reverse Engineering to Fabricate a New Respirator Technology Compatible with the COVID-19 Pandemic" looks into reverse engineering and repurposing a respirator for CV-19 rehabilitation purposes. Given the limitations in supply chain and delays incurred in the delivery of critical medical equipment, this study proposes 3D printing/scanning and PCB prototyping to offer a low-cost quick solution for the provision of life critical medical equipment such as the COVID-19 respirator. Chapter "Exploiting Egocentric Cues for Action Recognition for Ambient Assisted Living Applications" sheds the light on ambient assisted living applications to help elderly people to extend their independent lifestyle through the prediction of mental health issues that could seriously harm their independence. The chapter focuses on the key enablers of these applications, in particular the egocentric cameras and action recognition techniques for the analysis of egocentric videos. Chapter "Pulmonary Fibrosis Progression Prediction Using Image Processing and Machine Learning" investigates the use of image processing and machine learning techniques for identifying the progression of the COVID-19 disease. The chapter presents a conducted study aimed at modelling the severity levels of the disease and argues the importance of biological data compared to the ordinary CT scans for predicting the degeneration of the COVID-19 infected lungs. Chapter "A Simulation-Based Method to Study the LQT1 Syndrome Remotely Using the EMI Model" employs the extracellular membrane-intracellular model to simulate the effects of the long QT syndrome. Interestingly, the simulations were conducted on data taken from healthy cells, cells that exhibit the syndrome and cells that have been treated to restore healthy cardiac function. The chapter argues that the obtained simulation results demonstrate that advances in biomedical engineering combined with computer simulations can enhance the applicability of telemedicine well beyond the state of the art.

Given this unique mix of diverse but complementary topical areas of bioinformatics focusing in particular on the relevance and applicability to contemporary real-world challenges such as COVID-19, this book will prove an essential guide to the use of enabling technologies to provide modelling solutions, machine learning disease classification and identification techniques and reverse engineering schemes for optimising the time required for prototyping new designs of essential medical equipment. This book will make an interesting read to a large audience of researchers in a broad range of disciplines from both Engineering and Medical backgrounds and will enrich the experience of readers from both the academic research community and the biomedical industry.

I take pleasure in introducing this book to the targeted audience and am confident it will appeal to large segments of readers.

Yours sincerely,

December 2020

Prof. Abdul Hamid Sadka, Ph.D, CEng, FHEA, FIET, FBCS
Director of the Institute of Digital Futures
Founding Head of the Media Communications Research Group
Former Head of the Department of Electronic
and Electrical Engineering
Brunel University London
Uxbridge, England, UK

Introduction

This book on Emerging Technologies in Biomedical Engineering and Sustainable Telemedicine consists of 12 chapters on recent trend and applications in the field from different perspectives. Contributors from various experts present their findings in an incremental manner. Telemedicine is not in competition with the traditional system and services of healthcare. However, it should improve the quality of services offered by contributing to the homogenization of medicine without any geographical barriers. Telemedicine transforms local hospitals, with limited services, into a node of an integrated network. In this manner, these nodes start to play an important role in preventive medicine and in high-level management of chronic diseases. The main challenge in telemedicine development in a country consists of creating human capacity in "health informatics" and in "e-health management". The field includes synchronous and asynchronous telemedicine with e-health applications; virtual medical assistance, real-time virtual visits, digital telepathology, home health monitoring, medication adherence, wearable sensors, tele-monitoring hubs and sensors, and augmented and virtual reality. The book addresses the main challenges the health sector is facing and sheds the light on the existing gap between traditional and telemedicine healthcare. It can be an excellent reference for students and researchers interested in this field to discover the new applications and theories on the Internet of Medical things, fog and cloud computing, artificial intelligence and machine learning in health informatics, face analysis, coronavirus pandemic impact, rehabilitation, ambient assisted living applications, and coronavirus pandemic. All the chapters have been peer reviewed by experts in the field and selected accordingly. We hope that the readers will find this book highly valuable and can open new horizons for future research and applications.

Prof. Jihad Alja'am
Prof. Somaya Al-Maadeed
Dr. Osama Halabi

Contents

Internet of Medical Things (IoMT) Applications in E-Health Systems Context

An Overview and Research Challenges

Kayo Monteiro, Élisson Silva, Émerson Remigio, Guto Leoni Santos, and Patricia Takako Endo

Abstract

The Internet of Things (IoT) has been adopted by several areas of society, such as smart transportation systems, smart cities, smart agriculture, smart energy, and smart healthcare. Healthcare is an area that takes a lot of benefits from IoT technology (composing the Internet of Medical Things (IoMT)) since low-cost devices and sensors can be used to create medical assistance systems, reducing the deployment and maintenance costs, and at the same time, improving the patients and their family quality of life. However, only IoT is not able to support the complexity of e-health applications. For instance, sensors can generate a large amount of data, and IoT devices do not have enough computational capabilities to process and store these data. Thus, the cloud and fog technologies emerge to mitigate the IoT limitations, expanding the IoMT applications' capacities. Cloud computing provides virtually unlimited computational resources, while fog pushes the resources closest to the end-users, reducing the data transfer latency. Therefore, the IoT, fog, and cloud computing integration provides a robust environment for e-health systems deployment, allowing plenty of different types of IoMT applications. In this paper, we conduct a systematic mapping with the goal to overview the current state-of-the-art in IoMT applications using IoT, fog, and cloud infrastructures.

K. Monteiro · É. Silva · É. Remigio · P. T. Endo (✉)
Universidade de Pernambuco, Programa de Pós-Graduação em Engenharia de Computação, Recife, Brazil
e-mail: patricia.endo@upe.br

K. Monteiro
e-mail: khcm@ecomp.poli.br

É. Silva
e-mail: esr2@ecomp.poli.br

É. Remigio
e-mail: ers2@ecomp.poli.br

G. L. Santos
Universidade Federal de Pernambuco, Recife, Brazil
e-mail: guto.leoni@gprt.ufpe.br

1　Introduction

According to a study performed by the World Health Organization (WHO) [53], we will have the largest number of older people in history by 2020, and at the first time, it will surpass the number of children up to 5 years old. The same study also says that the life expectancy will reach 90 years by 2030, and up to 80% of the elderly population will live in low- and middle-income countries. The academic and business communities are devoting many efforts to develop new applications that promote quality of life, not only for this portion of the population but also for all those who need constant caring; services, such as vital signs monitoring, fall detection systems, heart attacks, among others, are increasingly in evidence [35]. The greater demand for long-term patient health care and the need of controlling health care expenditures require the efficient use of low-cost technologies in order to apply them in the best possible way.

Most of these e-health systems rely on the Internet of Things (IoT) infrastructure (or specifically the Internet of Medical Things (IoMT)). Smartphones and smart devices are very popular and cheaper than medical specialized devices. With these IoT devices, it is possible to collect different vital signals, such as heart rate, body temperature, blood pressure, or still identify if the user has suffered some accident, such as a fall, by using accelerometer sensor data. However, commonly the IoT devices do not provide good computational processing, long-term storage, neither guarantee of the quality of service (QoS) due to their hardware capacity limitations. So, to mitigate this issue, IoT has two major allies to provide e-health applications with high availability and quality: cloud and fog computing.

As the cloud architectures were not designed to operate integrated to IoT, there are some transversal requirements that

© Springer Nature Switzerland AG 2021
J. Alja'am et al. (eds.), *Emerging Technologies in Biomedical Engineering and Sustainable TeleMedicine*,
Advances in Science, Technology & Innovation, https://doi.org/10.1007/978-3-030-14647-4_1

should be complied with, such as scalability, interoperability, flexibility, reliability, efficiency, availability, and security, as well as specific computation, storage, and communication needs [46]. On the other hand, fog computing has emerged between the cloud and the IoT devices, providing data management and also communication services to facilitate the execution of relevant IoT applications through intermediary compute elements (fog nodes) [23].

In this paper, we provide an overview of IoMT applications in e-health systems, through a systematic mapping, focusing on the integrated infrastructure with IoT, fog, and cloud, the methods used in the literature to evaluate them, and the main research challenges opportunities in this area.

The reaming of this work is organized as follows: Sect. 2 describes the methodology applied to perform the systematic mapping study; Sect. 3 presents and discuss the results obtained in the study; Sect. 4 highlights the main research challenges found in the literature; and Sect. 5 concludes the work.

2 Systematic Mapping Methodology

In this paper, we follow the methodology presented by [39] to conduct a systematic mapping. Fig. 1 shows the process steps and the respective outcomes. For details about the methodology, see [39].

2.1 Definition of Research Questions

According to [39], the main goal of a systematic mapping *"is to provide an overview of a given research area, and identify the quantity and type of research available within it."* Often, a systematic map can also be used to map the frequencies of publication over time to see trends.

These goals are described as following four research questions (RQs):

- **RQ 1**: What is the current state-of-the-art in e-health applications using fog-to-cloud computing infrastructure?
- **RQ 2**: What are the most common e-health applications using fog-to-cloud computing infrastructure?
- **RQ 3**: What are the most common methods (simulation, modeling, or prototype) used to evaluate e-health applications?
- **RQ 4**: What are the main challenges for implementing e-health applications that rely on fog-to-cloud computing?

2.2 Conduct Search for Primary Studies

According to [39], the primary studies *"are identified by using search strings on scientific databases or browsing manually through relevant conference proceedings or journal publications."*

In this work, we performed the primary studies identification by using search string on relevant databases. The search string used was *("e-health" OR "ehealth" OR healthcare) AND ("cloud" OR "fog") AND ("Internet of things" OR "IoT")*; and the scientific databases were IEEE,[1] ACM,[2] and Springer.[3] We retrieved 83 papers from IEEE, 1 from ACM and 81 from Springer.

2.3 Screening of Papers for Inclusion and Exclusion

As we can find many papers that are not strictly related to our research questions (or can not answer our research questions), we should define inclusion and exclusion criteria. Table 1 shows the inclusion and exclusion criteria we used in this systematic map.

As IoT, fog computing and cloud computing are very embracing terms, they are often used in abstracts but not necessarily are addressed further in the paper. So the application of the inclusion and exclusion criteria is done manually, and in order to avoid bias, when doubt appeared, more than one researcher classified the paper. After the screening, we kept 38 papers from IEEE and 12 from Springer (see Appendix).

2.4 Keywording of Abstracts

In this step, we made a little adaptation proposed by [39]. Originally, authors use keywording to *"reduce the time needed in developing the classification scheme and ensuring that the scheme takes the existing studies into account"* by reading the abstract and keywords of the selected papers. If the abstract is poor of information quality, they take into consideration the introduction and the conclusion of the paper.

In our systematic map, we are not considering the two steps separately (read the abstract and keywords, and then the introduction); we are reading the abstract, the introduction, and the conclusions of the paper to provide the classification. The Fig. 2 shows our keywording step (gray squares) adapted from [39] (dot line squares are not being used in our work).

From the keywording step, we focused on defining the main contribution facets of the papers, as described in Table 2, considering infrastructure, application, monitoring type, and evaluation method.

---

[1] https://ieeexplore.ieee.org/Xplore/home.jsp.
[2] https://dl.acm.org/.
[3] https://www.springer.com/gp.

Process steps

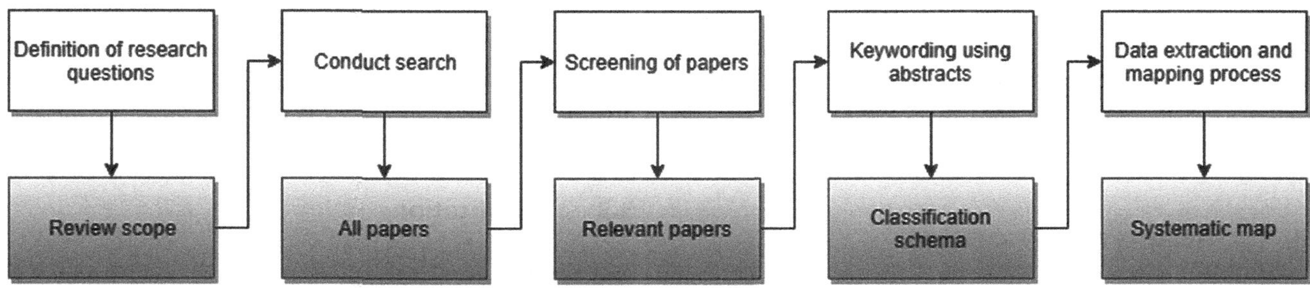

Outcomes

Fig. 1 Systematic map schema from [39]

Table 1 Inclusion and exclusion criteria to select relevant papers

Inclusion	The abstract explicitly mentions e-health applications on fog or IoT or cloud computing context. We consider papers from the conference, journals, and chapter books
Exclusion	The paper lies outside the e-health application on fog or IoT or cloud computing. e-health is a common application, however, some papers do not deal with this integrated infrastructure, so they are not considered in our systematic map

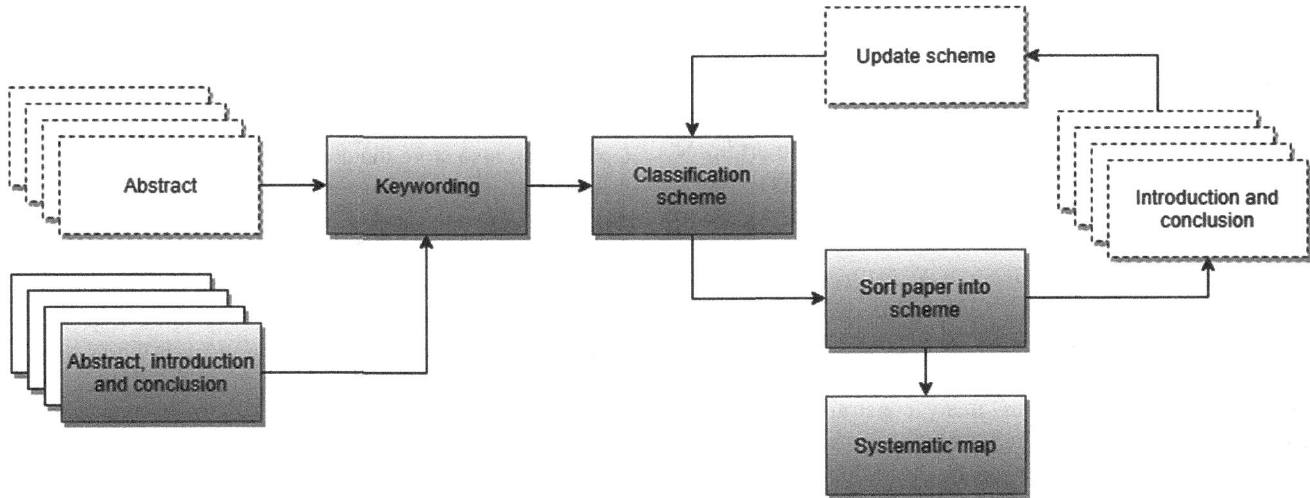

Fig. 2 Keywording of abstract adapted from [39]

Table 2 Contribution facets of the papers

Category	Description
Infrastructure	Describe what kind of scenario the IoMT application is deployed, as well as the infrastructure used (combination of IoT, fog, and cloud)
Application	Specify the IoMT application
Monitoring target	Describe how and what is being monitored by the IoMT application presented in the work
Evaluation	Describe how the proposal was evaluated in the work

2.5　Data Extraction and Mapping of Papers

After having the classification scheme produced in the previous step, the relevant articles are sorted, and the actual data extraction takes place [39]. The results of the systematic mapping are presented in the next section.

3　Results and Discussions

Based on the systematic mapping methodology, this section presents the works classified according to the Table 2: infrastructure, application, monitoring target, and evaluation.

3.1　Infrastructure

Usually, IoMT applications generate a big amount of data that must be processed and stored for several purposes: help doctors in diagnoses, alert the patient family in emergency cases, identify patterns of patients with a certain disease, and so on.

However, IoT devices are not able to deal with big data, and additional infrastructures with high performance and availability are needed. We found papers that present e-health systems that integrate IoT devices with cloud and fog infrastructures. We classify the works according to the context where the e-health system is used: personal use, hospital, smart home, and generic (no specific context defined in paper). Table 3 presents a summary of the papers classified by infrastructure configuration and context.

According to [55], *the rising of the IoT technology pushes the ambient intelligence forward by expanding the scale and scope of the healthcare domain significantly,* creating innovative non-invasive health monitoring solutions. However, as said previously, there are many constraints inherent to IoT devices, such as limited memory, power supply, and processing capabilities that negatively influence the performance of the networks [7,17], making them commonly cloud infrastructure-dependent. This fact is reflected in the works found in the literature, where the predominant infrastructure configuration is the integrated cloud + IoT with 75,51%. When we consider only the hospital context, the integrated cloud + IoT infrastructure is used by all solutions.

Another observation from the results is about the recent studies on the integrated cloud + fog + IoT infrastructure. From the 50 papers observed, 56% are dated from 2017 or 2018, however, when analyzing only the papers that rely on the cloud + fog + IoT infrastructure, this number increases to approximately 83%. Based on this result, we can reconfirm that fog computing is playing its role as the technology that "glues" IoT and cloud resources, especially when the IoMT applications are the focus, providing a quick action when is needed (such as push notification for fall, pulse abnormality, gas leak…) [19]. According to [9], *"local processing is mandatory in order to reduce the network data traffic […]. For this reason, we are trying to perform data processing as near as possible to the device that is generating the data,"*

3.2　Applications

As described previously, there is an infrastructure diversity when deploying healthcare systems, and this diversity also impacts the IoMT applications. In our study, we identified some groups of applications according to the infrastructure configuration, as described in Table 4. Each application group uses different types of monitoring.

Next, we briefly describe the applications found during our systematic mapping study.

Patient monitoring at hospitals: Several IoMT applications were found aimed at the patients who are hospitalized, ranging from bed monitoring as described in [18,33] to more complex applications, such as [49], where the sedation levels of the patients in the surgical block are monitored.

Patients monitoring in daily activities: The IoMT applications that provide follow-up of patients during their daily activities are commonly used by patients who are accompanied by physicians but need constant monitoring of their vital signs, such as blood pressure and heart rate. These applications also store the collected data at clouds for future checks or analysis, and in case of any abnormality the application can generate some alert for the doctor who follows up [2,5,12,17,20,22,25,26,28,31,32,34,40,43]. Among these applications, it is interesting to note one proposed by [52], where daily follow-up of patients is performed during the period of 30 days after their discharge from the hospital to avoid recurrence of the patient with the same problem.

Patient with respiratory diseases monitoring: This IoMT application is focused on patients who have chronic respiratory diseases and need to use oxygen cylinders, as described in [33]. The solution intends to offer a better quality of life to people who present this need. Originally, this application was designed to be used in a personal use context, following the patient during his or her daily activities; however, this IoMT application can also be used in hospitalizations because through the IoT devices, it can measure the amount of oxygen that is circulating through the patient's blood.

Elderly monitoring: With the life expectancy increasing [53], a number of IoMT applications that monitor the elderly have emerged, ranging from monitoring blood pressure, [22,29,32] to daily activities monitoring with the use of digital image processing techniques [31]. Among the applications found during this study, authors in [34] present a solution to avoid the thermal shock that is one of the biggest causes of

Table 3 Commonly infrastructure configurations used by IoMT applications

Infrastructure	Context	Paper
Cloud + IoT	Personal use	[10,12,15,16,25,34,38,40,42–44]
	Hospital	[3,4,8,18,20,21,26,28,31,36,37]
	Smart Home	[17,27,41,48,54]
	Generic	[1,5,6,22,29,32,50–52]
Cloud + Fog + IoT	Personal use	[2,9,19,33]
	Smart Home	[14,49]
	Generic	[7,11,13,24,30,55]

Table 4 IoMT application and monitoring

Application	Monitoring	Paper
Patient follow-up in hospital	Temperature; blood pressure; heart rate; glucose level	[18,33,49]
Follow-up of patients in daily activities	Temperature; blood pressure; heart rate	[2,5,12,17,20,22,25,26,28,31,32,34,40,43, 52]
Follow-up of patients with respiratory diseases	Heart rate; volume of oxygen in the blood	[33]
Follow-up the elderly	Temperature; blood pressure; heart rate; glucose level; digital image processing	[22,29,32,34]
Patient follow-up during rehabilitation	Motion sensors; digital image processing	[4]
Detection of variation of artificial light	Digital image processing	[11]
Detection of diseases through the iris	Digital image processing	[2]
Detection of heart attacks	Heart rate	[12,20,44]
Fall detection	Digital image processing; accelerometer; gyroscope; motion sensors	[4,30,55]
Realization and evaluation of electrocardiogram	Blood pressure; heart rate	[9,25,28]

deaths of the elderly in Japan, in this application the authors use sensors spread by the house and a sensor next to the elderly all of them interconnected to a center that controls the temperature of the environment, during the locomotion of the elderly by the house the system goes heating the surroundings closer to avoid the shock thermal.

Patient monitoring during rehabilitation: Daily monitoring of the patient during rehabilitation in order to measure and follow-up the progress in real time is possible through the IoMT application proposed by [4], that monitors through digital image processing and motion sensors.

Detection of variation of artificial light: In [11], authors present an IoMT application for detection of health risks by the variation of artificial light. The application consists of image processing to identify which risks the user is being exposed to the light oscillation at frequencies of approximately 3 to 70 Hz, may cause seizures in highly sensitive individuals while moderate scintillation frequencies, from about 100 Hz to up to 500 Hz, can lead to the indirect perception of strobe effects.

Detection of diseases through the iris: Authors in [2] propose a solution that also is based on image processing, where through an image of the patient's iris, the application can identify possible diseases, besides making the monitoring of the patient's mood.

Detection of heart attacks: IoMT applications for detection of heart attacks, as presented by [2], make use of several types of wearable devices, for example, smartwatch and smartphone, where through the application it is possible to monitor the patient and identify when an attack occurs and generate a notification to the nearest hospital. In our systematic mapping study, we found other three applications that detect heart attacks: [12,20,44].

Human fall detection: We found human fall detection applications in [4,30,55]. These IoMT applications can use different data sources, such as unmask motion sensors used in devices connected to the body, accelerometer and gyroscope data, images, videos, and so on. After the fall detection, an alert is generated for the patient's emergency contacts (family members, caregivers, or medical staff).

Electrocardiogram exam: During the study were found some IoMT applications that deal with electrocardiogram data: [9,25,28]. From these applications, it is interesting to note the one presented by [9]; it is an application used to provide quality medical services to patients who live in remote locations, where through an IoT device, it is possible to do the electrocardiogram, and then the data is sent to the cloud, where medical specialists can evaluate it.

3.3 Target of Monitoring

IoT devices play an important role in the development of e-health systems. By having a great diversity of devices, one can monitor several aspects related to patients' health. During our research, we found the following targets of monitoring: temperature, blood pressure, heart rate, glucose level, humidity, and room temperature, vibration, luminosity, sound, digital image processing, accelerometer, gyroscope, motion sensors, electromyography (EMG), and volume of oxygen in the blood.

The IoMT applications presented in the previous section require devices to collect the data, and these devices are segmented according to the target of the monitoring, as described next.

Temperature: The monitoring of body temperature is collected through the sensors interconnected to the patient's body. These data are used to feed patient monitoring applications. Through these applications, the data can be accessed by the family or doctors who follow the patient. These applications are described in [5,22,34,43]. This type of monitoring is also used in hospital patient follow-up applications as presented in [18,33].

Blood pressure: Sensors that monitor blood pressure are used in patient follow-up applications in hospitals [18,33], realization and evaluation of electrocardiogram [9], and follow-up of patients in daily activities [12,17,26,43].

Heart rate: The heart rate is a vital sign used in patient's follow-up during their daily activities [2,5,17,20,25,28,31, 32,43], patient follow-up applications in hospitals [18,49]. In addition, authors in [9] also collect heart rate to perform cardiologic exams in patients who live in more distant places.

Glucose level: The monitoring of the glucose level was found in some IoMT applications whose main objective is the monitoring of the patient who has chronic diseases that suffer glucose influence [15,24,51].

Humidity and room temperature: Relative humidity and ambient temperature levels are monitored in e-health systems targeting smart homes and hospitals, where control over the environment is required [6,7,18,38,40,47,51]. In [34], authors use the temperature of the environment as the main factor of the e-health system since the proposal is an intelligent air conditioning system to prevent the elderly from suffering a thermal shock and end up having health complications or even to die.

Digital image processing: Some IoMT applications use digital image processing from data collected by IP cameras and Kinect. Through image processing, it is possible to identify the patient's rehabilitation process [55], evaluate the risks of artificial light variation [11] and also diagnose possible diseases through iris [13].

Accelerometer and gyroscope: Accelerometer and gyroscope data are used for human fall detection applications, where through the data it is possible to identify if the patient has suffered a fall [4,30,55]. The collection of this data is usually done through wearable devices, such as smartwatches or smartphones.

Motion sensors: The use of data collected through motion sensors is of paramount importance for patient monitoring applications during the rehabilitation process [4] and is also used in fall detection applications [55].

Electromyography (EMG): It is commonly used to diagnose disorders, such as muscular neuropathy and myopathy, as proposed in [17]

Volume of oxygen in the blood: As described in [33], this IoMT application monitors the amount of oxygen in the blood to follow-up patients suffering from respiratory diseases.

3.4 Evaluation Method

Fig. 3 shows the main evaluation methods used in the works found in this systematic mapping study. Most of the authors use prototype to evaluate their solutions (41%). These prototypes implement a sort of applications, such as patient monitoring at hospitals [18,33,49], patients monitoring in daily activities [2,5,12,17,20,22,25,26,28,31,32,34,40,43,52], patient with respiratory diseases monitoring [33], elderly monitoring [22,29,31,32,34], patient monitoring during rehabilitation [4], detection of variation of artificial light

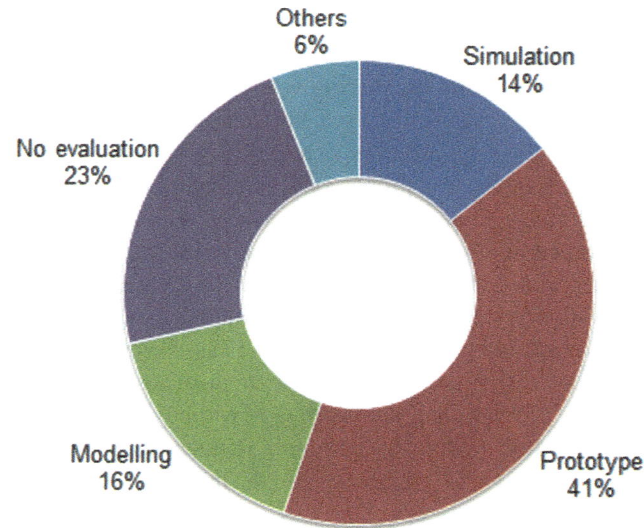

Fig. 3 Evaluation methods used by authors for proposal's validation

[11], detection of diseases through the iris [2], detection of heart attacks [2,12,20,44], human fall detection [4,30,55], electrocardiogram exam [9,25,28].

We realize that works using modeling and simulation methods usually aim for helping or creating a technology to solve part of the problem, they are not applications that can be implemented and used as we see in prototype kind. There are two exceptions: e-health monitoring signs for people in environment work [5], and an application for detecting diseases through the iris [13].

Even with sensors' variety for prototypes, simulation, and modeling, some works have not done any evaluation. So, we investigate and find that 82% of these "No evaluation" works are "Survey" type that is a more qualitative approach, this explains the high number without evaluation. In addition, we have some works classified as "Others" by having a single way (among selected works by our filter) to evaluate their solution, such: Carley eight-steps technique [24], prototype assumption [33], and critical points analysis [29].

In order to analyze what is implemented in the applications, we present the infrastructure from modeling, simulation, and prototype evaluation methods in Fig. 4. These infrastructures are classified into four types: cloud; IoT; cloud and IoT; and cloud, fog, and IoT.

Figure 4a shows infrastructures used in modeling method where cloud, fog, and IoT are used by 60% of applications. When it change for simulation method on Fig. 4b, fog is present in 33.3% of infrastructures, and for prototype method (Fig. 4c) is only 18%. This indicates in a scenario where there is an application running (prototype) is still a complex task to integrate cloud, fog, and IoT. However, to solve a specific problem or in a more theoretical rather than a practical approach, it was more used (simulation and modeling).

4   Research Challenges and Opportunities

Despite many advantages, IoMT also brings many challenges. In this section, we describe some research challenges and opportunities found in IoMT applications deployed in the e-health system context.

4.1   Limited IoT Devices' Capacity

The IoT devices are the main actors in this context, and as mentioned before, they are commonly characterized by heterogeneity and compact size, limiting some of their resources, such as computing, storage, and battery. Despite technological advances, most of the IoT devices are still computationally limited, and this impacts not only on their computational task capacity per si but also on networking aspects, such as latency and communication with other devices [17].

Depending on the IoMT application, the IoT device should be able to connect with other devices at the same time and synchronize the data constantly, as presented in [25,44]. Moreover, one also should take into consideration the amount of data collected by the IoT devices and decide where to process and store them (IoT device, fog, or cloud?), and analyze the bandwidth (and other network resources) needed to transfer them from the IoT device to the cloud, if or when necessary.

Due to the constant sensing task, battery life can be also a critical issue, especially when dealing with healthcare systems [40]. To overcome this problem, the system could also monitor the resource usage of the IoT devices, and generate notifications to recharge or replace the device, for instance. In this case, the healthcare system should be improved; instead, generate only patient health alarms, it can also take care of the IoT devices' health to prevent system unavailability.

In [7,41], the energy consumption of the IoT devices is monitored, however no management system is applied; and in [40], the authors uses a standby cyclic system to save energy.

4.2   System Availability

The availability of e-health systems is critical to ensure the sensing and integrity of vital information collected from the user [24,52]. For instance, in [52], authors focused on the usage of sensors to provide vital data as soon as the patient is discharged from the hospital, and they state that the availability of the cloud and IoT devices is a critical aspect in this scenario.

However, not only do the devices (at software and hardware levels) play an important role regarding the availability aspect, the network connection also needs to be highlighted. Considering that communication link is not always available, authors in [47] exploited the Delay-Tolerant Networking (DTN) approach, storing the data locally and conducting updates as soon as a network connection becomes available.

To improve the healthcare system availability as a whole, computational modeling could be used to predict faults in the IoT devices (at hardware and software levels), to find system bottlenecks, and to suggest redundant resource placements [45]. By using those kinds of models, one can also analyze the robustness and the scalability of the solution.

For instance, authors in [45] combined availability and performance modeling using Reliability Block Diagram (RBD) and Stochastic Petri Nets (SPNs) to present a more robust evaluation of an IoT-to-cloud (I2C) healthcare system, crossing from edge devices, fog devices, and cloud system. From their results, the authors identified that the sensors and the fog devices are the components that most impact the availability of the e-health monitoring system. The authors in [45] also realize that cloud-based e-health systems have their performance impacted by the cloud data center geo-location.

Fig. 4 Infrastructure used by evaluation methods

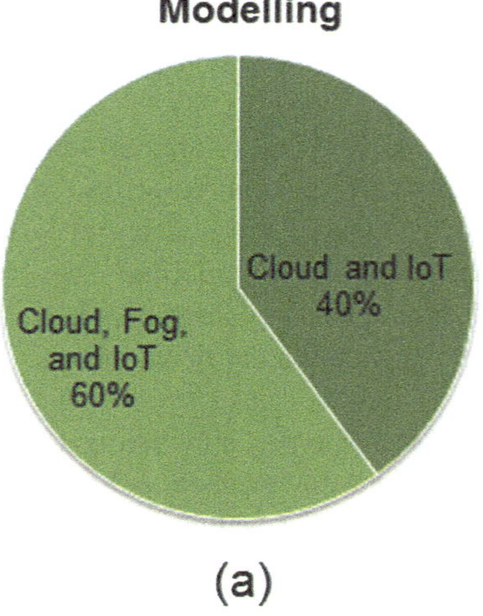

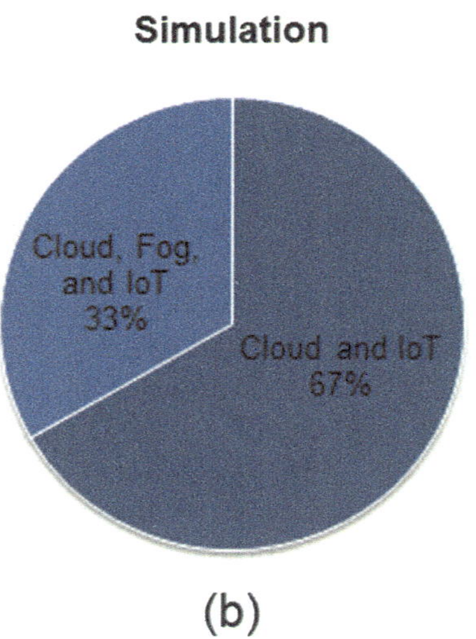

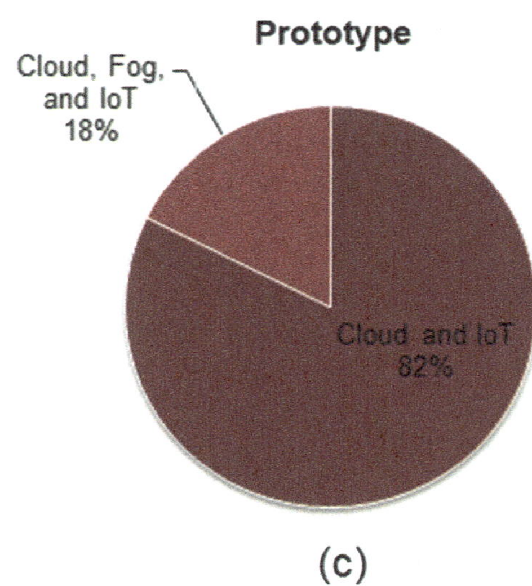

4.3   Integration, Interoperability, and Standardization

According to [55], several challenges remain concerning the interoperability among different sensors with specific communication technologies and different types of information collected by them. Moreover, each user is different, and they will vary in how, when, and why they use such systems [48].

Commonly, middleware is presented as a flexible interoperability solution. For instance, in [55], authors propose an IoT middleware to address this challenge. The main goal is to provide the infrastructure to transparently and seamlessly glue heterogeneous resources and services together, by accessing sensors and actuators across different protocols, platforms, and locations over the Internet stack. Authors in [48] also proposed a middleware as systems-glue, highlighting the requirements of such a real-time healthcare system, based on multi-device data production, multiple communication support, data security, and dynamic configuration.

In [31], authors state that the majority of current IoMT solutions rely on isolated systems that face interoperability problems, and present some efforts done to develop a standardized and open Personalized Health Systems (PHS), such as Continua Alliance (CA),[4] Active and Assisted Living (AAL)[5] and European Patients Smart Open Services (epSOS).[6] They proposed an open-source cloud-based e-health solution designed for monitoring people with chronic diseases or some frailty. Authors argue that the open-source approach brings several advantages, such as transparency, usage of open standards, and avoidance of vendor lock-in.

---

[4]http://www.pchalliance.org/.

[5]http://www.aal-europe.eu/.

[6]http://www.epsos.eu/home.html.

4.4 Data Security

Using an IoMT application based on cloud and fog infrastructure allows long-term storing and easy remote access to medical data [3,52]. With these information, it is possible to provide a comprehensive view of the patient's health history, supporting the decision-making and planning more personalized processes [14].

According to [54], protection of privacy and data security of such medical data assume higher pronounce and priority, since the data may be very sensitive, and may be linked to the life of patients. However, as described previously, IoT devices present constraints on computation and communication resources, and this feature poses challenges in terms of security mechanisms that can be deployed on such systems.

For example, authors in [9] present an IoMT application to perform an electrocardiogram exam, and they report the patient's data security as one of the main challenges. In [16], the authors present a reference design for services based on IoT, where they state that one of the biggest drawbacks in this scenario is security and privacy, as well as data access control since, in addition to the low computational power of the IoT devices, the data collected goes through a long infrastructure [35]. The authors have used cryptographic techniques in [14] to ensure the protection and privacy of patient medical records data.

5 Final Considerations

With the great effort of academic and business communities in the healthcare field, several IoMT applications are being developed and deployed in different contexts, such as personal use, hospital, or smart home. The IoMT technology has been presented as a great ally, providing the capacity to collect data through low-cost devices and sensors. However, due to their resource limitations, IoMT needs other technologies to help it to achieve high availability, high processing power, and rapid delivery of data analysis.

In this work, we performed a systematic mapping in order to obtain an overview of IoMT applications developed in e-health systems, analyze the different infrastructure configurations, and identify the most used evaluation methods, and delineate main research challenges and opportunities in this area.

It was observed the great usage of the cloud + IoT infrastructure configuration in 62% of the papers, but in the last 2 years, 2017 and 2018, there was a growing in researches with the integrated cloud + fog + IoT infrastructure. Through the systematic mapping, it was also possible to identify the main IoMT applications that are being developed; the monitoring of patients in daily activities and monitoring of elderly people are the applications most used in the works. Regarding elderly monitoring, there are several IoMT application types, ranging from common daily monitoring to more specific applications, such as the one proposed by [34] to avoid thermal shock in elderly people living in Japan. As a consequence of the mapping, it was found that the two most common targets of monitoring used are Heart rate with 12 papers and Humidity and Room Temperature with 09 papers. 42% of the works found in this systematic mapping study used prototyping for proposal evaluation, 16% modeling, 14% simulation, and another 28% did not evaluate the proposal.

To conclude the study, we presented some common research challenges and opportunities in IoMT application area, highlighting the IoT devices' limitations, the system availability, the standardization process, and data security.

Acknowledgements This work was partly funded by the Coordenação de Aperfeiçoamento de Pessoal de Nível Superior—Brasil (CAPES)—Finance Code 001.

List of Papers of the Systematic Mapping

See Table 5.

Table 5 A List of papers of the systematic mapping

Title	References
Mobile caching-enabled small cells for delay-tolerant e-Health apps	Radwan et al. [43]
Exploiting the FIWARE cloud platform to develop a remote patient monitoring system	Fazio et al. [15]
Implementation of e-health care system using web services and cloud computing	Dhanaliya and Devani [12]
Reference design for smart collaborative telehealth and telecare services based on iot technologies	Gerdes et al. [16]
Integrating wireless sensor network into cloud services for real-time data collection	Piyare et al. [40]
Intercloud platform for connecting and managing heterogeneous services with applications for e-health	Radu et al. [42]
The device cloud-applying cloud computing concepts to the internet of things	Renner et al. [44]
Resource-Efficient Secure Data Sharing for InformationCentric E-Health System Using Fog Computing	Dang et al. [10]
Mobile cloud ECG intelligent monitoring and data processing system	Ji et al. [25]
An IoT-inspired cloud-based web service architecture for e-health applications	Pescosolido et al. [38]

(continued)

Table 5 (continued)

Title	References
Temperature management system to prevent heat shock in households for elderly people	Matsui and Choi [34]
eWALL: An Open-Source Cloud-Based eHealth Platform for Creating Home Caring Environments for Older Adults	Kyriazakos et al. [31]
A Cloud-IoT based sensing service for health monitoring	Neagu et al. [36]
Remote health monitoring system through IoT	Ghosh et al. [18]
Experimental characterization of mobile iot application latency	Pereira et al. [37]
ThriftyEdge: Resource-Efficient Edge Computing for Intelligent IoT Applications	Chen et al. [8]
Health monitoring using wearable sensor and cloud computing	Joshi et al. [26]
Distributed performance management of Internet of Things as a service for caregivers	Ha and Lindh [20]
A Patient-centered medical environment with wearable sensors and cloud monitoring	Ko et al. [28]
Cloud based patient prioritization as service in public health care	Bagula et al. [3]
Mobile phone-based internet of things human action recognition for E-health	Bao et al. [4]
Cost-effective resource provisioning for multimedia cloud-based e-health systems	Hassan [21]
Cloud-assisted IoT-based health status monitoring framework	Ghanavati et al. [17]
Efficient large-scale medical data (ehealth big data) analytics in internet of things	Plageras et al. [41]
New Engineering Method for the Risk Assessment: Case Study Signal Jamming of the M-Health Networks	Karoui and Ftima [27]
IT applications in healthcare management: a survey	Yamin [54]
On middleware for emerging health services	Singh and Bacon [48]
A Health Gateway for Mobile Monitoring in Nursing Home	Li et al. [32]
Live Demonstration: An IoT Cloud-Based Architecture for Anesthesia Monitoring	Stradolini et al. [50]
Managing criticalities of e-health iot systems	Kotronis et al. [29]
Effective ways to use Internet of Things in the field of medical and smart health care	Ullah et al. [51]
Constructing ideas of health service platform for the elderly	Huaxin et al. [22]
An IoT approach for Wireless Sensor Networks applied to e-health environmental monitoring	Cabra et al. [6]
Influencing data availability in IoT enabled cloud based e-health in a 30 day readmission context	Vargheese and Viniotis [52]
The application of internet of things in healthcare: a systematic literature review and classification	Ahmadi et al. [1]
Exploring Temporal Analytics in Fog-Cloud Architecture for Smart Office HealthCare	Bhatia and Sood [5]
Real-time heart attack mobile detection service (RHAMDS): An IoT use case for software-defined networks	Ali and Ghazal [2]
The use of IoT technologies for providing high-quality medical services	Corotinschi and Găitan [9]
CC-fog: Toward content-centric fog networks for E-health	Guibert et al. [19]
Fog-to-cloud Computing (F2C): the key technology enabler for dependable e-health services deployment	Masip-Bruin et al. [33]
IoT for Telemedicine Practices enabled by an Android™ Application with Cloud System Integration	Stradolini et al. [49]
A new computing environment for collective privacy protection from constrained healthcare devices to IoT cloud services	Elmisery and Aborizka [14]
Internet of medical things: Architectural model, motivational factors and impediments	Irfan and Ahmad [24]
A fog-enabled IoT platform for efficient management and data collection	Charalampidis et al. [7]
A Model-based Approach for Managing Criticality Requirements in e-Health IoT Systems	Kotronis et al. [30]
Application of IoT in detecting health risks due to flickering artificial lights	Das et al. [11]
Score level multibiometrics fusion approach for healthcare	El-Latif et al. [13]
WITS: an IoT-endowed computational framework for activity recognition in personalized smart homes	Yao et al. [55]
Multidisciplinary approaches to achieving efficient and trustworthy eHealth monitoring systems	Sawand et al. [47]

References

[1] Ahmadi, H., Arji, G., Shahmoradi, L., Safdari, R., Nilashi, M., Alizadeh, M.: The application of internet of things in healthcare: a systematic literature review and classification. Universal Access in the Information Society pp. 1–33 (2018)

[2] Ali, S., Ghazal, M.: Real-time heart attack mobile detection service (rhamds): An iot use case for software defined networks. In: Electrical and Computer Engineering (CCECE), 2017 IEEE 30th Canadian Conference on, pp. 1–6. IEEE (2017)

[3] Bagula, A., Lubamba, C., Mandava, M., Bagula, H., Zennaro, M., Pietrosemoli, E.: Cloud based patient prioritization as service in public health care. In: ITU Kaleidoscope: ICTs for a Sustainable World (ITU WT), 2016, pp. 1–8. IEEE (2016)

[4] Bao, J., Ye, M., Dou, Y.: Mobile phone-based internet of things human action recognition for e-health. In: Signal Processing (ICSP), 2016 IEEE 13th International Conference on, pp. 957–962. IEEE (2016)

[5] Bhatia, M., Sood, S.K.: Exploring temporal analytics in fog-cloud architecture for smart office healthcare. Mobile Networks and Applications pp. 1–19 (2018)

[6] Cabra, J., Castro, D., Colorado, J., Mendez, D., Trujillo, L.: An iot approach for wireless sensor networks applied to e-health envi-

ronmental monitoring. In: 2017 IEEE International Conference on Internet of Things (iThings) and IEEE Green Computing and Communications (GreenCom) and IEEE Cyber, Physical and Social Computing (CPSCom) and IEEE Smart Data (SmartData), pp. 578–583. IEEE (2017)

[7] Charalampidis, P., Tragos, E., Fragkiadakis, A.: A fog-enabled iot platform for efficient management and data collection (2017)

[8] Chen, X., Shi, Q., Yang, L., Xu, J.: Thriftyedge: Resource-efficient edge computing for intelligent iot applications. IEEE Network **32**(1), 61–65 (2018)

[9] Corotinschi, G., Găitan, V.G.: The use of iot technologies for providing high-quality medical services. In: System Theory, Control and Computing (ICSTCC), 2017 21st International Conference on, pp. 285–290. IEEE (2017)

[10] Dang, L., Dong, M., Ota, K., Wu, J., Li, J., Li, G.: Resource-efficient secure data sharing for information centric e-health system using fog computing. In: 2018 IEEE International Conference on Communications (ICC), pp. 1–6. IEEE (2018)

[11] Das, S., Ballav, M., Karfa, S.: Application of iot in detecting health risks due to flickering artificial lights. In: Advances in Computing, Communications and Informatics (ICACCI), 2015 International Conference on, pp. 2331–2334. IEEE (2015)

[12] Dhanaliya, U., Devani, A.: Implementation of e-health care system using web services and cloud computing. In: Communication and Signal Processing (ICCSP), 2016 International Conference on, pp. 1034–1036. IEEE (2016)

[13] El-Latif, A.A.A., Hossain, M.S., Wang, N.: Score level multibiometrics fusion approach for healthcare. Cluster Computing pp. 1–12 (2017)

[14] Elmisery, A.M., Aborizka, M.: A new computing environment for collective privacy protection from constrained healthcare devices to iot cloud services

[15] Fazio, M., Celesti, A., Marquez, F.G., Glikson, A., Villari, M.: Exploiting the fiware cloud platform to develop a remote patient monitoring system. In: 2015 IEEE Symposium on Computers and Communication (ISCC), pp. 264–270. IEEE (2015)

[16] Gerdes, M., Reichert, F., Nytun, J.P., Fensli, R.: Reference design for smart collaborative telehealth and telecare services based on iot technologies. In: 2015 International Conference on Computational Science and Computational Intelligence (CSCI), pp. 817–820. IEEE (2015)

[17] Ghanavati, S., Abawajy, J.H., Izadi, D., Alelaiwi, A.A.: Cloud-assisted iot-based health status monitoring framework. Cluster Computing **20**(2), 1843–1853 (2017)

[18] Ghosh, A.M., Halder, D., Hossain, S.A.: Remote health monitoring system through iot. In: 2016 International Conference on Informatics, Electronics and Vision (ICIEV), pp. 921–926. IEEE (2016)

[19] Guibert, D., Wu, J., He, S., Wang, M., Li, J.: Cc-fog: Toward content-centric fog networks for e-health. In: e-Health Networking, Applications and Services (Healthcom), 2017 IEEE 19th International Conference on, pp. 1–5. IEEE (2017)

[20] Ha, M., Lindh, T.: Distributed performance management of internet of things as a service for caregivers. In: e-Health Networking, Applications and Services (Healthcom), 2017 IEEE 19th International Conference on, pp. 1–6. IEEE (2017)

[21] Hassan, M.M.: Cost-effective resource provisioning for multimedia cloud-based e-health systems. Multimedia Tools and Applications **74**(14), 5225–5241 (2015)

[22] Huaxin, S., Qi, X., Xiaodong, L., Baoyan, L., Shusong, M., Xuezhong, Z.: Constructing ideas of health service platform for the elderly. In: e-Health Networking, Applications and Services (Healthcom), 2012 IEEE 14th International Conference on, pp. 526–529. IEEE (2012)

[23] Iorga, M., Feldman, L., Barton, R., Martin, M.J., Goren, N., Mahmoudi, C.: Draft sp 800-191, the nist definition of fog computing. NIST Special Publication **800**, 800–191 (2017)

[24] Irfan, M., Ahmad, N.: Internet of medical things: Architectural model, motivational factors and impediments. In: Learning and Technology Conference (L&T), 2018 15th, pp. 6–13. IEEE (2018)

[25] Ji, C., Liu, F., Wang, Z., Li, Y., Qi, C., Li, Z.: Mobile cloud ecg intelligent monitoring and data processing system. In: e-Health Networking, Applications and Services (Healthcom), 2017 IEEE 19th International Conference on, pp. 1–6. IEEE (2017)

[26] Joshi, J., Kurian, D., Bhasin, S., Mukherjee, S., Awasthi, P., Sharma, S., Mittal, S.: Health monitoring using wearable sensor and cloud computing. In: Cybernetics, Robotics and Control (CRC), International Conference on, pp. 104–108. IEEE (2016)

[27] Karoui, K., Ftima, F.B.: New engineering method for the risk assessment: Case study signal jamming of the m-health networks. Mobile Networks and Applications pp. 1–20 (2018)

[28] Ko, Y.J., Huang, H.M., Hsing, W.H., Chou, J., Chiu, H.C., Ma, H.P.: A patient-centered medical environment with wearable sensors and cloud monitoring. In: Internet of Things (WF-IoT), 2015 IEEE 2nd World Forum on, pp. 628–633. IEEE (2015)

[29] Kotronis, C., Minou, G., Dimitrakopoulos, G., Nikolaidou, M., Anagnostopoulos, D., Amira, A., Bensaali, F., Baali, H., Djelouat, H.: Managing criticalities of e-health iot systems. In: 2017 IEEE 17th International Conference on Ubiquitous Wireless Broadband (ICUWB), pp. 1–5. IEEE (2017)

[30] Kotronis, C., Nikolaidou, M., Dimitrakopoulos, G., Anagnostopoulos, D., Amira, A., Bensaali, F.: A model-based approach for managing criticality requirements in e-health iot systems. In: 2018 13th Annual Conference on System of Systems Engineering (SoSE), pp. 60–67. IEEE (2018)

[31] Kyriazakos, S., Prasad, R., Mihovska, A., Pnevmatikakis, A., op den Akker, H., Hermens, H., Barone, P., Mamelli, A., de Domenico, S., Pocs, M., et al.: ewall: An open-source cloud-based ehealth platform for creating home caring environments for older adults living with chronic diseases or frailty. Wireless Personal Communications **97**(2), 1835–1875 (2017)

[32] Li, Y., Liu, P., Cai, Q., Guo, J., Zhou, Z., Yan, H., Qian, M., Yu, F., Yuan, K., Yu, J.: A health gateway for mobile monitoring in nursing home. Wireless Personal Communications pp. 1–15 (2018)

[33] Masip-Bruin, X., Marín-Tordera, E., Alonso, A., Garcia, J.: Fog-to-cloud computing (f2c): the key technology enabler for dependable e-health services deployment. In: Ad Hoc Networking Workshop (Med-Hoc-Net), 2016 Mediterranean, pp. 1–5. IEEE (2016)

[34] Matsui, K., Choi, H.: Temperature management system to prevent heat shock in households for elderly people. In: 2017 IEEE SmartWorld, Ubiquitous Intelligence & Computing, Advanced & Trusted Computed, Scalable Computing & Communications, Cloud & Big Data Computing, Internet of People and Smart City Innovation (SmartWorld/SCALCOM/UIC/ATC/CBDCom/IOP/SCI), pp. 1–6. IEEE (2017)

[35] Monteiro, K., Rocha, É., Silva, É., Santos, G.L., Santos, W., Endo, P.T.: Developing an e-health system based on iot, fog and cloud computing. In: 2018 IEEE/ACM International Conference on Utility and Cloud Computing Companion (UCC Companion), pp. 17–18. IEEE (2018)

[36] Neagu, G., Preda, Ş., Stanciu, A., Florian, V.: A cloud-iot based sensing service for health monitoring. In: E-Health and Bioengineering Conference (EHB), 2017, pp. 53–56. IEEE (2017)

[37] Pereira, C., Pinto, A., Ferreira, D., Aguiar, A.: Experimental characterization of mobile iot application latency. IEEE Internet of Things Journal **4**(4), 1082–1094 (2017)

[38] Pescosolido, L., Berta, R., Scalise, L., Revel, G.M., De Gloria, A., Orlandi, G.: An iot-inspired cloud-based web service architecture for e-health applications. In: Smart Cities Conference (ISC2), 2016 IEEE International, pp. 1–4. IEEE (2016)

[39] Petersen, K., Feldt, R., Mujtaba, S., Mattsson, M.: Systematic Mapping Studies in Software Engineering. In: 12th Int. Conference

on Evaluation and Assessment in Software Engineering, p. 10. BCS Learning & Development Ltd., Italy (2008). http://dl.acm.org/citation.cfm?id=2227115.2227123

[40] Piyare, R., Park, S., Maeng, S.Y., Park, S.H., Oh, S.C., Choi, S.G., Choi, H.S., Lee, S.R.: Integrating wireless sensor network into cloud services for real-time data collection. In: ICT Convergence (ICTC), 2013 International Conference on, pp. 752–756. IEEE (2013)

[41] Plageras, A.P., Stergiou, C., Kokkonis, G., Psannis, K.E., Ishibashi, Y., Kim, B.G., Gupta, B.B.: Efficient large-scale medical data (ehealth big data) analytics in internet of things. In: Business Informatics (CBI), 2017 IEEE 19th Conference on, vol. 2, pp. 21–27. IEEE (2017)

[42] Radu, A., Costan, A., Iancu, B., Dadarlat, V., Peculea, A.: Intercloud platform for connecting and managing heterogeneous services with applications for e-health. In: 2015 Conference Grid, Cloud High Performance Computing in Science (ROLCG), pp. 1–4 (2015). 10.1109/ROLCG.2015.7367229

[43] Radwan, A., Domingues, M.F., Rodriguez, J.: Mobile caching-enabled small-cells for delay-tolerant e-health apps. In: Communications Workshops (ICC Workshops), 2017 IEEE International Conference on, pp. 103–108. IEEE (2017)

[44] Renner, T., Kliem, A., Kao, O.: The device cloud-applying cloud computing concepts to the internet of things. In: Ubiquitous Intelligence and Computing, 2014 IEEE 11th Intl Conf on and IEEE 11th Intl Conf on and Autonomic and Trusted Computing, and IEEE 14th Intl Conf on Scalable Computing and Communications and Its Associated Workshops (UTC-ATC-ScalCom), pp. 396–401. IEEE (2014)

[45] Santos, G.L., Endo, P.T., da Silva Lisboa, M.F.F., da Silva, L.G.F., Sadok, D., Kelner, J., Lynn, T., et al.: Analyzing the availability and performance of an e-health system integrated with edge, fog and cloud infrastructures. Journal of Cloud Computing 7(1), 16 (2018)

[46] Santos, G.L., Ferreira, M., Ferreira, L., Kelner, J., Sadok, D., Albuquerque, E., Lynn, T., Endo, P.T.: Integrating iot+fog+cloud infrastructures: System modeling and research challenges. Fog and Edge Computing: Principles and Paradigms pp. 51–78 (2019)

[47] Sawand, A., Djahel, S., Zhang, Z., Naït-Abdesselam, F.: Multidisciplinary approaches to achieving efficient and trustworthy ehealth monitoring systems. In: Communications in China (ICCC), 2014 IEEE/CIC International Conference on, pp. 187–192. IEEE (2014)

[48] Singh, J., Bacon, J.M.: On middleware for emerging health services. Journal of Internet Services and Applications 5(1), 6 (2014)

[49] Stradolini, F., Tamburrano, N., Modoux, T., Tuoheti, A., Demarchi, D., Carrara, S.: Iot for telemedicine practices enabled by an android™application with cloud system integration. In: Circuits and Systems (ISCAS), 2018 IEEE International Symposium on, pp. 1–5. IEEE (2018)

[50] Stradolini, F., Tamburrano, N., Modoux, T., Tuoheti, A., Demarchi, D., Carrara, S.: Live demonstration: An iot cloud-based architecture for anesthesia monitoring. In: Circuits and Systems (ISCAS), 2018 IEEE International Symposium on, pp. 1–1. IEEE (2018)

[51] Ullah, K., Shah, M.A., Zhang, S.: Effective ways to use internet of things in the field of medical and smart health care. In: Intelligent Systems Engineering (ICISE), 2016 International Conference on, pp. 372–379. IEEE (2016)

[52] Vargheese, R., Viniotis, Y.: Influencing data availability in iot enabled cloud based e-health in a 30 day readmission context. In: Collaborative Computing: Networking, Applications and Worksharing (CollaborateCom), 2014 International Conference on, pp. 475–480. IEEE (2014)

[53] World health organization. https://goo.gl/XAYvnq. Accessed: 2018-09-27

[54] Yamin, M.: It applications in healthcare management: a survey. International Journal of Information Technology pp. 1–7 (2018)

[55] Yao, L., Sheng, Q.Z., Benatallah, B., Dustdar, S., Wang, X., Shemshadi, A., Kanhere, S.S.: Wits: an iot-endowed computational framework for activity recognition in personalized smart homes. Computing 100(4), 369–385 (2018)

Artificial Intelligent and Machine Learning Methods in Bioinformatics and Medical Informatics

Noor A. Jebril and Qasem Abu Al-Haija

Abstract

Recently, the machine learning techniques have been widely adopted in the field of bioinformatics and medical informatics. Generally, the main purpose of machine learning is to develop algorithms that can learn and improve over time and can be utilized for predictions in hindcast and forecast applications. Computational intelligence has been significantly employed to develop optimization and prediction solutions for several bioinformatics and medical informatics techniques in which it utilized various computational methodologies to address complex real-world problems and promises to enable computers to help humans in analyzing large complex data sets. Its approaches have been widely applied in biomedical fields, and there are many applications that use the machine learning, such as genomics, proteomics, systems biology, evolution and text mining, which are also discussed. In this chapter, we provide a comprehensive study of the use of artificial intelligent and machine learning methods in bioinformatics and medical informatics, including AI and its learning processes, machine learning and its applications for health informatics, text mining methods, and many other related topics.

Glossary

AI	Artificial intelligence.
IT	Information technology.
ML	Machine learning.
NN	Neural networks.
EHR	Electronic health records.
ANI	Artificial narrow intelligence.
AGI	Artificial general intelligence.
NLP	Natural language processing.
SR	Speech recognition.
ES	Expert systems.
AI-R	Artificial intelligence for robotics.
PML	Probabilistic machine learning.
MLD	Machine learning data.
aML	automated Machine Learning.
iML	interactive Machine learning.
HCI	Human–computer interaction.
KDD	Knowledge discovery/data.
RNA	Ribonucleic acid.
DNA	Microarray deoxyribonucleic acid.
cDNA	complementary Microarray deoxyribonucleic acid.
mRNA	messenger ribonucleic acid.
MIAME	Minimum information about a microarray experiment.
FGED	Functional Genomics Data Society.
FRG/BKG	Foreground/background.
MS	Mass spectrometry.
SVM	Support vector machine.
RBF	Radial basis function.
CART	Classification and regression tree.
OOB	Out of the bag.
TM	Text mining.
IR	Information retrieval.
DC	Document classification.
NER/NEN	Named entity recognition/normalization.
ART	Adaptive resonance theory.
DNN	Deep neural network.

N. A. Jebril
Department of Computer Sciences, King Faisal University, Hufof, Al-Ahsa, Saudi Arabia

Q. Abu Al-Haija (✉)
Department of Computer Information and Systems Engineering, Tennessee State University, Nashville, TN, USA
e-mail: qasem.abualhaija@uop.edu.jo

© Springer Nature Switzerland AG 2021
J. Aljaâ am et al. (eds.), *Emerging Technologies in Biomedical Engineering and Sustainable TeleMedicine*,
Advances in Science, Technology & Innovation, https://doi.org/10.1007/978-3-030-14647-4_2

1 Introduction

Due to the rapid advances in the digital computing technology where computers become core parts of any modern industry and automated applications, it becomes a necessity to involve the machine with latest trend in the current industry. This in turn led to moving ahead toward the smart industry by adopting intelligent machines and computational systems that can replace or reduce the human intervention at several points of execution or production. Thus, the *artificial intelligence (AI)* can be interpreted naturally as the work of a machine that a human could have done using his intelligence [1, 2]. Currently, the artificial intelligence is gaining an appreciated amount of interest as almost all major IT companies are spending millions on the development and implementation of the artificial intelligence considering its criticality to their future situation. Providing personal relationships with machines is the latest trend in product-based industries and is believed to be booming more recently [3].

Artificial intelligence (AI) occupies significant part of computer science applications that use algorithms, inference, pattern matching, grammar, deep learning and cognitive computing for approximate results without direct human input. Even though the artificial intelligence can determine meaningful relationships in raw data, however, the use of artificial intelligence creates a non-easy challenge for researchers which can face complex troubles that are hard to fix or almost impossible to fix. Nevertheless, it can be used to support the diagnosis, treatment and prediction of outcomes in many medical situations which increased the possibility for artificial intelligence to be applied in almost every scoop of medical fields, including drug expansion, patient observation and personalized patient processing plans.

Artificial intelligence can be designed in a way that mimics the task of *neural networks (NN)* in the human brain. This was made possible by utilizing multiple layers of nonlinear processing units to "teach" itself how to comprehend data/record classification or make predictions. Thus, artificial intelligence can synthesize electronic health records (EHR) data and unstructured data to build predictions about patient health. For instance, artificial intelligence software can speedily read a retinal image or flag cases for follow-up when multiple manual reviews would be too heavy. Doctors benefit from having more time and concise data to make better patient decisions. Artificial intelligence solutions for healthcare currently run toward enhancing outcomes of patients and decreasing healthcare budgets. Figure 1 illustrates the amount of market spending on AI application in the healthcare sector during the period from 2013 to the mid of 2018 [4]. According to the figure, it can be clearly seen that the healthcare AI is increasingly gaining a significant funding as it accumulated around 4300 million USD from 2013 to 2018 through 576 deals which pushed it on top of among AI-based industries.

The adoption of artificial intelligence in medicine started early since 1972, where the researchers at Stanford University developed the MYCIN program, which is an early expert system, or artificial intelligence (AI) program, for treating blood infections. This project has been revisited again in the 1980s, where people at Stanford University resumed the work with artificial intelligence for medical care via developing newer version of their medical expert system via the Stanford University Medical Experimental Computer —Artificial Intelligence in Medicine (SUMEX-AIM) project. Indeed, AI has acquired its importance as *"the next big thing"* for decades but its widespread practical uses have only begun to take off in the 2000s; for instance, AI has attracted more than \$17 billion in investments since 2009 and is likely to reach \$36.8 billion by 2025 [5].

AI neural networks have been used efficiently to handle raw data blocks and learn how to organize those data using the most important variables in predicting health outcomes. Today, artificial intelligence techniques such as IBM Watson are used at Memorial Sloan-Kettering Cancer Center to support diagnosis and create management plans for oncological patients [5]. Watson is achieving these plans by collecting millions of medical reports, patient records, clinical trials and medical journals. Watson's findings routinely refer to "medical patients" in certain cases [5]. IBM also joined CVS Health in the treatment of chronic diseases using artificial intelligence technology. Johnson & Johnson and IBM AI is used to analyze scientific research to find new links to drug development [5].

Other examples of AI currently used in medicine include patient care in radiology [5]. AI can quickly search and interpret billions of data points—text or images—inside the patient's electronic medical record. It can be done using other patient-like conditions and through the latest medical research. In genomics [5], AI can extract unstructured data from peer-reviewed literature to continuously improve its knowledge base. It gives various information and modern clinical content—based on the latest approved handling options, including targeted options, immune cells, occupational guidance and clinical trial options based on biological indicators, genome databases and related publications.

In a more realistic way, the best way of achieving AI in medical care applications is by adoption of the *machine learning,* which is a method of data analysis that automates analytical model building. Machine learning (ML) is an artificial intelligence field in which the system depends on learning from the data, identifying patterns, taking the decisions with minimal involvement of human and then determining or predicting a set of events. Recently, machine learning (ML) research focuses more on the selection or

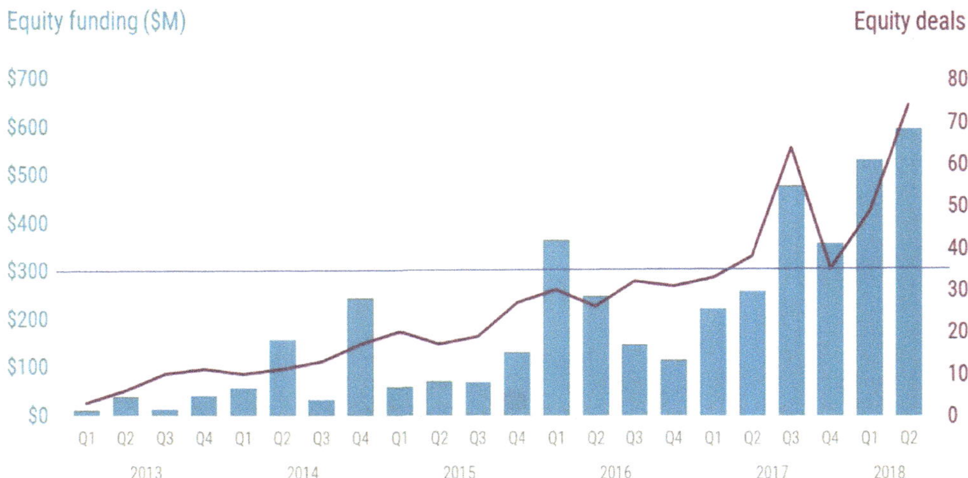

Fig. 1 Funding of artificial intelligence of healthcare hit a historic high in second quarter of 2018 (Q2'18), disclosed equity funding, Q1'13–Q2'18

improvements of algorithms that learn how to make data-based predictions and implement experiments on the basis of such algorithms [6] which resulted in several emerging applications in the field of bioinformatics.

Bioinformatics deals with computational and mathematical methods for understanding and manipulating biological data [7]. Prior to the development of machine learning algorithms, bioinformatics algorithms had to be programmed by hand, which, for problems such as protein structure prediction, proved to be very difficult [8]. The recent machine learning techniques such as deep learning algorithms employ learning automatic features, which means that based on the data set alone, the ability of the algorithm is to learn how to integrate multiple features of input data into a more abstract set of features that are further learned [9]. This multilayered approach to learning patterns in input data allows these systems to make fully complex predictions when trained on large data sets. In recent years, the size and number of available biological data sets has increased, enabling biotechnological researchers to benefit from these automated learning systems [9].

2 Artificial Intelligence and Machine Learning

Artificial intelligence (AI), the term first formulated by John McCarthy, is the field of science that concerned with the development of computer systems to accomplish missions that would need human intelligence. It includes things like planning, understanding language, recognizing objects and sounds, learning and problem-solving [10]. The technology of artificial intelligence passes through three levels of integration: artificial narrow intelligence (ANI), artificial general intelligence (AGI) and artificial super intelligence (ASI). The emergence of these levels is illustrated in Fig. 2. ANI is the first level that can decide only in one field; AGI is the second level and it can reach the intelligence level of a human, i.e., it can imagine, plan, solve problems, think abstractly, understand the complicated ideas, learn quickly and learn from experience [11]; and the last level is ASI. It is much smarter than the best human brain in practically every area, including scientific creativity, general wisdom and social skills [12].

The artificial intelligence has been used efficiently to develop solutions for wide range of applications, especially those based on human thinking to provide a proper decision. AI is contributing to several fields with many significant relation and commonalities between them. The most common fields AI being used nowadays are shown in Fig. 3, including the machine learning (ML) approaches, natural language processing (NLP) applications, speech recognition (SR) techniques, expert systems (ES), AI for robotics (AI-R), which provides solutions for optimization and planning as well as scheduling problems, and also provide artificial algorithms for machine vision applications.

In addition, the artificial intelligence has been employed for the last couple of years to develop significant solutions in even more sensitive situations such as the medical care applications where it can develop the course of care for patients with chronic diseases and suggests accurate treatments for complex diseases and improves adherence to substances in clinical trials [5]. Artificial intelligence can be used in a variety of ways in medicine, and the following are four examples:

- Clinical data annotated: Almost 80% of healthcare data is unorganized, and AI can read and understand unorganized data. AI's ability to address natural language allows for clinical text to be read from any source, medical, social concepts, classification and coding.

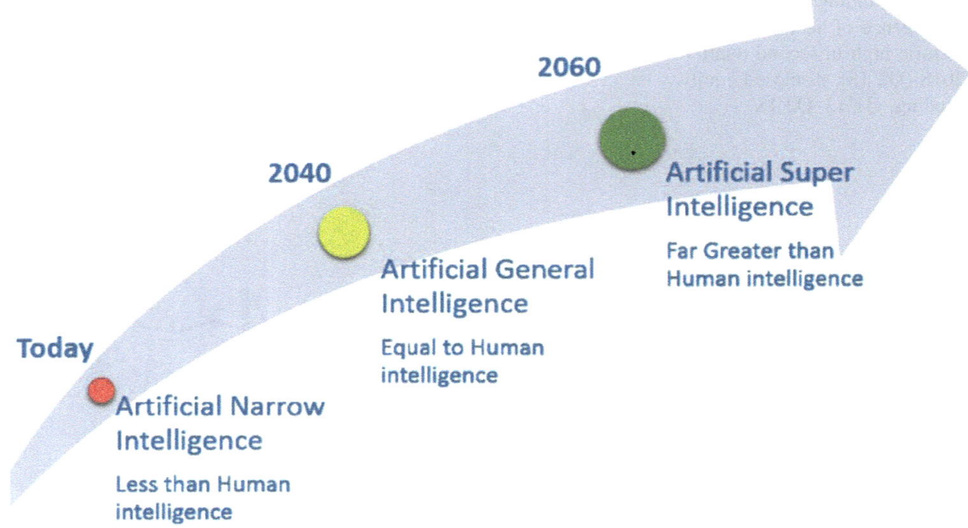

Fig. 2 Future evolution of artificial intelligence

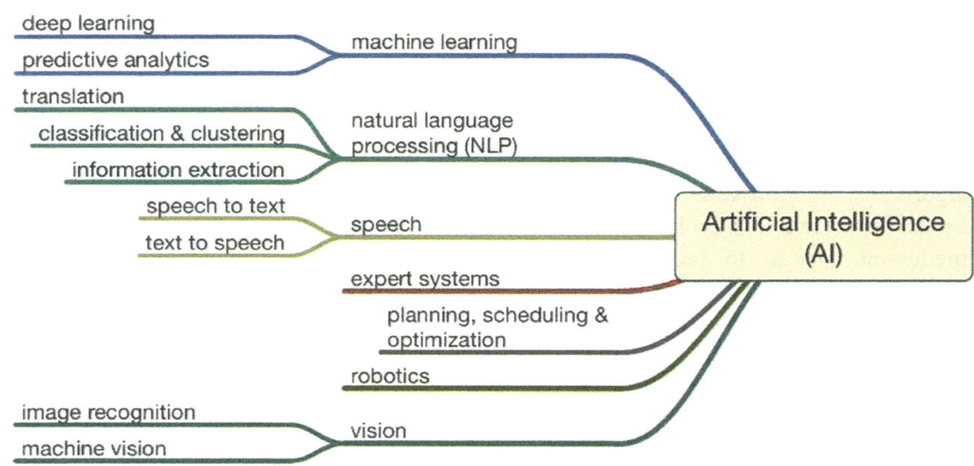

Fig. 3 Fields of artificial intelligence

- Visions for patient data: Artificial intelligence can identify problems in historical medical records of patients—whether in structured or unstructured text. It summarizes the history of their care about these problems and can provide a concise summary of patient records.
- Patient similarity: AI can determine the clinical similarity measure among patients. This allows researchers to create dynamic patient groups rather than fixed patient groups. It also allows understanding what the path of care works best for a group of patients.
- Medical visions: Using AI techniques, researchers can find information in uneducated medical literature to support hypotheses—assist to find new insights. AI can access a full area of medical literature, such as Medellin, and identify documents that are medically linked to any combination of medical concepts.

In more realistic situations, the AI for machine learning field provided more precise methods for medical applications that are heavily based on the data analysis that automates analytical model building. The applicable machine learning algorithms fall into four main categories that are briefly illustrated in Fig. 4. The techniques used in these categories differ mainly in the learning process rule which defines the mathematical models of updating the weights and bias levels of the neural network when a network is simulated in a specific data environment.

2.1 Supervised Learning

In this technique, the learning process depends on the comparison between the calculated outputs and the desired (i.e., expected) outputs since the desired output is already

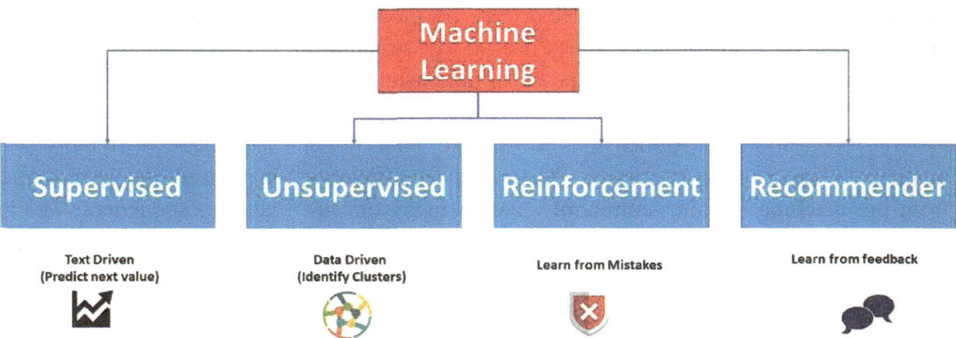

Fig. 4 Types of machine learning

known prior to the initialization of learning process, i.e., learning refers to the calculation of the error and then adjusts the error to achieve the expected output. Supervised learning is the main methodology in machine learning and it also has central importance in the processing of multimedia data [13].

2.2 Unsupervised Learning

In this technique, the desired output is not known before the starting of the learning process, i.e., unsupervised learning, and thus the network learns by its own and that is done by discovering and adopting based on the input pattern. If the data are split into various clusters and then the learning is called a clustering algorithm such as Google News (*news.-google.com*), which is a well-known example where clustering is used and where in Google News, the network groups new stories on the web and puts them into collective news stories [6].

2.3 Reinforcement Learning

In this technique, the reinforcement learning process depends on the output with how an agent will take behavior in an environment to maximize some notion of long-term reward. A reward is given for the correct output and a penalty is issued for the incorrect output. Reinforcement learning is different from the supervised learning problem in that correct input/output pairs are never presented, nor sub-optimal actions explicitly corrected [6].

2.4 Recommender Systems

In this technique, the recommender systems learning process depends on the online users who can customize their sites to check customer desires. There are mainly two approaches: content-based recommendation and collaborative recommendation, which assist the user for getting and mining data, producing intelligent and novel recommendations, ethics. Most e-commerce site uses this system [14].

3 Machine Learning for Health Informatics

The area of *machine learning* (ML) has emerged very fast as a development technical domain at the interchange of informatics and statistics [15, 16] closely associated with data science and knowledge discovery, especially the *probabilistic machine learning* (PML) that is highly helpful for health informatics where most problems include treatment with uncertainty. The theoretical fundamental of probabilistic machine learning [17, 18] was first initiated by the mathematician, Thomas Bayes (1701–1761), and since then, probabilistic inference has widely affected the artificial intelligence and statistical learning methods while the inverse probability allowed to conclude unknowns, learn from data and make predictions [19, 20].

The recent advances in machine learning have been driven by the expansion of new learning algorithms and theory that can accommodate the newer technologies raised from the constant collapse of data, meanwhile, reduced computation. The adoption of data-intensive *machine learning data algorithms (MLD)* can be found in all areas of health informatics employment and is specifically useful for brain information from the basic research of intelligence understanding [21] to a more complex domain of certain brain informatics research [22]. Implementation of machine learning methods in biomedical and health has enabled to drive to more evidence-based decisions making and assist in going to personal medicine [23]. Indeed, the realization of any scientific area can be discussed by the questions it studies, for instance, the machine learning area trying to answer the question: "*How can we construct algorithms that automatically get better through experience? What are the primary laws that control all learning processes?*" [24].

The challenge in almost all machine learning techniques is to find the related structural patterns/temporal patterns (i.e., knowledge) in such data, which are often hidden and unavailable to the human expert. However, the problem is that majority of biomedical data sets are poorly structured and unmanaged [25], with most data are in dimensions well above three, and although human experts are excellent at pattern recognition for dimensions <= 3, like data build manual analysis is often impossible. Therefore, most fellows from the machine learning community are focusing on *automated machine learning* (aML) with the great goal of getting humans out of the loop and a realistic example of best practice can exist in autonomous vehicles [26]. Nevertheless, biomedical data sets are full of uncertainty and incompleteness [27] and may include missing data, noisy data, dirty data, undesirable data, and most of all, some medical problems are difficult, which makes it difficult to implement the complete automated approaches.

Another noticeable issue is the complexity of advanced machine learning algorithms which has been arrested by non-experts from the application of these solutions. Thus, the integration of knowledge from the area expert and the interaction of the area expert with the data can be greatly enhanced by the strengthening of pipeline knowledge discovery process. Hence, the *interactive machine learning* (iML) places the "human-in-the-loop" to authorize what a human nor a computer could not do on their own. This concept is supported by a synergistic combination of two field methodologies that provide ideal conditions for solving such problems: Human–computer interaction (HCI) and knowledge discovery/data mining (KDD), in order to support human intelligence with machine intelligence to find new insights unknown in data HCI-KDD approach [28].

The enormous growth of the amount of available biological data raises two problems: the first is the efficient storage and management of information, and the second problem is the extraction of useful information from such data. The second trouble is one of the major challenges in computer biology, which demand the development of tools and methods that can transform all these heterogeneous data into biological information about the underlying mechanism. These tools and methods must enable us to go further than describing data and providing knowledge in the form of testable models to be able to gain system predictions.

There are many biological fields where machine learning techniques can be implemented to extract knowledge from data. Figure 5 displays a diagram for the major biological problems in which arithmetic methods are applied. The problems are categorized into six different areas: genomics, proteomics, microarrays, systems biology, evolution and text mining. The category named "Other application groups" combines the remaining issues. These categories should be understood in a very general way, particularly, genomics and proteomics, which in this review are considered a study of nucleotide chains and proteins, respectively.

3.1 Genomics

Genomics is one of the most substantial fields in bioinformatics. According to Fig. 6, the number of available sequences is steadily growing where these data must be processed in order to gain useful information. Using the genome sequences, we can extract the location and structure of the genes [29] and recently, regulatory elements [30–32] and irregular ribosomal genes [33] have been specified from an accounting point of view. Sequencing information is also used in gene function and prediction of secondary ribonucleic acid (RNA) structure. If genes include information, proteins are the factor that converts this information into life. Proteins play a very important part in the life process, and their three-dimensional (3D) structure is a major feature of their functions.

In the area of proteomic, the major application of arithmetic methods is to predict protein structure. *Proteins* are massive complex molecules containing thousands of atoms and boundaries. Thus, the number of potential structures is huge. This makes predicting of protein structure a very complicated fusion problem where optimization techniques are required. In proteomics, as in genomics, machine learning techniques are implemented to predict protein function.

3.2 Microarray

Another interesting application of computational methods in biology is complicated, experimental data management. *Microarray* articles are the best known (but not the only) domain where this type of data is collected. Microarrays can be utilized to define gene expression patterns in a specific cell or tissue. *Microarray deoxyribonucleic acid* (DNA) is a set of microscopic DNA sequences (oligos) connected to a solid surface. These sequences appear as part of a large library of genes in the cell [34].

The states of the gene as shown in Fig. 7 can be classified according to these points [34]:

- If the gene is active within the cell, then the complementary DNA (cDNA) (resulting from the transcript of the messenger RNA (mRNA)) will bind to its complementary oligo.
- If the cDNA has been characterized by fluoridation, it can determine the complementary oligo (along with the gene it represents).
- If cDNA is classified from healthy and diseased cells with different fluorophores, comparisons of gene expression can be made.
- Only active genes in a diseased or natural state will be of particular interest to scientists.

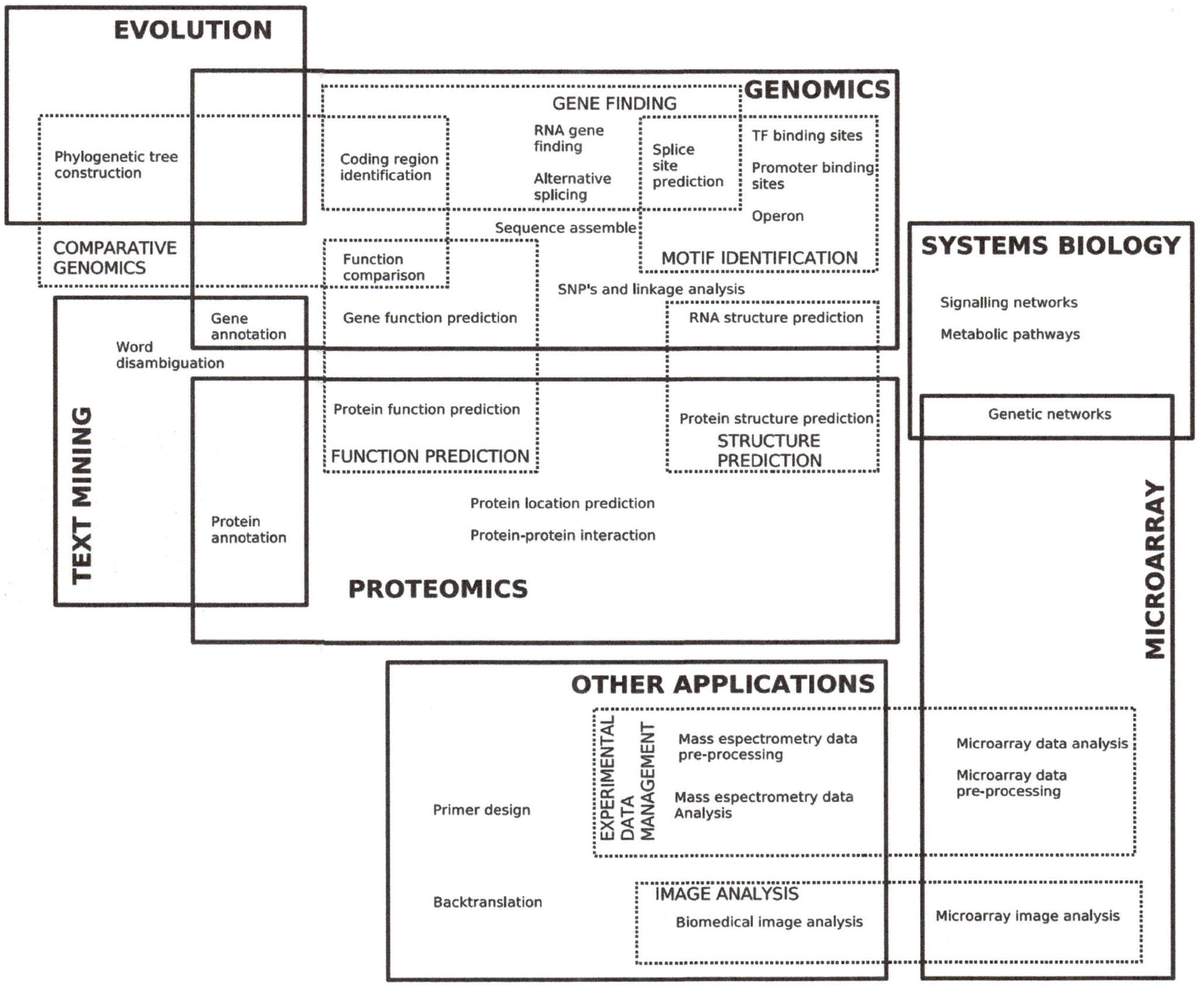

EVOLUTION

Phylogenetic tree construction

COMPARATIVE GENOMICS

GENOMICS

GENE FINDING

RNA gene finding

Alternative splicing

Coding region identification

Splice site prediction

TF binding sites

Promoter binding sites

Operon

Sequence assemble

MOTIF IDENTIFICATION

Function comparison

SNP's and linkage analysis

Gene function prediction

RNA structure prediction

Gene annotation

Word disambiguation

TEXT MINING

SYSTEMS BIOLOGY

Signalling networks

Metabolic pathways

Genetic networks

Protein function prediction

FUNCTION PREDICTION

Protein structure prediction

STRUCTURE PREDICTION

Protein location prediction

Protein-protein interaction

Protein annotation

PROTEOMICS

MICROARRAY

OTHER APPLICATIONS

Primer design

Backtranslation

EXPERIMENTAL DATA MANAGEMENT

Mass espectrometry data pre-processing

Mass espectrometry data Analysis

IMAGE ANALYSIS

Biomedical image analysis

Microarray data analysis

Microarray data pre-processing

Microarray image analysis

Fig. 5 Classification of the topics where machine learning methods are applied

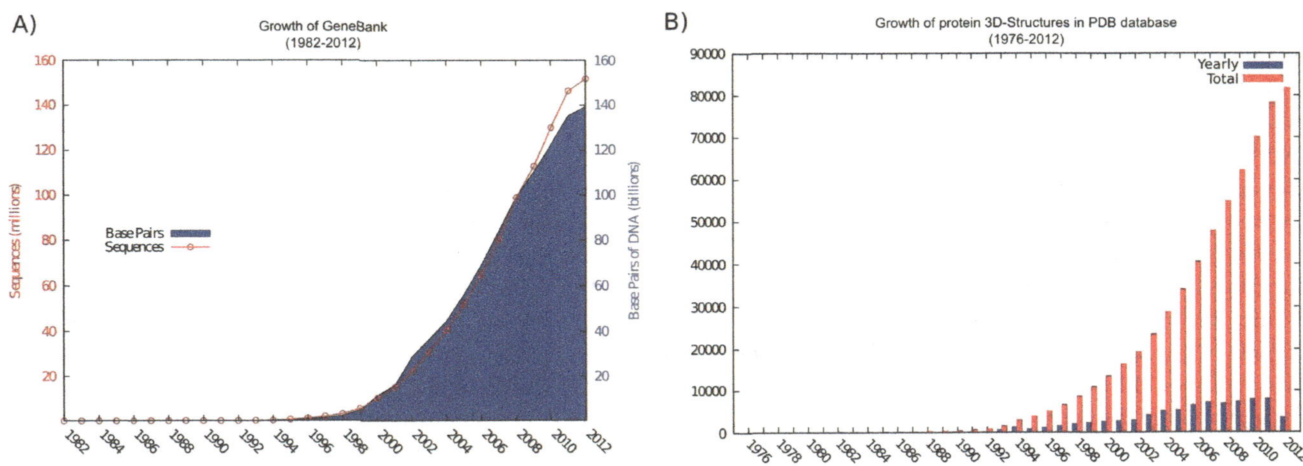

Fig. 6 Growth of public databases: **A** Evolution of the GenBank database size and **B** 3D structures of proteins

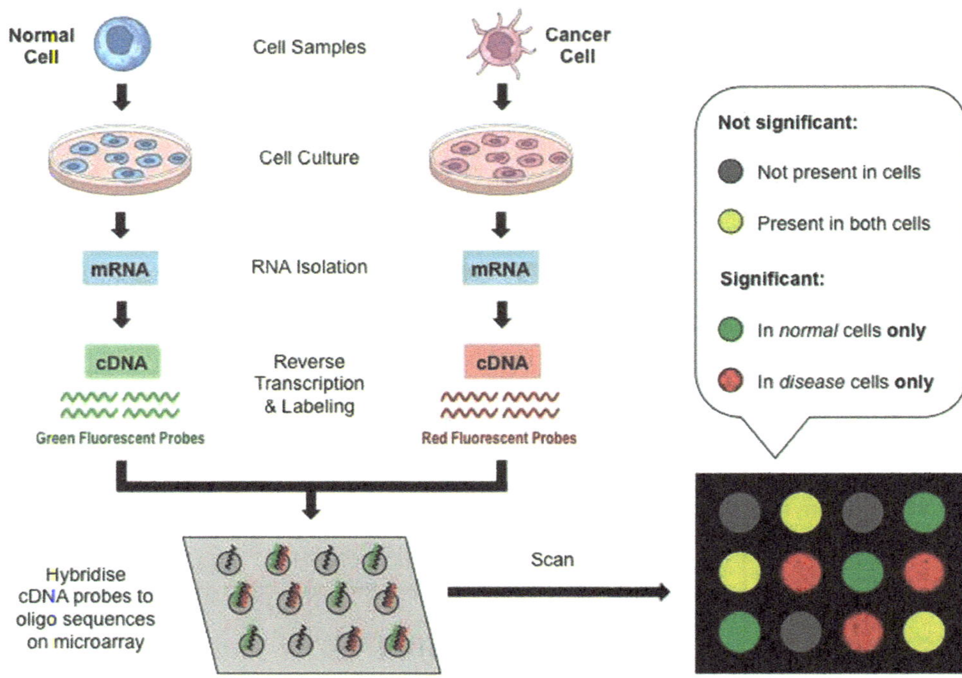

Fig. 7 DNA microarray overview [34]

Complicated empirical data raise two different troubles. First, data must be processed in advance, i.e., modified data to be used appropriately by machine learning algorithms. Second is data analysis, which relies on what we are looking for. In the case of microarray data, the most popular application is to determine the pattern of expression, classification and induction of the genetic network. Microarray framework for data management is shown in Fig. 8. Generally, the objective of microarray image analysis is to extract density descriptors from each point representing the levels of gene expression and input properties for the upcoming analysis and then the biological results are plotted using the data mining and statistical results of all extracted features. The DNA microarray image analysis components include grid alignment problem, foreground separation, quality assurance, quantification and normalization [35].

In addition, management of data should satisfy to a *minimum information about a microarray experiment* (MIAME), which is a standard created by the Functional Genomics Data Society (FGED) for reporting microarray experiments [36]. It is prepared to assign all the information needed to unambiguously understand the results of the experiment and to potentially reproduce the experiment. While the standard determines the content required for compliant reports, it does not specify the format in which this data should be presented; there are several file formats for representing this data, both public and subscription-based repositories for such experiments [37].

In short, the process in Fig. 8 can be summarized as follows: it starts by the laser scanning of the images (data) which generates accurate 2D microarray-DNA images. Then, the outcome is automatically derived from the data (a machine learning perspective) to subsequent model fitting, and the alignment of the microarray grid produces a set of cut-off rows at each point that realize a correct introduction as well as the separation of the foreground, which are the main processing steps of DNA microarray images that impact the quality of the gene expression information, and therefore affect the confidence in any biological conclusions derived from the data. Thus, understanding the microarray data processing steps becomes crucial for optimal data analysis in the microarray. Then the unreliable microarray cells are eliminated. Finally, an image of the average sample values in each grid cell is extracted using a special mask and colored in a red, green and blue space with the color assigned to each cluster/pixel. The statistics for each cluster can be found in the text area. Finally, the output of all steps is the statistical behavior of measurements and thus the test of the hypotheses or knowledge must be performed automatically from the data (machine learning perspective) for subsequent model fitting and draw biologically meaningful conclusions [35].

The microarray data processing framework contains issues related to data management (MIAME-compliant database) [38]; however, the main concern is of mechanism by which all stains should be reliably determined without any human intervention dependent on human preparation once. One-time setup is to incorporate any prior knowledge of microarray image layout into network alignment algorithms in order to reduce their parameter search

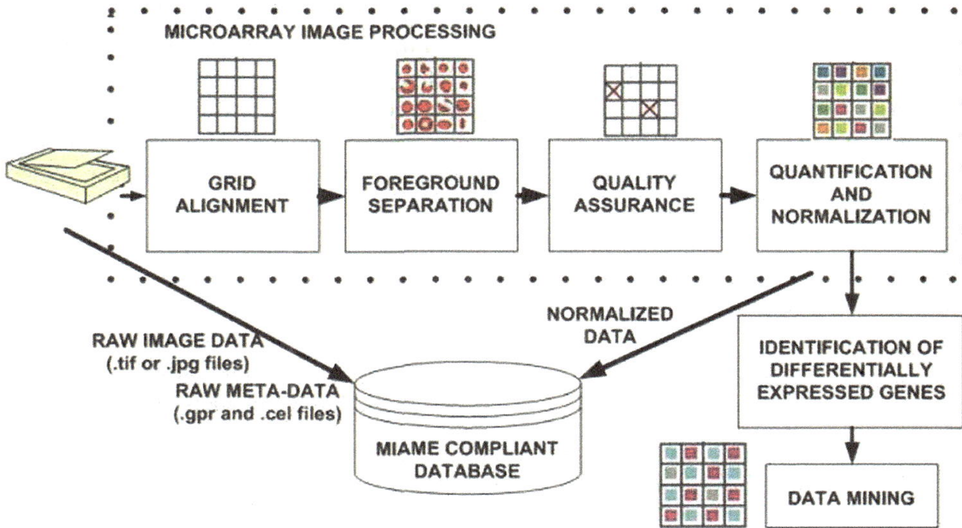

Fig. 8 Microarray data processing workflow [35]

space. This method is usually data-driven and has multiple internal arithmetic coefficients improved in the parameter search area to compensate for differences in microarray image [35].

Grid Line Algorithm

The grid line algorithm [39] is the first step of microarray data processing workflow. It is based on data and it aims to find a set of mutually orthogonal lines intersecting at the center of each grid cell obtained from DNA microarray scanners. The points generally have two states: the varying radii and their position deviates from a perfect grid placement. The grid cell is defined as a one-point area that is part of a set of two-dimensional arrays of points.

Foreground Separation Algorithm

The foreground separation algorithm [35] is the second step of microarray data processing workflow. It can be implemented by several methods, including foreground separation using spatial templates [40], foreground separation using intensity-based clustering [41], foreground using intensity-based segmentation [42], foreground separation using spatial and intensity information (hybrid methods) [43], and foreground separation from multichannel microarray images [35].

Quality Assurance Process

The quality assurance process is the third step of microarray data processing workflow where the spot quality assessment is implemented to identify grid cells that include valid spots and to eliminate invalid spots from further analysis. It is also used to determine the invalid or defective spots, for example, as deviations from the "ideal" microarray image and the deviation threshold values separating valid and invalid spot

categories. Indeed, there are two types of background variation criteria: local and global background variability. The local metrics can detect the existence of noise in a grid cell while global standards provide indicators of differences across a complete microarray slide. The quality metric q for background according to the designed formulas at [44]:

$$q_{BKG}^{LOC\&GLOB1} = \frac{\mu_{BKG}^{GLOBAL}}{\mu_{BKG}^{LOCAL} + \mu_{BKG}^{GLOBAL}} ; q_{BKG}^{LOC\&GLOB2}$$
$$= \frac{m_{BKG}^{GLOBAL}}{m_{BKG}^{LOCAL} + m_{BKG}^{GLOBAL}} \qquad (1)$$

where q the quality is metric, m is a median and μ is a mean. The notations, *FRG* refers to foreground and *BKG* to background.

Quantification and Normalization

After a set of valid spots and two sets of image pixels labeled as foreground and background each spot is calculated, and the descriptors are extracted to evaluate the gene regulation in a process called *data quantification* [45] (also called spot feature extraction), where the feature should be directly proportional to the mRNA quantity in the solution that was deposited in a spot and should perform as the deposited gene expression level. During the step of data preparation, the fluorescent intensity measurements are assessed or distorted differently according to some linear or nonlinear functions. Thus, a normalization process for the descriptors of extracted points is desirable.

In general, spot descriptors are split into two classes: the absolute-relative descriptors and the statistical-deterministic descriptors. It is important to understand the experimental structure of the microarray in expression of the outcome of the gene expression. The intensity of the raw microarray cannot be explained as an absolute measurement due to the random and systematic fluctuations in microarray image data preparation. Thus, in the experiments of cDNA, one is concerned with the statistical difference in the levels of gene expression between the probe and the target (also referred to as the test and reference) which is a hybrid mRNA mixture to the array and library in the array. Based on these considerations, the relative statistics descriptions will focus on the forms of microarray spot descriptors by using ratio or logarithmic ratio provided as follows [46]:

$$des_{RATIO}^{X} = \frac{X_{FRG}^{CHANNEL\ 0}}{X_{FRG}^{CHANNEL\ 1}} \quad (2)$$

$$des_{LOG\ RATIO}^{X\ WRT\ BKG} = \log_2\left(\frac{X_{FRG}^{CHANNEL\ 0} - X_{BKG}^{CHANNEL\ 0}}{X_{FRG}^{CHANNEL\ 1} - X_{BKG}^{CHANNEL\ 1}}\right) \quad (3)$$

where X is the symbol for sample mean or median or mode, the subscripts FRG and BKG refer to foreground and background, respectively, and the superscript $CHANNEL$ refers to red or green microarray laser scans. While Eq. (1) represents a direct ratio of absolute values, Eq. (2) is a logarithmic ratio of relative differences ($XWRTBKG$ stands for X with respect to background). Also, the normalization via statistical descriptors is common technique that can be applied by either division or subtraction of statistical descriptors in which Z-transformation would normalize intensities but would not compensate for labeling nonlinearity. This method is modeled in Eq. (4) where μ is the mean and σ is the standard deviation of an entire image [46]:

$$I_{Z-TRANSFORM}^{NORM\ STAT}(row, col) = \frac{I(row, col) - \mu}{\sigma} \quad (4)$$

3.3 Proteomics

One of the major aims of late biology is to know the relationships between the context of the structure and function of genomic information. Different *mass spectrometry* (MS) techniques attempt to provide qualitative results that describe relationships. The isotope labeling and fluorescent labeling techniques have been used in the quantitative analysis of proteins. However, researchers are turning to non-discriminatory methods because they are faster and simpler [47–49].

Peptides are produced by enzymatic digestion of the protein mixture and then the development of these peptides for training [50]. The label-free method makes use of several peptides to characterize MS tryptic observations to estimate the relative amount of protein [51]. However, the spectral count of the possibility of a peptide can be confused to be observed [52, 53]. A series of studies have found that we can

determine the protein based on one note or a few peptides that have been detected preferentially [47]. Some research has also found that different types of peptide likelihood detection may differ from others. Peptide physicochemical properties can affect the discovery of final MS due to many factors such as peptide length, mass, average flexibility indices, net charge and other properties that can affect peptide compliance [54]. This variation must be considered to estimate the quantity; otherwise errors may occur in the assessment of abundance of protein.

To estimate the quantity of protein, we can use the number of peptides detected to indicate abundance, and two classifiers can be used to classify peptides into two types called *proteotypic* and *unposerved*. The peptides are produced through different platforms and must be classified separately. The likelihood of each peptide can be deduced for its original protein and then if we are trying to identify a new protein and quantify it, the likelihood can be very useful for accurate prediction. Some peptides are more readily identified than others that can be observed from the experiments given in Table 1. Thus, the preferentially observed peptides are called as *proteotypic peptides* and therefore, the main two question regarded to proteotypic peptides are: (1) *"What characteristics distinguishing the frequently observed peptides from peptides in the same protein sample but remain unknown?"* and (2) *"What peptide characteristic can be applied to all living organisms?"*. Moreover, if we find the characteristics of the outside, is it possible to predict whether the peptide is *proteotypic* using the protein's sequence. To implement these targets, the *proteotypic* peptides are taken from four different platforms and distinguished with physicochemical properties [55].

To determine the characteristic that controls a peptide's proteotypic inclination, 544 different parameters of the physicochemical properties of amino acids is evaluated, including the water-resistant index, containing hydrophobicity index, residue volume and transfer-free energy to surface [54]. Given that both the total and the average value can contribute to the inclination at the same time, we used a value to describe the peptides, resulting in 1088-dimension property vector in the peptide. There are two methods used in this approach: Support vector machine and random forests. *Support vector machine* (SVM) sets a hyper-plane to classify the given pattern; its basic idea is given in Fig. 9. In addition, this approach used transformation method for getting better performance and kernel functions. The input features vector space can be converted by nonlinear function applications to a high-dimensional space where the best hyper-plane level can be learned which can resolve more complex classification among set that have not been identified at all in the original space [56, 57].

Figure 9 displays two state of vectors that are separated by hyper-plane: the white circle which presents the positive

Table 1 The genuine and imposter distance distribution [54]

Peptide example		K	L	I	G	D	Total	Average
1	Amino acid composition	0.68	0.98	1.02	0	0.76	3.44	0.688
2	Relative mutability	6.6	7.4	4.5	8.4	5.5	32.4	6.48
3	Melting point	56	40	96	49	106	347	69.4
4	Optical rotation	224	337	284	290	270	1405	281
5	Steric parameter	14.6	−11	12.4	0	5.05	21.05	4.21

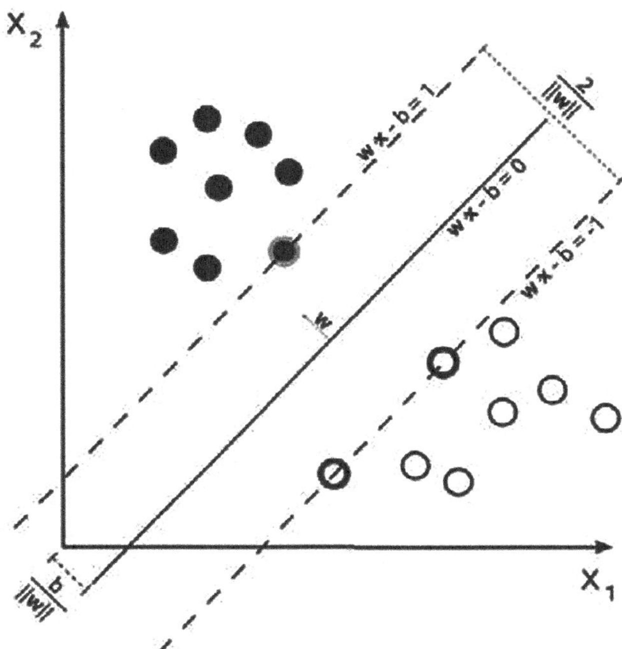

Fig. 9 Support vector machine

vectors and the black presents the negative vectors. The kernel function is used to avoid the overlap circles that called overfitting, which convert the input space to a higher dimensional space. The kernel function plays an important role in assigning the input space implicitly to a larger dimension space for features, and in this situation, the separation can be better in that the original model will lead to overfitting learning. There are many types of kernel functions [56, 57], such as the polynomial kernel function that is widely used. The function is:

$$K(x_i^T + x_j + 1)^p, \text{ where } p \text{ is a positive constant} \quad (5)$$

Or the Gaussian radial basis function (RBF) kernel given by

$$K(x_i + x_j) = \exp\left(-\gamma \|x_i + x_j\|^2\right) \quad (6)$$

Sometimes parameterized using:

$$\gamma = 1/2\sigma^2 \quad (7)$$

where $\sigma > 0$ is a constant that defines the kernel width. Furthermore, there are some other kernel functions that can be used into various states such as the hyperbolic tangent function. Under the use of kernel function, the discriminant function in an SVM classifier is:

$$f(x) = \sum_{i=1}^{N} \alpha_i y_i K(x_i, x) + b \quad (8)$$

where $K(xi, x)$ is the kernel function, are the support vectors specified from the training data, is the class indicator (e.g., +1 and −1 for a two class problem) related with each , N is the number of supporting vectors specified through training process and b is a scalar representing the perpendicular distance of the hyper-plane from origin. The data of the training set are support vectors that are used by SVM classifier to make the decision and predict the label (positive or negative) of samples. In fact, they consist of those training examples that are most difficult to classify.

The features in Table 1 are used to extract different vector data and then generate an input space. These vectors can be described as positive or negative, representing traditional and non-observed peptides. There are two parts of vectors separated by SVM: the first part is applied for training and the second part is applied to predict the performance of the training model. For each peptide in the training set, the vectors have 1088 features as a representation, for example, considering the sample of the amino acid composition of peptides varies from 0 to 4 while the melting point can vary up to several hundred centigrade. As a result of these different ranges, the corresponding features of the rating may dominate the classification and invalidate the effects of other features.

To avoid this problem, each feature vector is normalized to [−1, 1] and after calculating the features, matrix is generated. Suppose: $X = (x_1, x_2, \ldots, x_k)$, where k is the number of features, $X_k = (x_{1k}, x_{2k}, \ldots, x_{nk})$, where n is the number of peptides in training set and $\max(X_k)$ is the maximum value in x_k and $min(x_k)$ is the minimum value in x_k. The normalization method is shown as below:

$$x_{(i,k)} = -1 + 2 \frac{x_{(i,k)} - \min(x_k)}{\max(x_k) - \min(x_k)} \quad (9)$$

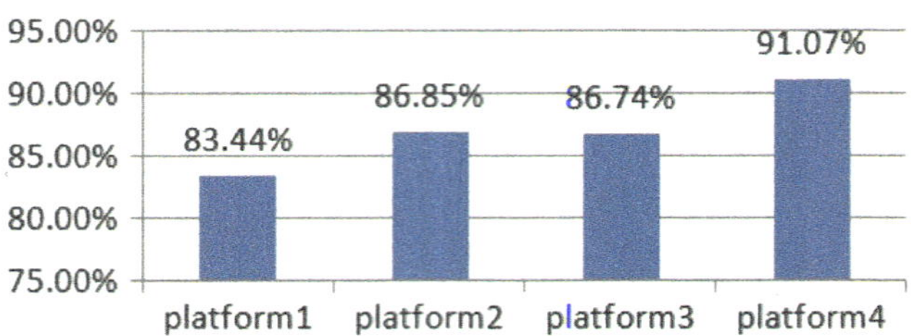

Fig. 10 The accuracy under the SVM classification [55]

After normalization, we categorized the classification, and prediction accuracy is used to define the performance of the trainer model. The four-accuracy platforms are as given in Fig. 10 which shows that the accuracy of training model has an impressive performance in peptide identification and some additions can improve it to better results: parameter selection. Parameter set is evaluated to get the best classification under the grid search of cost and gamma and thus the cross-validation accuracy for four platforms varies from 85 to 90%.

Figure 11 illustrates the parameter chosen for platform 4 with g representing gamma for radial basis function (RBF) kernel function and c represents cost function of SVM classification. In this optimum parameter's selection, the best $c = 4$ and $g = 0.0039$, and the best accuracy is 89%. In this case, the best model has the best robustness. In conclusion, the classification of SVM can lead to high accuracy in prediction of approximately 90%, and the process of parameterization can improve its performance.

Random forests is the other method used in Proteomics where it consists of many individual classification trees [58].

Each tree gives a single classification and the final result relies on how the results of these trees are classified. *Breiman procedure* [59] must conform to the following algorithms: assume that the training set number is N, and the experiment with n cases in the bootstrap method, which means a sample with the substitution. The number of sample training set is approximately $2/3$ to the original training set number. Construct classification and regression tree (CART) for each bootstrap training set. These trees are unknown. Assuming there are M features for each input vector, the best features of M is chosen for split use. M is the only parameter that can be modified.

Since each classification gives a result, then aggregate it and the mode of classification results is the final classification. One benefit of the bootstrap sampling method is that $1/3$ of the original training set is not selected and that these samples can be used in prediction. Random forests give discretionary error in training, which is called out of the bag (OOB) error. Berman [59] stated that the experience indicates an OOB error in an unbiased estimate as a cross-validation error. The random forest method is employed to train a classifier, and there are 100 trees trained to use in prediction and the m try was set to be 32 $(= \sqrt{1088}$Features. The results are listed in Fig. 12.

The accuracy of random forest is cross-checking accuracy [59]. Random forest accuracy is better than SVM prediction accuracy, which means that random forest is the most appropriate classifier for this condition. In addition, random forest classifier can give functionality to choose features, which is very useful for some classifications. However, in this case, the less features may reduce the accuracy and all

Fig. 11 The parameter selection for platform 4 [55]

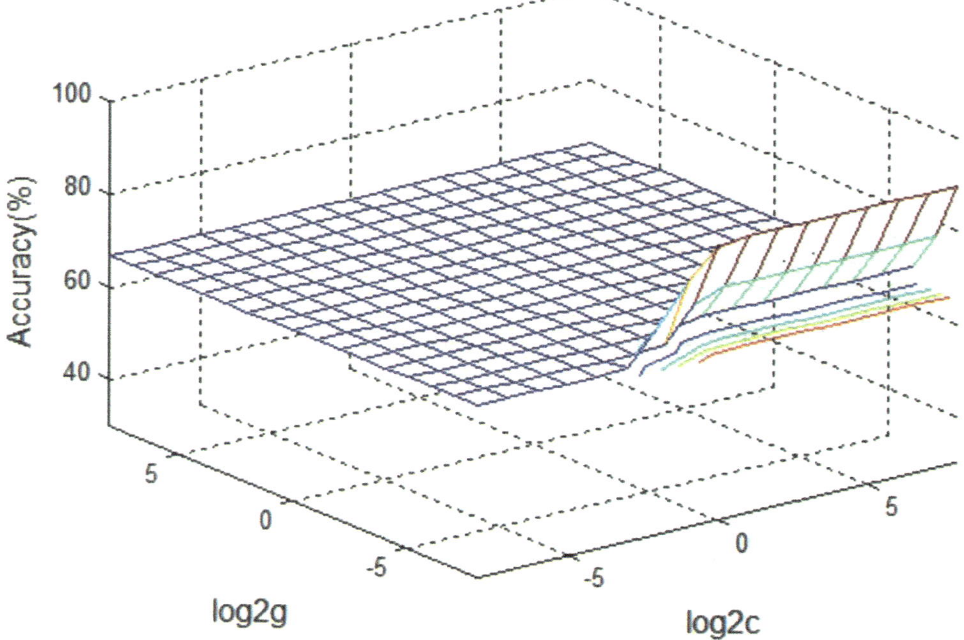

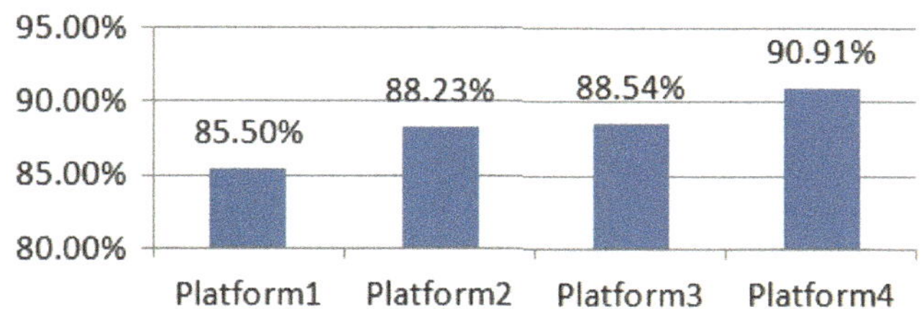

Fig. 12 The accuracy under the random forest classification [55]

1088 dimensions must be used. It is still very convenient because the computer is fully capable of solving the algorithm in a few hours. As the result for all the number of observed peptides is usually influenced by their physicochemical property, it makes the correction necessary for accurate prediction.

3.4 Text Mining Methods

Text mining (TM) is the process of exploring and analyzing large amounts of non-structural text data with the help of software that can identify concepts, patterns, subjects, keywords and other features in the data. One of the main objectives of text mining is to find the related information in the text by converting it into data that can be analyzed. However, this definition does not cover the real relevance, efficiency and role that text mining plays in bioinformatics. In the past decade, the research articles collected in public repositories, such as PubMed [60], are growing exponentially. Figure 13 shows that the number of publications per year on bioinformatics doubles in 2018 compared with 2001.

The applications of text mining require to achieve the linguistic analysis by using *natural language processing* (NLP) algorithms to resolve ambiguity in the human language. The NLP algorithms contain part-of-speech tagging, disambiguation and other fundamental methods that have been modified or better customized to classify text mining in bioinformatics and biomedical literature. Examples of the most text mining applications in bioinformatics include [60]:

- *Information retrieval* (IR) dedicated to obtaining related information from a set of information resources and user query.
- *Document classification* (DC) which defined one or more categories to a document.
- *Named entity recognition/normalization* (NER/NEN) dedicated to extracting the so-called machine-read or semi-structured entity.
- *Summarize* (SUM) which compiles the input text that covers all the contents of the analyzed documents.

In practice, there are several methods to be used to assess the text extraction applications that exist. For instance, ROUGE metric is used to evaluate text summarization systems to estimate the similarity of the resulting summary with the so-called gold summary at syntactic level by matching the n-grams, or at semantic level [61] by evaluating notion covered by the generated summary. There are many variables for ROUGE, where the next level comes with the scale that estimates the number of n-gram in both the gold and the summary that was created [60].

Fig. 13 The number of publications in PubMed on text mining

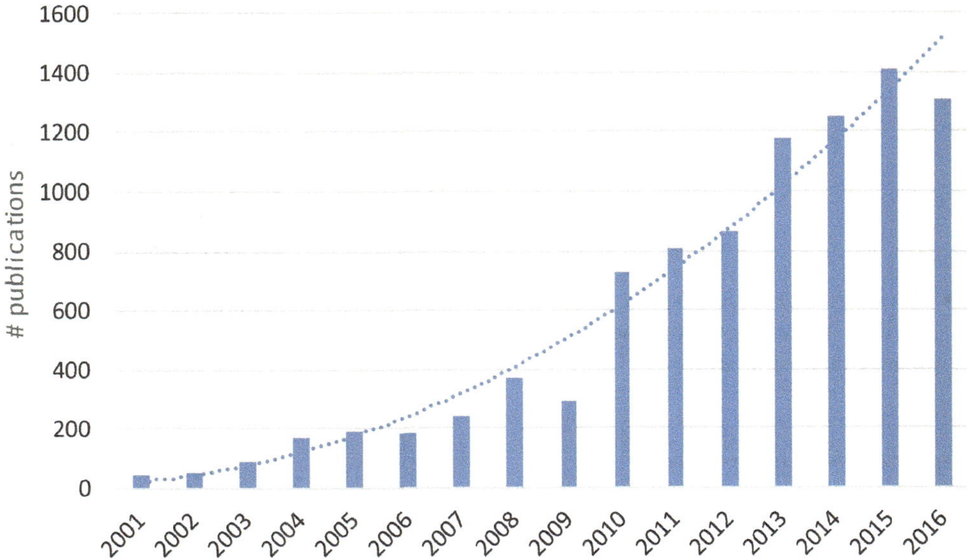

$$ROUGE = \frac{\#(\text{relevent n - gram retrieved in Generate Summaries})}{\#(\text{relevent n - gram in Gold Summaries})}$$ (10)

However, the most commonly used measures to evaluate information retrieval, document classification, NER and other applications can be summarized as follows [62]:

- *Precision (P)* which is a part of all recovered documents that have been labeled as relevant

$$Precision = \frac{\#(\text{relevant items retrieved})}{\#(\text{retrieved items})}$$
$$= P(\text{relevant}|\text{retrieved})$$ (11)

- *Recall (R)* which is a part of all relevant documents that have been retrieved effectively:

$$Recall = \frac{\#(\text{relevant items retrieved})}{\#(\text{relevant items})}$$
$$= R(\text{retrieved}|\text{relevant})$$ (12)

For those two measures (i.e., precision and recall), their relevancy can be judged according to the confusion or error matrix provided in Table 2, then:

$$P = \frac{tp}{(tp+fp)} R = \frac{tp}{(tp+fn)}$$ (13)

- *Balanced F-measure (F)* which attempts to reduce precision and recall to a single measurement.

$$F = 2\frac{(PR)}{(P+R)}$$ (14)

- *Accuracy (A)* which is the number of correct answers divided by the total number of answers. In terms of matrix confusion above

$$Accuracy = \frac{(tp+tn)}{(tp+fp+fn+tn)}$$ (15)

- *Error (E)* which is the proportion of incorrectly identified instances:

$$Error = 1 - Accuracy \; or \; E = 1 - A \; (\%)$$ (16)

3.5 Systems Biology

It has been a while when the relationship between biology and the field of machine learning started; indeed it's a historical and long-complex relationship. Early technique for machine learning called perceptron [63] was an attempt to plot the actual neurological behavior and the field of artificial neural network (ANN) design emerged from this attempt. More artificial neural network architecture has been inspired, such as adaptive resonance theory (ART) [64] and neocognitron [65] inspired from the organization of the visual nervous system. In the intervening years, the flexibility of machine learning techniques has grown along with mathematical frameworks to measure their reliability, and hopefully that machine learning methods will improve the efficiency of discovery and understanding on increasing the size and complexity of biological data.

Supervised and unsupervised learning methods of machine learning are used in applications of biology. In *supervised learning*, objects are grouped into a particular group using a set of attributes or features. The result of a classification process is a set of rules that specify object assignments for existing categories only to attribute values. In a biological context, examples of object-to-class assignments are images of the embodiment of genetic tissues into a group of diseases and the sequence of the protein into its secondary structures. Figure 14 shows the main difference between supervised and unsupervised learning by illustrating data samples for both cases. According to the figure, the features in these samples are levels of term of individual genes measured in tissue samples and the presence/absence

Table 2 The confusion matrix		Relevant	Non-relevant
	Retrieved	*True Positive (tp)*	*False Positive (fp)*
	Non-retrieved	*False Negative (fn)*	*True Negative (tn)*

of a specific amino acid code at a given position in the protein sequence, respectively.

The aim of supervised learning is to create a system that can accurately predict the membership of the new object category based on available features. In addition to predicting class properties such as class label (like classical discriminant analysis), supervised techniques can also be applied to predict continuous object properties (like regression analysis). In any supervised learning application, it would be helpful for the classification algorithm to return a "doubt" value (indicating that it is not obvious which one of several possible categories the object should be assigned to) or "externally" (indicating that this object is different from anything previously observed such that the appropriateness of any decision on class membership is questionable). In contrast to the supervised framework, in *unsupervised learning*, there are no predefined labels for the objects and in this case the unsupervised learning aims to search data and find similarities between objects. Similarities are utilized to identify groups of objects, referred to as *clusters*. In other words, unsupervised learning aims to reveal natural groups in the data. Thus, the two models can vary informally as follows: In supervised learning, the data comes with class labels and how to associate labeled data with classes; but in unsupervised learning, all data is unlabeled, and the learning procedure consists of both identify labels and link things to them.

In some applications, such as protein structure classification, only a few labeled samples (protein sequences with a known structural class) are available, while many other samples (sequences) with an unknown class are also available. In such status, *semi-supervised techniques* can be implemented to get a best classifier than can be gained if the labeled samples are used only [66]. This is potential, for instance, by making the cluster assumption, that is, class labels can be reliably divert from labeled to unlabeled objects that are "nearby" in feature space. Life science applications of unsupervised and/or supervised machine learning techniques abound in literature. For instance, gene expression data were used successfully to classify patients in different clinical groups and distinguish new disease groups [67–70] while allowing the genetic code to predict the structure of the secondary protein [71]. Continuous variable prediction was used with machine learning algorithms to estimate bias in microarray data [72].

Finally, Fig. 15 provides a machine learning workflow [73] that shows the difference between supervised and unsupervised learning in biological cases in which the whole process can be summarized in four steps labeled in the figure from **(A) to (D)**.

A. Data preparation stage includes four steps: data preprocessing, feature extraction, model learning and evaluation. It is common to refer to a single data sample including all common variables and features such as x input (vector of numbers) and distinguish it from the output response variable y (one number) when available.

B. The learning method: supervised machine learning methods relate input features x to an output label y, whereas unsupervised method learns factors about x without observed labels. The goals of supervised machine learning model are to learn a function $f(x) = y$ from a list of training pairs $(x_1, y_1), (x_2, y_2)$ for which data are listed. One model application in biology is to predict the sensitivity of a cancer cell line when exposed to a selection drug [73].

C. Raw input data is of high dimensions and associated with the corresponding label in a complex manner which challenges many classical machine learning algorithms (left plot). Alternatively, higher-level features extracted using a deep model may be better able to distinguish between layers (right plot). As the x inputs, calculated from raw data, appear what the "model sees around the world", their choice is highly problem-specific.

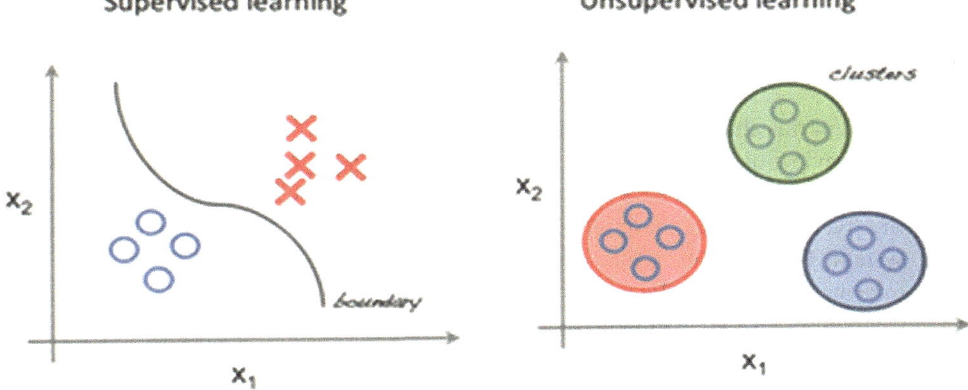

Fig. 14 Supervised versus unsupervised learning in a biological context

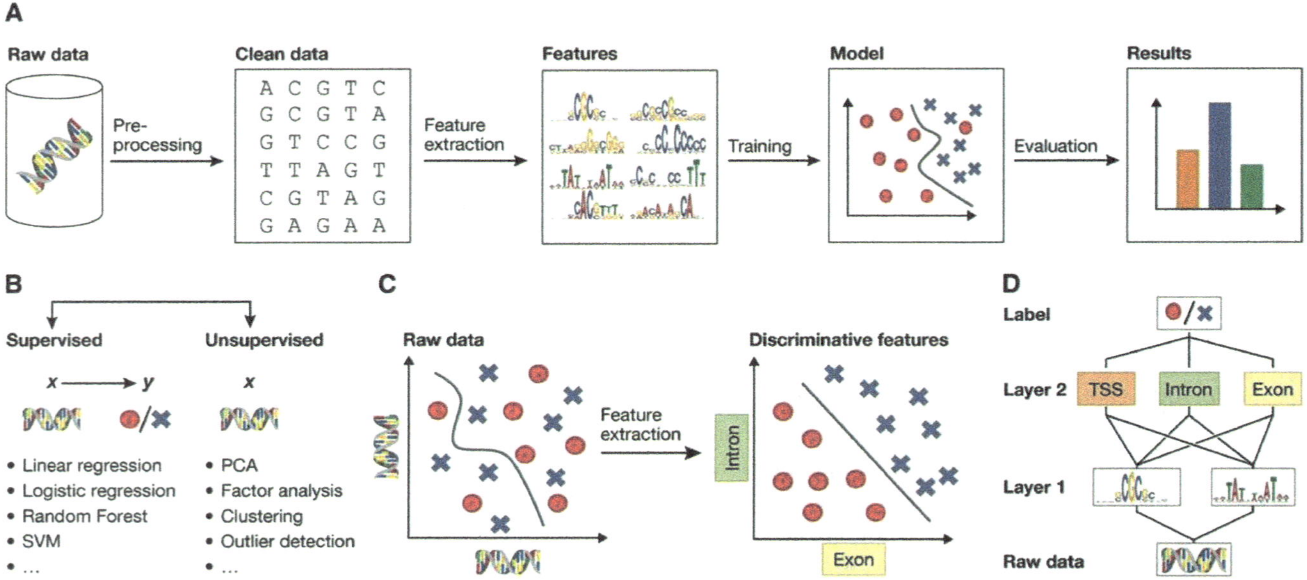

Fig. 15 The complete framework of machine learning workflow for biological applications

D. Deep networks utilize a hierarchical structure to learn abstract representations of raw data increasingly. The discovery of most informative features is fundamental to the performance, but the process can be labor-intensive and need knowledge of the field. This bottleneck is particularly limited by high-dimensional data; even methods of selecting arithmetic properties are not scaled to assess the advantage of the large number of possible input combinations. A major advance in machine learning is the automation of this critical phase by learning an appropriate representation of data with deep artificial neural networks [74]. In short, the *deep neural network* transfers the raw data in the lower layer (input) and converts it into increasingly simulated representations by sequentially combining the output from the previous layer in a data-based way and encapsulating the very complex tasks in the process.

4 Review Questions

By the end of this chapter, you are encouraged to answer the following review questions:

1. Briefly, describe each of the following concepts: Expert system, Bioinformatics, Recommender systems, Reinforcement learning, Probabilistic machine learning, Genomics, MIAME, Support vector machine.

2. What are the three levels of integration for artificial intelligence?

3. What is the distinction between bioinformatics and biomedical engineering fields?

4. What is the distinction between artificial intelligence and machine learning fields?

5. Discuss the importance of Stanford applications in the field bioinformatics?

6. Provide one practical example for each of the following: natural language processing, AI for robotics, AI for speech processing, AI for clinical data annotated and AI for patient similarity

7. List two differences between supervised and unsupervised learning. Give two examples for each.

8. How can we construct algorithms that automatically get better through experience?

9. What are the primary laws that control all learning processes?

10. What is the distinction between automated machine learning (aML) and interactive machine learning (iML)?

11. What are the major biological problems in which arithmetic methods are applied as an AI solution?

12. Why predicting the protein structure is a very complicated problem?

13. Explain in steps how the DNA microarray works?

14. Develop a mathematical numerical example for the quality metric q for background quality assurance process of microarray process?

15. Why do we need a normalization process for the quantified data of microarray process? Justify your answer with numerical examples.

16. What characteristics distinguishing the frequently observed peptides from peptides in the same protein sample but remain unknown?

17. What peptide characteristic can be applied to all living organisms?

18. What is meant by text mining process? Explain by example its role in bioinformatics?

19. List six examples of text mining applications in bioinformatics?

20. Given the following values: Precision = 90% and Recall = 75%. Calculate the information retrieval error percent and the balanced F-measure.

21. Discuss the semi-supervised techniques data classification for bioinformatics applications?

22. What is the main purpose of deep neural network (DNN) in the machine learning workflow for biological applications?

References

1. Brunette E.S, Flemmer RC, Flemmer CL, (2009). *A review of artificial intelligence*. Proceedings of 4th International Conference on Autonomous Robots and Agents (ICARA 2009), pp: 385–392.
2. Boden M.A (1998). *Creativity and artificial intelligence*. Artificial Intelligence 103: 347–356.
3. Müller V.C, Bostrom N. (2014). *Future progress in artificial intelligence*. AI Matters 1: 9–11.
4. Research Report. (2018). *The AI Industry Series: Top Healthcare AI Trends to Watch*. Retrieved online: https://www.cbinsights.com/research/report/.
5. IBM Watson Health (2018). Artificial Intelligence in medicine. Technical Report. Retrieved online: https://www.ibm.com/watson-health/learn/.
6. Sumit D. et. al. (2015): *Applications of Artificial Intelligence in Machine Learning: Review and Prospect*. International Journal of Computer Applications, Vol. 115, No. 9, April 2015.
7. Rahul C. Deo. (2018). *Machine Learning in Medicine*. Circulation. 2015 Nov 17; 132(20): 1920–1930. https://doi.org/10.1161/circulationaha.115.001593.
8. Yuedong Y. (2016). *Sixty-five years of the long march in protein secondary structure prediction: the final stretch*. Briefings in Bioinformatics, Volume 19, Issue 3, 1 May 2018, Pages 482–494, https://doi.org/10.1093/bib/bbw129.
9. Pedro. L. (2006). Machine learning in bioinformatics. Briefings in Bioinformatics, Volume 7, Issue 1, 1 March 2006, Pages 86–112, https://doi.org/10.1093/bib/bbk007.
10. Stuart R., Peter N. (2009). *Artificial Intelligence: A Modern Approach*. Pearson; 3 edition (December 11, 2009).
11. Linda S. G. (1997). *Mainstream Science on Intelligence: An Editorial With 52 Signatories*. Ablex Publishing Corporation.
12. Nick B. (2006). *How long before superintelligence?* Linguistic and Philosophical Investigations, 2006. - pp. 11–30.
13. Padraig C, Matthieu C., Sarah J.D Delany. (2008). *Supervised Learning: Machine Learning techniques for Multimedia*. Springer, Case studies on Organizational and retrieval.
14. Ricci F., Rokach L., Shapira B. (2010). *Recommender Systems Handbook*. Boston, MA: Springer. ISBN 9780387858197.
15. Jordan MI, Mitchell TM (2015). *Machine learning: trends, perspectives, and prospects*. Science, Vol. 349 No. 6245, P. p. 255–260.
16. LeCun Y, Bengio Y, Hinton G (2015). *Deep learning*. Nature, Vol. 521, No. 7553, P.p.:436–444.
17. Bayes T. (1763). *An essay towards solving a problem in the doctrine of chances (posthumous communicated by Richard Price)*. Philosophical Transactions of the Royal Society of London 53 (1763), 370–418.].
18. Barnard GA, Bayes T (1958). *Studies in the history of probability and statistics: IX. Thomas Bayes's essay towards solving a problem in the doctrine of chances*. Biometrika, Volume 45, Issue 3–4, 1 December 1958, Pages 293–295, https://doi.org/10.1093/biomet/45.3-4.293.
19. Hastie T, Tibshirani R, Friedman J (2009). *The elements of statistical learning: data mining, inference, and prediction*. 2nd edition. Springer, New York.
20. Murphy KP (2012). *Machine learning: a probabilistic perspective*. MIT press, Cambridge.
21. Silver D, et. al. (2016). *Mastering the game of go with deep neural networks and tree search*. Nature, Vol. 529, No. 7587, P.p. 484–489.
22. Zhong N, et. al. (2007). *Web intelligence meets brain informatics*. Zhong N, Liu JM, Yao YY, Wu JL, Lu SF, Li KC (eds) Web intelligence meets brain informatics., Lecture Notes in Artificial Intelligence 4845, Springer, Berlin, pp 1–31.
23. Holzinger A (2014). *Trends in interactive knowledge discovery for personalized medicine: cognitive science meets machine learning*. IEEE Intelligence Inform Bull 15(1):6–14.
24. Mitchell TM (1997). *Machine learning*. McGraw Hill, New York.
25. Holzinger A, Dehmer M, Jurisica I. (2014). *Knowledge discovery and interactive data mining in bioinformatics-state-of-the-art, future challenges and research directions*. BMC Bio inform 15 (S6):I1.
26. Spinrad N. (2014). *Google car takes the test*. Nature, Vol. 514, No.7523, P.p. 528–528.
27. Holzinger A (2014). *Biomedical informatics: discovering knowledge in big data*. Springer, New York.
28. Holzinger A (2013). *Human–computer interaction and knowledge discovery (HCI-KDD): what is the benefit of bringing those two fields to work together?* Multidisciplinary research and practice for information systems., Springer Lecture Notes in Computer Science LNCS 8127Springer, Heidelberg, pp 319–328.
29. Mitchell, T. (1997). *Machine Learning*. McGraw-Hill.
30. Ohler, W., Liao, C., Niemann, H. & Rubin, G. M. *Computational analysis of core promoters in the Drosophila genome*. Genome Biol. 3, RESEARCH0087 (2002).

31. Degroeve, S., Baets, B. D., de Peer, Y. V. & Rouzé, P. *Feature subset selection for splice site prediction*. Bioinformatics 18, S75–S83 (2002).

32. Bucher, P. (1990). *Weight matrix description of four eukaryotic RNA polymerase II promoter elements derived from 502 unrelated promoter sequences*. J. Mol. Biol. 4, 563–578.

33. Heintzman, N. et al. (2007). *Distinct and predictive chromatin signatures of transcriptional promoters and enhancers in the human genome*. Nature Genet. 39, 311–318.

34. BioNinja. *Microarrays*. Retrieved online: http://ib.bioninja.com.au/higher-level/topic-7-nucleic-acids/72-transcription-and-gene/.

35. Peter B, Lei L. and Mark B. (2007). *DNA Microarray Image Processing*. DNA Array Image Anal. Nuts Bolts (Nuts Bolts Ser), Pages 1–77.

36. Adams R. M, B. Stancampiano, M. McKenna and D. Small. (2002). *Case Study: A Virtual Environment for Genomic Data Visualization*. IEEE Transactions on Visualization, Boston, MA, USA (published as CD).

37. Affymetrix Inc., *Gene Chip Arrays*. Retrieved online: http://www.affymetrix.com/index.affx.

38. Brazma A., et. al, (2001). *Minimum Information About a Microarray Experiment (MIAME)–toward standards for microarray data*, Nat. Genet. 29, 365–371, December 2001.

39. Whitfield CW, Cziko AM, Robinson GE. (2003). *Gene expression profiles in the brain predict behavior in individual honey bees*. Science. Vol. 302, pages 296–9.

40. Jain A. N., et. al. (2002). *Fully Automated Quantification of Microarray Image Data*. Genome Research, Vol. 12, No. 2, Feb 2002, pp. 325–332.

41. Steinfath M., et. al. (2001). *Automated image analysis for array hybridization experiments*. Bioinformatics, Vol. 17, pages 634–641.

42. Russ J. (1999). *The Image Processing Handbook: Third Edition*. CRC Press with IEEE Press. Published by CRC Press LLC. 1999.

43. Liew A W-C., H. Yan, and M. Yang. (2003). *Robust Adaptive Spot Segmentation of DNA Microarray Images*. Pattern Recognition 36, pages 1251–1254.

44. Axon Instruments Inc., *GenePix Pro*. Retrieved Online at: http://www.axon.com/GN_Genomics.html.

45. Dodd L. E., et. al., (2004). *Correcting Log Ratios for Signal Saturation in cDNA Microarrays*. Bioinformatics, Vol. 20, No. 16, pp. 2685–2693.

46. Kamberova G., S. Shah (editors) (2002). *DNA Array Image Analysis - Nuts and Bolts*. Data Analysis Tools for DNA Microarrays, DNA Press LLC, MA, 2002.

47. P. Mallick, et. al. (2007). *Computational prediction of proteotypic peptides for quantitative proteomics*. Nat Biotech, 25(I): I 25-I 31.

48. W. H. Zhu, J. W Smith and C. M. Huang (2010). *Mass Spectrometry-Based LabelFree Quantitative Proteomics*. Journal of Biomedicine and Biotechnology, vol. 2010, article ID: 840518.

49. S. E. Ong and M. Mann (2005). *Mass spectrometry-based proteomics turns quantitative*. Nature Chemical Biology, vol. 1, pp. 252–262.

50. R. Aebersold and M. Mann. (2003). *Mass spectrometry-based proteomics*. Nature, 422, pp. 198–207.

51. L. N. Mueller, M. Y. Brusniak, D. R. Mani and R. Aebersold (2008). *An Assessment of Software Solutions for the Analysis of Mass Spectrometry Based Quantitative Proteomics Data*. J. Proteome Res., 7 (01), pp. 51–61.

52. P. Lu, C. Vogel, R. Wang, X. Yao and E. M. Marcotte. (2007). *Absolute protein expression profiling estimates the relative contributions of transcriptional and translational regulation*. Nature Biotechnology, 25, pp. 117–124.

53. J. C. Braisted, et. al., (2008) The Apex Quantitative Proteomics Tool: Generating protein quantitation estimates from LC-MS/MS proteomics results, BMC Bioinformatics 9:529.

54. S. Kawashima and M. Kanehisa. (2000). *AA_index: amino acid index database*. Nucleic Acids Res.vol. 28, no. 374.

55. Biao H., Baochang Z., Yan. F., (2013). *Discovery of Proteomics based on Machine Learning*. Quantitative Biology > Quantitative Methods.

56. B. M. Webb-Robertson, et. al., (2008). *A support vector machine model for the prediction of proteotypic peptides for accurate mass and time proteomics*, Bioinformatics Corrigendum, vol.26, no.13, pp. 1677–1683.

57. C. Cortes and V. Vladimir. (1995). *Support-Vector Networks*, Machine Learning, Vol. 20, Issue. 3, pp. 273–297.

58. E. Alpaydin (2004). *Introduction to Machine Learning*, MIT Press.

59. L. Brieman (2001). *Random Forest*, Machine Learning, vol.45 issue.1, pp. 5–32.

60. Fie. Z., et. al, (2013). Biomedical text mining and its applications in cancer research. Journal of Biomedical Informatics 46 (2013) 200–211.

61. Frawley W.J, Piatetsky S.G, Matheus C. J. (1992). *Knowledge discovery in databases: an overview*. AI Mag 1992;13:57–70.

62. Agarwal S, Liu F, Yu H. (2011). *Simple and efficient machine learning frameworks for identifying protein–protein interaction relevant articles and experimental methods used to study the interactions*. BMC Bioinformatics 2011;12 (Suppl.8):S10.

63. Rosenblatt F (1958) The perceptron: A probabilistic model for information storage and organization in the brain. Psychol Rev 65: 386–408.

64. Carpenter GA, Grossberg S (1988). *The art of adaptive pattern recognition by a self-organizing neural network*. Computer 21: 77–88.

65. Fukushima K (1980). *Neocognitron: A self-organizing neural network model for a mechanism of pattern recognition unaffected by shift in position*. Biol Cybern 36: 193–202.

66. Weston J, et al. (2005) *Semi-supervised protein classification using cluster kernels*. Bioinformatics 21: 3241–3247.

67. Alizadeh A.A, et al. (2000). *Distinct type of diffuse large B-cell lymphoma identified by gene expression profiling*. Nature, Vol. 403, pages 503–510.

68. Perou CM, et. al. (1999). *Distinctive gene expression patterns in human mammary epithelial cells and breast cancers*. Proc Natl Acad Sci U S A 96: 9212–9217.

69. Alon U, et al. (1999). *Broad patterns of gene expression revealed by clustering of tumor and normal colon tissues probed by nucleotide arrays*. Proc Natl Acad Sci U S A 96: 6745–6750.

70. Ross DT, et al. (2000). *Systematic variation in gene expression patterns in human cancer cell lines*. Nat Genet 24: 227–235.

71. Rost B, Sander C (1994) *Combining evolutionary information and neural networks to predict protein secondary structure*. Proteins 19: 55–72.

72. Tarca AL, Cooke JE, Mackay J (2005) *A robust neural networks approach for spatial and intensity-dependent normalization of cDNA microarray data*. Bioinformatics 21: 2674–2683.

73. Christof A., et. al., (2016). Deep learning for computational biology. Published online 29.07.2016 Molecular Systems Biology (2016) 12, 878, https://doi.org/10.15252/msb.20156651.

74. Tin-Chih T.C, Cheng L. L., Hong D. L., (2018). *Advanced Artificial Neural Networks*. MDPI, Algorithms 2018, 11, 102; https://doi.org/10.3390/a11070102.

Human Facial Age Estimation: Handcrafted Features Versus Deep Features

Salah Eddine Bekhouche, Fadi Dornaika, Abdelkrim Ouafi,
and Abdelmalik Taleb-Ahmed

Abstract

In recent times, human facial age estimation topic attracted a lot of attention due to its ability to improve biometrics systems. Recently, several applications that exploit demographic attributes have emerged. These applications include: access control, re-identification in surveillance videos, integrity of face images in social media, intelligent advertising, human–computer interaction, and law enforcement. In this chapter, we present a novel approach for human facial age estimation in facial images. The proposed approach consists of the following three main stages: (1) face preprocessing; (2) feature extraction (two different kinds of features are studied: handcrafted and deep features); (3) feeding the obtained features to a linear regressor. Also, we investigate the strength and weakness of handcrafted and deep features for facial age estimation. Experiments are conducted on three public databases (FG-NET, PAL and FACES). These experiments show that both handcrafted and deep features are effective for facial age estimation.

1 Introduction

Humans live a certain period of time. With the progress of time, the human appearance shows some remarkable changes due to the age progression. Predicting the age is a difficult task for humans and it is more difficult for computers, although, the accurate age estimation is very important for some applications. Recently, several applications that exploit the exact age or the age group have emerged. The person's age information can lead to higher accuracy in establishing the user identity for the traditional biometric identifiers which can be used in access control applications.

In this chapter, we propose an automatic human facial age estimation system that is composed of three parts: face alignment, feature extraction and age estimation.

The purpose of face alignment is to localize faces in images, rectify the 2D or 3D pose of each face and then crop the region of interest. This preprocessing stage is important since the subsequent stages depend on it and since it can affect the final performance of the system. The processing stage can be challenging since it should overcome many variations that may appear in the face image. Feature extraction stage extracts the face features. These features are extracted either by texture descriptors or deep networks. In the last stage, we fed the extracted features to a regressor to estimate the age.

The remaining of the chapter is organized as follows: In Sect. 2, we summarize the existing techniques of facial age estimation. We introduce our approach in Sect. 3. The experimental results are given in Sect. 4. In Sect. 5, we present the conclusion and some perspectives.

S. E. Bekhouche
Department of Electrical Engineering, University of Djelfa, Djelfa, Algeria

S. E. Bekhouche · F. Dornaika (✉)
University of the Basque Country UPV/EHU, San Sebastian, Spain
e-mail: fadi.dornaika@ehu.eus

F. Dornaika
IKERBASQUE, Basque Foundation for Science, Bilbao, Spain

A. Ouafi
Laboratory of LESIA, University of Biskra, Biskra, Algeria

A. Taleb-Ahmed
IEMN DOAE UMR CNRS 8520, UPHF, 59313 Valenciennes, France

© Springer Nature Switzerland AG 2021
J. Alja'am et al. (eds.), *Emerging Technologies in Biomedical Engineering and Sustainable TeleMedicine*,
Advances in Science, Technology & Innovation, https://doi.org/10.1007/978-3-030-14647-4_3

2 Background

Facial age estimation is an important task in the domain of facial image analysis. It aims to predict the age of a person based on his or her face features. The predicted age can be an exact age (years) or age group (year range) [1]. Predicting the age is a difficult task for humans and it is more difficult for computers, although, the accurate age estimation is very important for some applications. From a general perspective, the facial age estimation approaches can be categorized based on the face image representation and the estimation algorithm. Age estimation approaches can be divided into three main types anthropometric-based, handcrafted-feature-based and deep-learning-based approaches [2].

The anthropometry-based approaches mainly depend on measurements and distances of different facial landmarks. Kwon and Lobo [3] proposed an age classification method which classify input images into one of three age groups: babies, young adults, and senior adults. Their method is based on craniofacial development theory and skin wrinkle analysis. The main theory in the area of craniofacial research is that the appropriate mathematical model to describe the growth of a person's head from infancy to adulthood is the revised cardioidal strain transformation [4].

Handcrafted-feature-based approaches are ones of the most popular approaches for facial age estimation since a face image can be viewed as a texture pattern. Many texture features have been used like Local Binary Pattern (LBP), Histograms of Oriented Gradients (HOG), Biologically Inspired Features (BIF), Binarized Statistical Image Features (BSIF), and Local Phase Quantization (LPQ). LBP and its variants were also used by many works like in [5–8]. BIF and its variants are widely used in age estimation works such as [9,10]. Some researchers used multi-modal features. For instance, the work presented in [8] proposed an approach which uses LBP and BSIF extracted from Multi-Block face representation.

Deep learning approaches mainly use a Convolutional Neural Networks (CNN) which is a type of feed-forward artificial neural networks in which the connectivity pattern between its neurons is inspired by the organization of the animal visual cortex. Some approaches train the networks from scratch such as [11] and other do a transfer learning such as [12].

3 Proposed Approach

In this section, we present the different stages of our approach that estimates the human age based on facial images. Our approach takes a face image as input. A face preprocessing stage is first applied to the image in order to obtain a cropped and aligned face. In the second stage, a set of features are extracted across texture descriptor or a pre-trained CNN. Finally, these features will be fed to a linear SVR in order to predict the age.

3.1 Face Preprocessing

Firstly, we apply the cascade object detector that uses Viola-Jones algorithm [13] to detect people's faces. Then, we detect the eyes of each face using the ERT algorithm [14]. To rectify the 2D face pose in the original image, we apply a 2D transformation based on the eyes center to align the face. Unlike the work described in [15], the cropping parameters are set as follows: $k_{side} = 1.25$, $k_{top} = 1.75$ and $k_{bottom} = 2.25$. These parameters are multiplied by a rescaled inter-ocular distance in order to obtain the side margins, the top margin and the bottom margin. Figure 1 illustrates the steps of the face preprocessing stage.

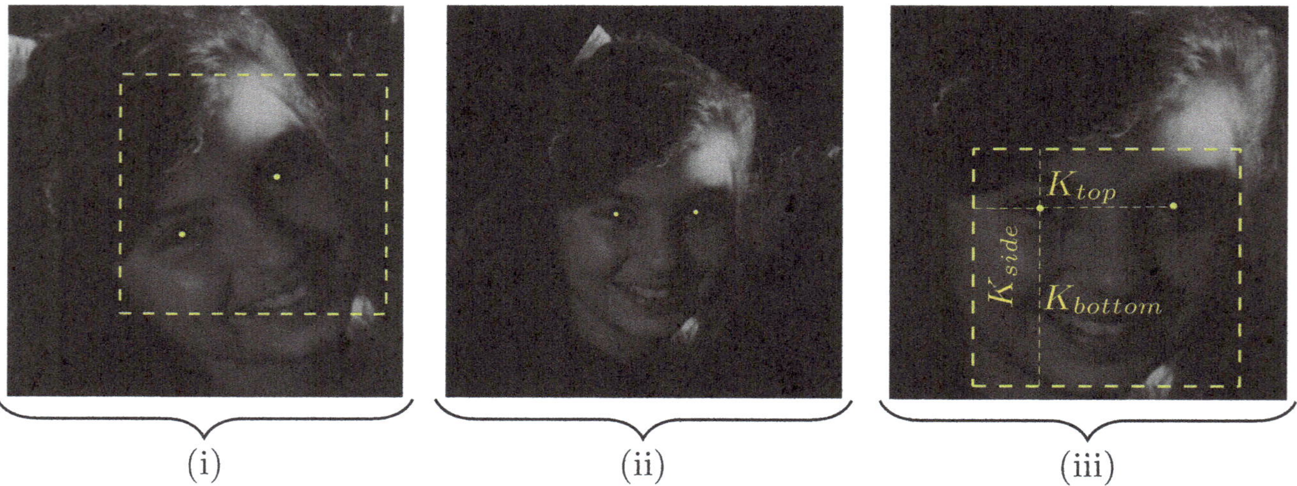

Fig. 1 Face preprocessing stage

3.2 Feature Extraction

Feature extraction stage has been the most studied topic among the rest stages due to its effective effect on the age estimation systems performance. In our approach, we studied two different kinds of feature extraction. The first one is based on handcrafted features or texture features and the second one is based on deep features which extracted using pretrained networks.

Handcrafted Features

Refer to the attributes derived using generic purpose texture descriptors which use the information present in the image itself. In our case, we used three types of texture descriptors LBP, LPQ and BSIF on a Pyramid Multi-Level (PML) face representation.

Local Binary Pattern (LBP) is a very efficient method for analyzing two dimensional textures. It used the pixels of an image by thresholding the neighborhood of each pixel and considers the result as a binary number. LBP was used widely in many image-based applications such as face recognition. The face can be seen as a composition of micro-patterns such as edges, spots and flat areas which are well described by the LBP descriptor [16].

Local Phase Quantization (LPQ) descriptor was proposed in [17]. It is based on the application of short-time Fourier transform (STFT). The advantage in STFT is that the phase of the low frequency coefficients is insensitive to centrally symmetric blur. The spatial blurring is represented by a convolution between the image intensity and a Point Spread Function (PSF).

Binarized statistical image feature (BSIF) is a new image texture descriptor proposed by Kannala and Rahtu [18]. It is inspired by LBP and LPQ texture descriptors. The idea behind BSIF is to automatically learn a fixed set of filters from a small set of natural images, instead of using handcrafted filters such as in LBP and LPQ, yet we consider it as a handcrafted descriptor.

The Pyramid Multi-Level (PML) representation adopts an explicit pyramid representation of the original image. It preceded the image descriptor extraction. This pyramid represents the image at different scales. For each such level or scale, a corresponding Multi-block representation is used. PML sub-blocks have the same size which is determined by the image size and the chosen level. In our work, we use 7 levels based on [15] observation. Figure 2 illustrates the PML face representation adopting three levels.

Deep Features

Refer to descriptors that are often obtained from a CNN. These features are usually the output of the last fully connected layer. In our work, we used the VGG-16 architecture [19] as well two variants of this architecture. We extract the deep features from the layer FC7 (fully connected layer) of this architecture, and the number of these features is 4096.

VGG-16 [19] is a convolutional neural network that is trained on more than one million images from the ImageNet database. The network is 16 layers deep and can classify images into 1000 object categories. As a result, the network has learned rich feature representations for a wide range of images. VGG-FACE [20] is inspired by VGG-16, it was trained to classify 2,622 different identities based on faces. DEX-IMDB-WIKI [12] was fine tuned on the IMDB-WIKI face database which has more than 500K images, yet it is also based on VGG-16.

In our empirical study, we use the following deep features: VGG-16, VGG-FACE, and DEX-IMDB-WIKI.

3.3 Age Estimation

The proposed method estimates the person age using a linear SVM regressor. This regressor was tuned to find the best configuration for its hyper-parameters.

4 Experiments and Results

To evaluate the performance of the proposed approach, we use FG-NET, PAL and FACES databases. The performance is measured by the Mean Absolute Error (MAE) and the Cumulative Score (CS) curve.

The MAE is the average of the absolute errors between the ground-truth ages and the predicted ones. The MAE equation is given by:

$$MAE = \frac{1}{N} \sum_{i=1}^{N} |p_i - gt_i| \qquad (1)$$

where N, p_i, and gt_i are the total number of samples, the predicted age, and the ground-truth age respectively.

The CS reflects the percentage of tested cases where the age estimation error is less than a threshold. The CS is given by:

$$CS(T) = \frac{N_{e \leq T}}{N} \% \qquad (2)$$

where T, N and $N_{e \leq T}$ are the error threshold (years), the total number of samples and the number of samples on which the age estimation makes an absolute error no higher than the threshold, T.

4.1 FG-NET

The FG-NET [21] aging database was released in 2004 in an attempt to support research activities related to facial aging.

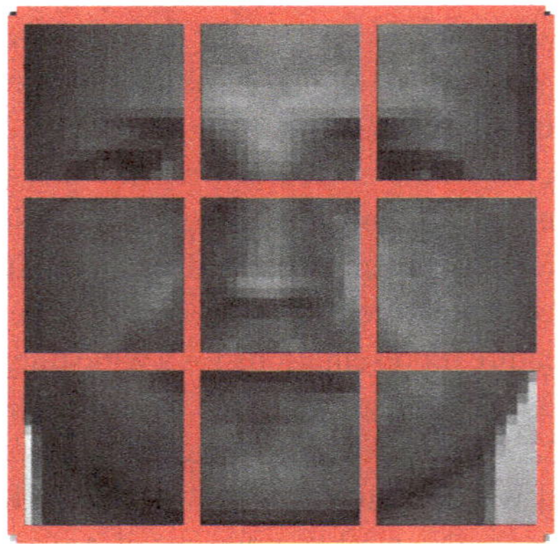
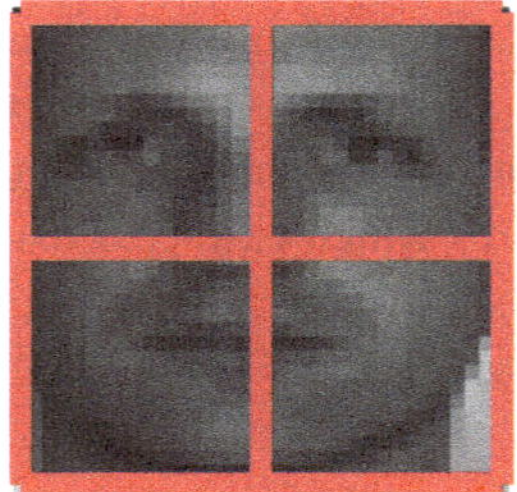
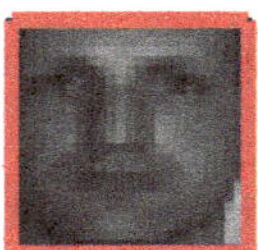

Fig. 2 PML face representation adopting three levels

Since then a number of researchers used the database for carrying out research in various disciplines related to facial aging. This database consists of 1002 images of 82 persons. On average, each subject has 12 images. The ages vary from 0 to 69. The images in this database have large variations in aspect ratios, pose, expression, and illumination. The Leave One Person Out (LOPO) protocol has been used due to the individual's age variation in this database, each time a person's images are put into a test set whereas the other persons' images are put in a train set. Figure 3 shows the cumulative score curves for the six features. We can observe that the PML-LPQ and PML-BSIF descriptors perform better than the deep features in term of CS which can be viewed as an indicator of the accuracy of the age estimators.

Table 1 illustrates the MAE of the proposed approach as well as of that of some competing approaches. From this table, we can observe that the best deep-features DEX-IMDB-WIKI and the best handcrafted features PML-LPQ outperform some

Table 1 Comparison with existing approaches on FG-NET database

Approach	MAE
IIS-LLD [22]	5.77
CA-SVR (2013) [23]	4.67
SVR+BSIF+LBP [8]	6.34
CS-LBFL (2015) [24]	4.43
CS-LBMFL (2015) [24]	4.36
AAM+GABOR+LBP (2016) [25]	4.87
SWLD (2017) [26]	5.85
PML-LBP	5.48
PML-LPQ	4.10
PML-BSIF	4.48
VGG16	6.15
VGG-FACE	4.41
DEX-IMDB-WIKI	**4.09**

of the existing approaches. Moreover, we can see that the DEX-IMDB-WIKI features give the best results, followed closely by the PML-LPQ features. Based on the CS curve of Fig. 3 and Table 1, we can see that the MAE and the CS are two different indicators that do not always highlight the same best approach.

Table 2 depicts the CPU time (in seconds) of features extraction stage and the training phase associated with 1002 images of FG-NET database. The experiments were carried out on a laptop DELL 7510 Precision (Xeon Processor E3-1535M v5, 8M Cache, 2.90 GHz, 64GB RAM, GPU NVIDIA Quadro M2000M, Windows 10). The handcrafted features significantly outperform the deep features in term of CPU time execution of the feature extraction stage knowing that the deep features are computed using the GPU instead of the CPU. On the other hand, the CPU time associated with the regressor training with the deep features is smaller than that of the regressor training using the handcrafted features. This

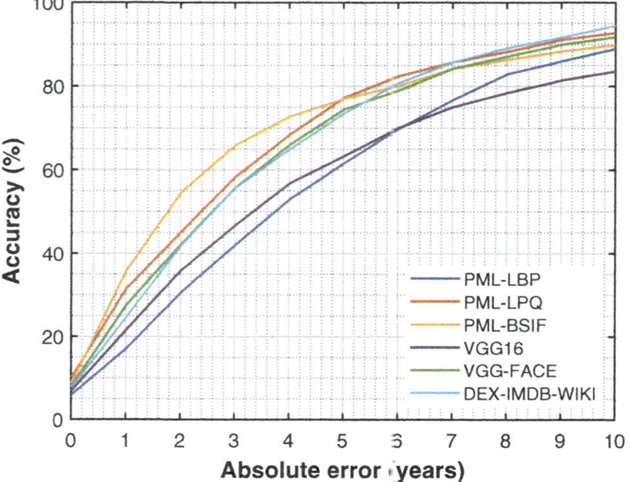

Fig. 3 Cumulative scores obtained by the proposed approach on the FG-NET database

Table 2 CPU time (in seconds) of extracting features and training stages on the FG-NET database

	Feature extraction	SVR training
PML-LBP	22.50	59.09
PML-LPQ	32.16	123.55
PML-BSIF	28.05	145.25
VGG-16	104.16	34.30
VGG-FACE	102.12	39.02
DEX-IMDB-WIKI	100.91	29.05

Table 3 Comparison with existing approaches on the PAL database

Approach	MAE
BIF (2012) [28]	8.93
BIF+MFA (2012) [28]	6.05
SVR+BSIF+LBP [8]	6.25
CS-LBFL (2015) [24]	5.79
CS-LBMFL (2015) [24]	5.26
AAM+GABOR+LBP (2016) [25]	5.38
SWLD (2017) [26]	6.68
PML+BSIF+LPQ (2017) [29]	5.00
LS-SVM (2018) [30]	5.26
PML-LBP	6.61
PML-LPQ	5.30
PML-BSIF	5.43
VGG16	6.31
VGG-FACE	5.64
DEX-IMDB-WIKI	**4.62**

is due to the fact that the size of the deep features is smaller than that of the handcrafted features.

4.2   PAL

The Productive Aging Lab Face (PAL) database from the University of Texas at Dallas [27] contains 1,046 frontal face images from different subjects (430 males and 616 females) in the age range from 18 to 93 years old. The PAL database can be divided into three main ethnicities: African-American subjects 208 images, Caucasian subjects 732 images and other subjects 106 images. The database contains faces having different expressions. For the evaluation of the approach, we conduct 5-fold cross-validation, our distribution of folds is selected based on age, gender and ethnicity. Figure 4 shows the cumulative score curves for the six different features. We can appreciate a change in the performance compared to FG-NET performance curve. It can be seen that the DEX-IMDB-WIKI features outperform the best handcrafted features which is PML-LPQ.

Table 3 illustrates the MAE of the proposed approach as well as of that of some existing approaches. These results show that the DEX-IMDB-WIKI features outperform most of the existing approaches on the PAL database.

4.3   FACES

This database [31] consists of 2052 images from 171 subjects. The ages vary from 19 to 80 years. For each subject, there are six expressions: neutral, disgust, sad, angry, fear, and happy. The database encounters large variations in facial expressions bringing an additional challenge for the problem of age prediction. Figure 5 shows the cumulative score curves for the six different features. The results considered all images in all expressions. We can observe that the DEX-IMDB-WIKI features outperform all the other features. It is followed by the PML-LPQ features.

Fig. 6 illustrates the cumulative score curves for the different facial expressions of the FACES database when using the DEX-IMDB-WIKI features. This figure shows that the neutral and sadness expressions correspond to the most accurate age estimation. In other words, among all tested expressions the neutral and sadness expressions are the ones that lead to the best age estimation.

Table 4 presents comparison with some existing approaches. This table confirms the idea that the neutral expression is the expression that provides the most accurate age estimation compared to other facial expressions.

5   Conclusion

This chapter presents a study about using handcrafted and deep features for facial age estimation. Using small number of images, the results showed that the handcrafted features

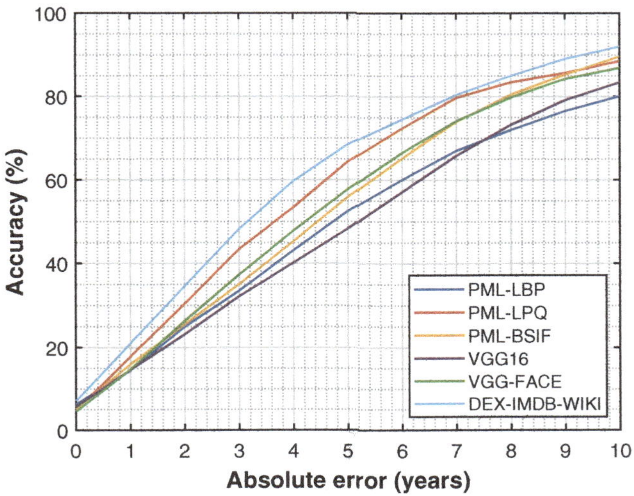

Fig. 4 Cumulative scores obtained by the proposed approach on the PAL database

Table 4 Comparison with existing approaches on FACES database

Approach	Neutrality	Anger	Disgust	Fear	Happiness	Sadness	Average
BIF (2012) [28]	9.50	13.26	13.23	12.65	10.69	10.78	11.68
BIF+MFA (2012) [28]	8.14	10.96	10.73	12.24	10.32	10.66	10.51
LS-SVM (2018) [30]	5.97	8.21	8.17	8.25	6.77	7.07	7.41
CS-LBFL (2015) [24]	5.06	6.94	7.15	6.32	6.53	6.27	6.38
DeepRank+ (2018) [32]	4.61	6.48	7.50	5.90	5.92	5.30	5.95
CS-LBMFL (2015) [24]	4.84	5.50	5.70	6.10	5.85	4.98	5.49
DLF (2018) [33]	–	–	–	–	–	–	5.18
LSDML (2018) [34]	3.88	3.87	4.41	5.10	3.49	4.09	4.14
PML-LBP	4.87	5.30	5.49	6.01	5.44	5.16	5.38
PML-BSIF	4.01	4.63	4.51	4.99	4.66	4.67	4.58
PML-LPQ	4.00	4.32	4.20	4.67	4.49	4.34	4.34
VGG16	5.45	6.69	6.16	5.83	6.26	5.54	5.99
VGG-FACE	4.27	5.21	5.67	5.17	4.65	4.81	4.96
DEX-IMDB-WIKI	3.49	3.82	4.51	3.99	3.93	3.52	**3.88**

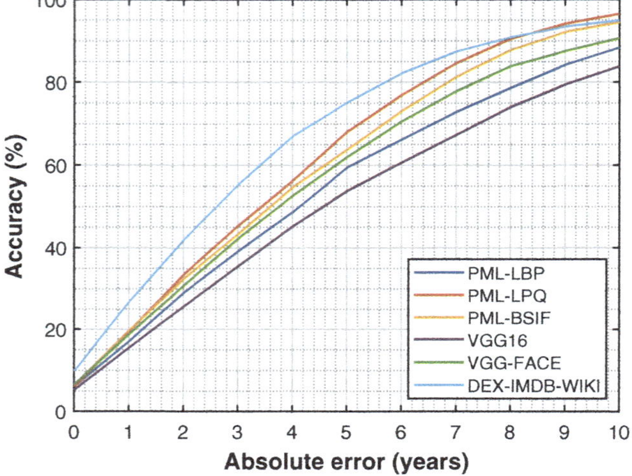
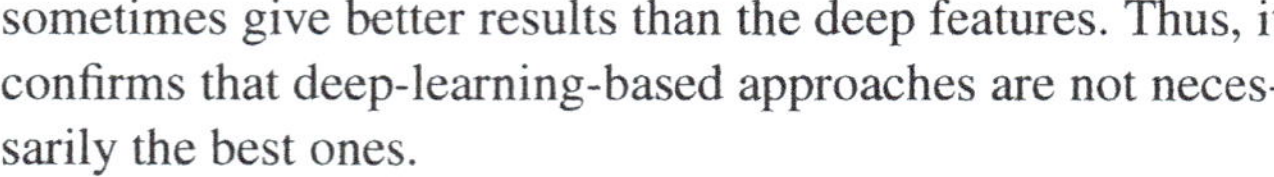

Fig. 5 Cumulative scores obtained by the proposed approach on the FACES database

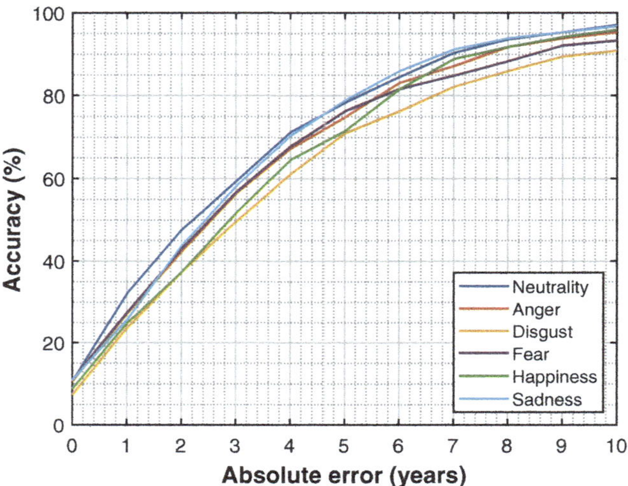

Fig. 6 Cumulative scores obtained by the DEX-IMDB-WIKI features for different expressions on the FACES database

sometimes give better results than the deep features. Thus, it confirms that deep-learning-based approaches are not necessarily the best ones.

As a future work, we envision the fine-tuning of new CNN architectures on face databases and creating new CNNs from scratch.

References

[1] Petra, G.: Introduction to human age estimation using face images. The Journal of Slovak University of Technology **21** (2013) 24–30

[2] Bekhouche, S.E.: Facial Soft Biometrics: Extracting demographic traits. PhD thesis, Faculté des sciences et technologies (2017)

[3] Kwon, Y.H., da Vitoria Lobo, N.: Age classification from facial images. Computer vision and image understanding **74**(1) (1999) 1–21

[4] Alley, T.: Social and Applied Aspects of Perceiving Faces. Resources for ecological psychology. Lawrence Erlbaum Associates (1988)

[5] Gunay, A., Nabiyev, V.V.: Automatic age classification with lbp. In: Computer and Information Sciences, 2008. ISCIS'08. 23rd International Symposium on, IEEE (2008) 1–4

[6] Shan, C.: Learning local features for age estimation on real-life faces. In: Proceedings of the 1st ACM international workshop on Multimodal pervasive video analysis, ACM (2010) 23–28

[7] Ylioinas, J., Hadid, A., Pietikäinen, M.: Age classification in unconstrained conditions using lbp variants. In: Pattern recognition (icpr), 2012 21st international conference on, IEEE (2012) 1257–1260

[8] Bekhouche, S., Ouafi, A., Taleb-Ahmed, A., Hadid, A., Benlamoudi, A.: Facial age estimation using bsif and lbp. In: Proceeding of the first International Conference on Electrical Engineering ICEEB'14. (2014)

[9] Guo, G., Mu, G., Fu, Y., Huang, T.S.: Human age estimation using bio-inspired features. In: Computer Vision and Pattern Recognition, 2009. CVPR 2009. IEEE Conference on, IEEE (2009) 112–119

[10] Sai, P.K., Wang, J.G., Teoh, E.K.: Facial age range estimation with extreme learning machines. Neurocomputing **149** (2015) 364–372

[11] Levi, G., Hassner, T.: Age and gender classification using convolutional neural networks. In: Proceedings of the IEEE Conference on Computer Vision and Pattern Recognition Workshops. (2015) 34–42

[12] Rothe, R., Timofte, R., Gool, L.V.: Dex: Deep expectation of apparent age from a single image. In: IEEE International Conference on Computer Vision Workshops (ICCVW). (December 2015)

[13] Viola, P., Jones, M.: Rapid object detection using a boosted cascade of simple features. In: Computer Vision and Pattern Recognition, 2001. CVPR 2001. Proceedings of the 2001 IEEE Computer Society Conference on. Volume 1. (2001) I–511–I–518 vol.1

[14] Kazemi, V., Sullivan, J.: One millisecond face alignment with an ensemble of regression trees. In: 2014 IEEE Conference on Computer Vision and Pattern Recognition. (June 2014) 1867–1874

[15] Bekhouche, S.E., Dornaika, F., Ouafi, A., Taleb-Ahmed, A.: Personality traits and job candidate screening via analyzing facial videos. In: Proceedings of the IEEE Conference on Computer Vision and Pattern Recognition Workshops. (2017) 10–13

[16] Ahonen, T., Hadid, A., Pietikainen, M.: Face description with local binary patterns: Application to face recognition. IEEE Transactions on Pattern Analysis & Machine Intelligence (12) (2006) 2037–2041

[17] Ojansivu, V., Heikkilä, J.: Blur insensitive texture classification using local phase quantization. In: International conference on image and signal processing, Springer (2008) 236–243

[18] Kannala, J., Rahtu, E.: Bsif: Binarized statistical image features. In: Pattern Recognition (ICPR), 2012 21st International Conference on, IEEE (2012) 1363–1366

[19] Simonyan, K., Zisserman, A.: Very deep convolutional networks for large-scale image recognition. arXiv preprint arXiv:1409.1556 (2014)

[20] Parkhi, O.M., Vedaldi, A., Zisserman, A., et al.: Deep face recognition. In: BMVC. Volume 1. (2015) 6

[21] Panis, G., Lanitis, A., Tsapatsoulis, N., Cootes, T.F.: Overview of research on facial ageing using the fg-net ageing database. Iet Biometrics **5**(2) (2016) 37–46

[22] Geng, X., Yin, C., Zhou, Z.H.: Facial age estimation by learning from label distributions. IEEE transactions on pattern analysis and machine intelligence **35**(10) (2013) 2401–2412

[23] Chen, K., Gong, S., Xiang, T., Change Loy, C.: Cumulative attribute space for age and crowd density estimation. In: Proceedings of the IEEE conference on computer vision and pattern recognition. (2013) 2467–2474

[24] Lu, J., Liong, V.E., Zhou, J.: Cost-sensitive local binary feature learning for facial age estimation. IEEE Transactions on Image Processing **24**(12) (2015) 5356–5368

[25] Günay, A., Nabiyev, V.V.: Age estimation based on hybrid features of facial images. In: Information Sciences and Systems 2015. Springer (2016) 295–304

[26] Günay, A., Nabiyev, V.V.: Facial age estimation using spatial weber local descriptor. International Journal of Advances in Telecommunications, Electrotechnics, Signals and Systems **6**(3) (2017) 108–115

[27] Minear, M., Park, D.C.: A lifespan database of adult facial stimuli. Behavior Research Methods, Instruments, & Computers **36**(4) (2004) 630–633

[28] Guo, G., Wang, X.: A study on human age estimation under facial expression changes. In: Computer Vision and Pattern Recognition (CVPR), 2012 IEEE Conference on, IEEE (2012) 2547–2553

[29] Bekhouche, S.E., Ouafi, A., Dornaika, F., Taleb-Ahmed, A., Hadid, A.: Pyramid multi-level features for facial demographic estimation. Expert Systems with Applications **80** (2017) 297–310

[30] Lou, Z., Alnajar, F., Alvarez, J.M., Hu, N., Gevers, T.: Expression-invariant age estimation using structured learning. IEEE Transactions on Pattern Analysis and Machine Intelligence **40**(2) (2018) 365–375

[31] Ebner, N.C., Riediger, M., Lindenberger, U.: Faces—a database of facial expressions in young, middle-aged, and older women and men: Development and validation. Behavior Research Methods **42**(1) (2010) 351–362

[32] Yang, H.F., Lin, B.Y., Chang, K.Y., Chen, C.S.: Joint estimation of age and expression by combining scattering and convolutional networks. TOMCCAP **14**(1) (2018) 9–1

[33] Kotowski, K., Stapor, K.: Deep learning features for face age estimation: Better than human? In: International Conference: Beyond Databases, Architectures and Structures, Springer (2018) 376–389

[34] Liu, H., Lu, J., Feng, J., Zhou, J.: Label-sensitive deep metric learning for facial age estimation. IEEE Transactions on Information Forensics and Security **13**(2) (2018) 292–305

Multi-scale Multi-block Covariance Descriptor for a Compact Face Texture Representation: Application to Kinship Verification

Abdelmalik Moujahid and Fadi Dornaika

Abstract

Division-based strategies for face representation are common methods for capturing local and global features and have proven to be effective and highly discriminative. However, most of these methods have been mainly considered for descriptors based only on one single type of features. In this chapter, we introduce an effective approach for face representation with application to kinship verification that relies on pyramid multi-level (PML) face representation, and which exploits second order statistics of several local texture features such as Local Binary Pattern (LBP), quaternionic local ranking binary pattern (QLRBP), gradients, and different color spaces. The proposed approach consists of two main components. First, we model the face image using a PML representation that seeks a multi-block-multi-scale representation where several local texture features are extracted from different blocks at each scale. Second, to achieve a global context information, we compute the covariance between local features characterizing each individual block in the PML representation. The resulting face descriptor has two interesting properties: (i) thanks to the PML representation, scales and face parts are explicitly encoded in the final descriptor without having to detect the facial landmarks, (ii) the covariance descriptor (second order statistics) encodes spatial features of any type allowing the fusion of several state-of-the art texture features. Experiments conducted on two challenging kinship databases provide results that outperform state-of-the-art Kinship verification algorithms.

1 Introduction

During the last decades, facial image analysis has become an important subject of study in the communities of pattern recognition and computer vision. In fact, facial images contain much information about the person they belong to: identity, age, gender, ethnicity, expression and many more. For that reason, the analysis of facial images has many applications in real world problems such as face recognition, age estimation, gender classification, facial expression recognition or kinship verification.

The task of deciding if two individuals are kin or not is known as kinship verification. It has been widely addressed in the field of neuroscience and psychology. Face similarity is thought to be one of the most important cues for kinship [9].

Kinship verification can be viewed as a typical binary classification problem, i.e., a face pair is either related by kinship or it is not [27,47,48,50]. Prior research works have addressed kinship types for which pre-existing datasets have provided images, annotations and a verification task protocol.

Visual kinship recognition is a relatively new research topic in the scope of facial image analysis. It is essential for many real-world applications (e.g., kinship verification [14,15,45], automatic photo management, social-media applications, genealogical research, image retrieval and annotation and more). However, nowadays there exist only a few practical vision systems capable to handle such tasks. Hence, vision technology for kinship-based problems has not matured enough to be applied to real-world problems. This leads to a concern of unsatisfactory performance when attempted on real-world datasets.

A. Moujahid
University of the Basque Country UPV/EHU, San Sebastian, Spain
e-mail: jibmomoa@gmail.com

F. Dornaika (✉)
University of the Basque Country UPV/EHU and Ikerbasque Foundation, San Sebastian, Spain
e-mail: fadi.dornaika@ehu.es

© Springer Nature Switzerland AG 2021
J. Alja'am et al. (eds.), *Emerging Technologies in Biomedical Engineering and Sustainable TeleMedicine*, Advances in Science, Technology & Innovation, https://doi.org/10.1007/978-3-030-14647-4_4

Previous efforts done to deal with these issues have argued that the performance of learning systems depends heavily on both the quality and type of the image descriptor, and the face image representation strategies adopted to extract local and global features. Recently, many division-based strategies have been proposed to extract not only the local features but also to get some global context information. Existing methods include multi-level representation used in the age estimation and gender classification topics [3,32], pyramid-based multi-scale representation reported for face recognition [43], and the pyramid multi-level (PML) representation proposed recently for facial demographic estimation [4].

In this chapter, we propose a simple and effective approach for kinship verification that relies on the PML face representation that exploits second order statistics of several local texture features such as LBP, QLRBP, gradients, and color information. Our main contribution is the introduction of the PML-based covariance descriptor and its use in the face analysis field (kinship verification). This face descriptor has two interesting properties: (i) thanks to the PML representation, scales and face parts are explicitly encoded in the final descriptor without having to detect the facial points, (ii) the covariance descriptor (second order statistics) encodes spatial features of any type, and thus the final descriptor naturally fuses several state-of-the art texture features. Previous finding from our group have already shown that the covariance descriptor can be used as a powerful discriminant texture descriptor [11]. To best of our knowledge, our work is the first one that uses the covariance descriptor for automatic kinship verification problem. According to our results, the performance of this descriptor is significantly higher than the state-of-the-art kinship verification algorithms (See Tables 1 and 2). The achieved performances are even better than those obtained with deep convolutional neural networks.

The remainder of the chapter is organized as follows. Section 2 briefly reviews some related works. Section 3 present some classic texture descriptors used in this work. Section 4 describes our proposed descriptor and scheme. This section presents the covariance descriptor, the Pyramid-Multi Level face representation, and the adopted scheme for using it for kinship verification. Experimental results are reported in Sect. 5. We conclude this work in Sect. 6.

2   Related Work

The work of [12] represents the first attempt for automating kinship verification. In that work, 150 pairs of parent-child face images have been characterized using low-level facial features (such as skin color, gray value, histogram of gradient, and facial structure information), and then classi-fied as "related" or "unrelated" (in terms of kinship) achieving an accuracy of 70.69%. Afterward, several algorithms have been proposed to solve automatic kinship verification. These can be classified into two categories: feature-based and model-based solutions. Feature-based methods relies in extracting discriminative features that represent the original facial images, and then performing supervised or unsupervised learning [6,7,16,33,42,44]. Model-based methods, however, aim to learn discriminative models using some statistical learning method to verify kin relationship from face pairs [14,28,45,49]. Very often, the model-based approaches takes the context of the kinship verification problem into account when they estimate the models and classifiers (e.g., [2,28,34]).

One of the promising methods is a neighborhood repulsed metric learning (NRML) method introduced by [27] which was also used as a baseline method in kinship verification in the wild evaluation [30]. This technique is a distance learning metric able to enhance the performance of kinship verification. The work of [34] adopted NRML method to evaluate kinship verification of periocular images. Further, the authors extract more discriminative information by extending the global NRML to a block-based NRML (BNRML). The work of [47] proposed a discriminative multi-metric learning (DMML) and a large margin multi-metric learning to jointly learn multiple distance metrics for multiple features.

The kinship verification problem has also been approached using other methods including genetic algorithm-based feature selection [2], ensemble similarity learning (ESL) based on sparse bilinear similarity function [50], gated autoencoder [10] or end-to-end solution based on deep convolutional neural network [48].

More recently, [19] introduced a new method called filtered contractive deep belief networks (fcDBN) where the relational information present in images is encoded using filters and contractive regularization penalty. In their research, a human study is conducted to understand the ability of humans in identifying kin, and to identify which face regions are the most relevant. Based on this study, they found three main relevant face regions: full face, eyes and mouth region (T face region), and non T face region. They learn high level representation of these three regions using two stages of fc-DBN with an external set of 600000 face images. They achieve state-of-the art result on the two public datasets KinfaceW-I and KinfaceW-II.

Tables 1 and 2 give an illustrative summary of the performance of existing kinship verification approaches over the last three years on two well-known face databases, namely, KinfaceW-I and KinfaceW-II. While the existing algorithms have achieved reasonable accuracies, there is a scope of further improving the performance.

Table 1 Results of the proposed framework compared to the recent state-of-the-art approaches on databases KinFaceW-I. The symbol * means that the approach takes outside data for training. Accuracy is shown as a percentage. Best results without using external data are shown in bold

	Publication	Method	F-S	F-D	M-S	M-D	Mean
1	Yan [46]	Neighborhood repulsed correlation metric learning (NRCML)$_{LE}$	66.1	61.1	66.9	73.0	66.3
2	Lan and Zhou [22]	Quaternion-Michelson Descriptor (QMD)	72.2	68.1	67.8	76.0	71.0
3	López et al. [26]	Simple scoring	69.9	65.7	70.7	79.6	71.4
4	Li et al. [24]	Similarity metric based convolutional neural networks (SMCNN)	75.0	75.0	68.7	72.2	72.7
5	Lan et al. [23]	Quaternionic weber local descriptor (QWLD)	73.7	69.7	72.8	78.0	73.6
6	Qin et al. [36]	Multi-view multi-task learning (MMTL)	–	–	–	–	73.7
7	Zhang et al. [48]	CNN-Basic	75.7	70.8	73.4	79.4	74.8
8	Puthenputhussery et al. [35]	SIFT flow based genetic Fisher vector feature (SF-GFVF)	76.3	74.6	75.5	80.0	76.1
9	Zhang et al. [48]	CNN-Points	76.1	71.8	78.0	84.1	77.5
10	Liu et al. [25]	Generalized inheritable color space (GInCS)	77.3	76.9	75.8	81.4	77.9
11	Zhou et al. [51]	Multiview scalable similarity learning (Multiview SSL)$_{HOG,LBP}$	82.8	75.4	72.6	81.3	78.0
12	Zhou et al. [50]	Ensemble similarity learning (ESL)$_{HOG}$	83.9	76.0	73.5	81.5	78.6
13	Patel et al. [34]	Block-based neighborhood repulsed metric learning (BNRML)$_{LTP}$	83.4	77.2	75.8	78.4	78.7
14	Fang et al. [13]	Sparse similarity metric learning (SSML)$_{HOG}$	84.6	75.0	76.3	82.3	79.6
15	Kumar [20]	Extended Harmonic Rule for Measuring the Facial Similarities (EHRMFS)	84.4	77.6	80.6	80.6	80.2
16	Alirezazadeh et al. [2]	Genetic Algorithm	77.9	78.0	81.4	87.9	81.3
17	Lu et al. [29]	Triangular Similarity Metric Learning (TSML)	83.0	80.6	82.3	85.0	82.7
18	Lu et al. [29]	Politecnico di Torino (Polito)	85.3	85.8	87.5	86.7	86.3
19	Kohli et al. [19]	Kinship Verification via Representation Learning (KVRL)	98.1	96.3	90.5	98.4	95.8*
	Ours	PML-COV-S	84.3	91.0	87.1	90.2	**88.2**

3   Face Descriptors: Background

In the past decades, texture analysis has been extensively studied. A wide variety of texture feature extraction methods have been proposed. Among the proposed approaches Local Binary Pattern (LBP) [33] has been known as one of the most successful statistical approaches due to its efficacy, robustness against illumination changes and relative fast calculation. Texture analysis and image feature extraction have been effectively used in face images. Since then several texture descriptors have been proposed (e.g., [5,8,37]). Many of them were also applied to face representation such as binarized statistical image features [17] and local ternary patterns [40].

In this section, we briefly present LBP, LPQ, and HOG descriptors. In the next section, we present our proposed face descriptor as well as the scheme for kinship verification based on that descriptor.

3.1   Local Binary Patterns (LBP) Descriptor

The original LBP operator replaces the value of the pixels of an image with decimal numbers, which are called LBPs or LBP codes that encode the local structure around each pixel [1]. Each central pixel is compared with its eight neighbors; the neighbors having smaller value than that of the central pixel will have the bit 0, and the other neighbors having value equal to or greater than that of the central pixel will have the bit 1. For each given central pixel, one can generate a binary number that is obtained by concatenating all these binary bits in a clockwise direction, which starts from the one of its top-left neighbor. The resulting decimal value of the generated binary number replaces the central pixel value. The histogram of LBP labels (the frequency of occurrence of each code) calculated over a region or an image can be used as a texture descriptor of that image.

Quaternionic Local Ranking Binary Pattern (QLRBP)

Several extensions of LBP to color have been proposed. The most well-known is the Opponent Color LBP. It describes color and texture jointly [31]. In recent times, the work described in [21] proposed the Quaternionic Local Ranking Binary Pattern to represent color images by quaternion notations (i.e., pure imaginary quaternions). Then, they use a reference quaternion (reference color) in order to retrieve a similarity score between the current pixel color and the reference color. These similarities define a phase map on which classic LBP operator can be applied. For each reference color, there will be one phase map.

In our work, we are interested in the phase maps in order to use them as feature maps.

Table 2 Results of the proposed framework compared to the recent state-of-the-art approaches on databases KinFaceW-II. The symbol * means that the approach takes outside data for training. Accuracy is shown as a percentage. Best results without using external data are shown in bold. The acronyms of the different algorithms are defined in Table 1

	Publication	Method	F-S	F-D	M-S	M-D	Mean
1	Lan and Zhou [22]	QMD	77.2	71.6	79.0	73.4	75.3
2	Zhou et al. [50]	ESL_{HOG}	81.2	73.0	75.6	73.0	75.7
3	Zhou et al. [51]	Multiview $SSL_{HOG,LBP}$	81.8	74.0	75.3	72.5	75.9
4	Lan et al. [23]	QWLD	77.4	73.6	78.4	76.8	76.6
5	Qin et al. [36]	MMTL	–	–	–	–	77.2
6	Yan [46]	$NRCML_{LE}$	79.8	76.1	79.8	80.0	78.7
7	Li et al. [24]	SMCNN	75.0	79.0	78.0	85.0	79.3
8	López et al. [26]	Simple scoring	78.2	73.2	84.2	88.2	80.1
9	Kumar [20]	EHRMFS	80.6	84.4	77.6	84.4	80.2
10	Fang et al.[13]	$SSML_{HOG}$	85.0	77.0	80.4	78.4	80.2
11	Patel et al. [34]	$BNRML_{LTP}$	84.0	79.0	79.2	80.0	80.5
12	Liu et al. [25]	GInCS	85.4	77.0	81.6	81.6	81.4
13	Lu et al. [29]	Polito	84.0	82.2	84.8	81.2	83.1
14	Zhang et al. [48]	CNN-Basic	84.9	79.6	88.3	88.5	85.3
15	Puthenputhussery et al. [35]	SF-GFVF	87.2	79.6	88.0	87.8	85.7
16	Lu et al. [29]	TSML	89.4	83.6	86.2	85.0	86.1
17	Alirezazadeh et al. [2]	Genetic algorithm	88.8	81.8	86.8	87.2	86.2
18	Zhang et al. [48]	CNN-Points	89.4	81.9	89.9	92.4	**88.4**
19	Kohli et al. [19]	KVRL	96.8	94.0	97.2	96.8	96.2*
	Ours	PML-COV-S	85.8	88.6	87.2	91.0	**88.2**

3.2 HOG Descriptor

Histogram of Oriented Gradients (HOG)[7] is a feature descriptor used to detect objects in computer vision and image processing. The HOG descriptor technique counts occurrences of gradient orientation in localized portions of an image—cells and blocks.

4 Proposed Scheme

This section presents our proposed scheme for image-based kinship verification problem. The scheme has three main components: (i) the covariance descriptor of face texture, (ii) the Pyramid-multi-level face representation; and (iii) pair image fusion scheme with an efficient filter method for feature selection.

4.1 Covariance Descriptor

The original covariance descriptor is a statistic based feature proposed by [41] for generic object detection and texture classification tasks. Instead of using histograms, they compute the covariance matrices among the color channels and gradient images. Compared with other descriptors, the covariance descriptor lies in a very low-dimensional space, and gives a natural way of fusing multiples types of features as long as they can be presented spatially. Thus, this descriptor can benefit from any progress made in image feature extraction. In addition, this descriptor lends itself nicely to efficient implementation whenever the image regions are rectangular by exploiting the integral image concept as it is described in [41].

Since its introduction the covariance descriptor has not received much attention by researchers despite its ability to incorporate a large number of existing and recent texture features. This motivates us to propose an extension of this descriptor that includes two new aspects. First, we compute the covariance matrices using texture descriptors such as LBP and LPQ images. Second, we exploit this covariance descriptor using a Pyramid-Multi Level (PML) face representation which allows a multi-level multi scale feature extraction. The PML representation will be described in the next section.

Given a color image, we start by extracting the local features that are represented in 2D maps having the same spatial gird as the original image. More precisely, we extract 20 different channels: (i) 6 channels corresponding to the color components in both RGB and HSV spaces; (ii) 8 channels for x and y coordinates and the first and second derivative of the image intensity with respect to x and y; (iii) 3 channels corresponding to three Local Binary Pattern images [1,33,39]

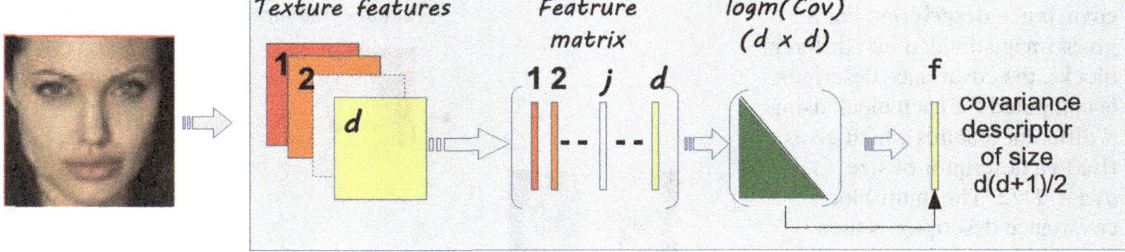

Fig. 1 A schematic representation of the covariance descriptor. The input face image is represented by a set of d texture and color features that will be fused in the final covariance descriptor

obtained by combining three different modes for 8 neighboring points at radius equal to 1; (iv) and finally 3 channels for the three LPQ phase images which have been computed following the work by [21].

This descriptor is computed as follows: let J denote a $M \times N$ intensity image, and V be the set of the $M \times N \times d$ dimensional feature images extracted from J (see Fig. 1 for a graphical illustration). Thus, V can be seen as a set of d 2D arrays (channels) where every array corresponds to a given image feature such as horizontal coordinate, vertical coordinate, color, image derivatives, and filter responses, etc. This multi-dimensional array can be written as $V(x; y) = \phi(J; x; y)$ where ϕ is a function that extracts image features. Figure 2(a) shows a visual representation of this descriptor.

For a given image region $\mathscr{R} \in J$ containing n pixels, let $\{\mathbf{v}_i\}_{i=1\ldots n}$ denote the d-dimensional feature vectors obtained by ϕ within $\mathscr{R}$. According to [41], the region $\mathscr{R}$ can be described by a $d \times d$ covariance matrix:

$$\Sigma_{\mathscr{R}} = \frac{1}{n-1} \sum_{i=1}^{n} (\mathbf{v}_i - \bar{\mathbf{v}})(\mathbf{v}_i - \bar{\mathbf{v}})^T, \qquad (1)$$

where $\bar{\mathbf{v}}$ is the mean vector of $\{\mathbf{v}_i\}_{i=1\ldots n}$. The matrix $\Sigma_{\mathscr{R}}$ represents the second order statistics of the d dimensional vectors $\{\mathbf{v}_i\}$ within the region $\mathscr{R}$.

Under the Log-Euclidean Riemannian metric, it is possible to measure the distance between covariance matrices. Given two covariance matrices Σ_1 and Σ_2, their distance is given by,

$$d(\Sigma_1, \Sigma_2) = ||log(\Sigma_1) - log(\Sigma_2)||_{\ell_2}, \qquad (2)$$

where $||.||_{\ell_2}$ is the ℓ_2 vector norm and $log(\Sigma)$ is the matrix logarithm of the square matrix Σ.

Thus, every image region, $\mathscr{R}$, can be characterized by the vectorized form of the matrix $log(\Sigma_{\mathscr{R}})$. Since this is a symmetric matrix, then the feature vector can be described by a $d \times (d + 1)/2$ where d is the number of channels. Since the number of channels used is 20, it follows that the covariance descriptor of each region is described by $20 * 21/2 = 210$ features. Figure 1 illustrates a schematic representation of the covariance descriptor applied to an input face image.

4.2 Pyramid Multi-Level (PML) Face Representation

The PML representation adopts an explicit pyramid representation of the original image. This pyramid represents the image at different scales. For each scale or level, a corresponding Multi-block representation is performed. Each image of the pyramid will be divided into an appropriate number of square blocks. The descriptor of each resulting block is then extracted using the steps described in the previous section. Figure 2 (Bottom) illustrates the PML principle for a pyramid of three levels associated with a face image.

Given the number of levels, ℓ, and the size of an individual square block ($b \times b$), the size of the resulting square image at level i is given by $i \times (b, b)$. The total number of blocks is given by $B = \sum_{i=1}^{\ell} i^2 = \ell(\ell+1)(2\ell+1)/6$. All blocks have a size of $b \times b$ pixels. At level 1 (the top of the pyramid), the whole image is reduced to one single block of $b \times b$ pixels.

Formally, the PML representation of an image is obtained as follows: Let f be an image of size $N \times N$. Let P be its pyramid representation with ℓ levels, $P = \{L_1, \ldots, L_\ell\}$ [38]. The size of the images L_i should meet the following. Each level L_i is represented by a partition of square blocks of size $\frac{N}{\ell} \times \frac{N}{\ell}, L_i = \{B_{i,1}, \cdots, B_{i,n_i}\}$, where $n_i = i^2$. Given a value ℓ, we pose $b = \frac{N}{\ell}$. Thus, the size of square blocks at all levels is $b \times b$. We point out that P_ℓ is f and $P_1 = B_{1,1}$ (coarsest resolution).

The pyramid representation of an image f by ℓ levels is the sequence $L_1, \ldots, L_\ell$ such that:

$$L_i = \{B_{i,1}, \ldots, B_{i,n_i}\} \quad \text{where } i = 1, \ldots, \ell \ \text{ and } \ n_i = i^2 \qquad (3)$$

4.3 PML Covariance Descriptor

Once the PML representation is obtained, the local features of each block at each level are described by the covariance descriptor as shown at the top part of Fig. 2. Concretely, the PML Descriptor at the level i ($i = 1, \ldots, \ell$) is given by:

$$COV(L_i) = COV(B_{i,1}) \| \cdots \| COV(B_{i,n_i})$$

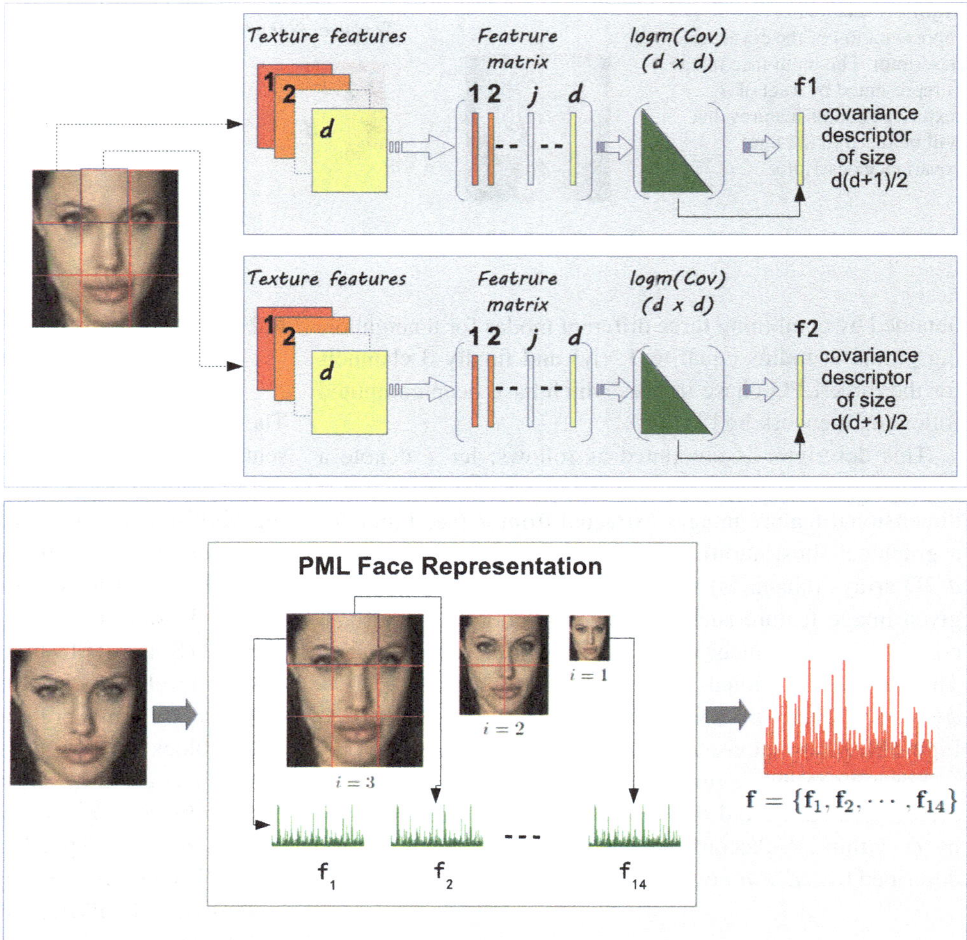

Fig. 2 (Top) **Multi-block covariance descriptor**. For a given image divided into different blocks, the covariance descriptor is computed for each block using d different features which gives rise to a descriptor of size $d(d+1)/2$. The multi-block covariance descriptor is then obtained by concatenating all the individual descriptors. (**Bottom**) **Pyramid Multi-Level (PML) covariance descriptor** for a pyramid of three levels. At each level i the image is divided into i^2 blocks resulting to a total number of blocks given by $B = \sum_{i=1}^{\ell} i^2 = \ell(\ell+1)(2\ell+1)/6$. For each block a regional multi-block covariance descriptor ($\mathbf{f_i}$) is extracted and finally the PML-based feature descriptor is obtained by concatenating all regional descriptors ($\mathbf{f} = \{\mathbf{f_1}, \mathbf{f_2}, \ldots, \mathbf{f_b}\}$)

where $\parallel$ denotes the concatenation operator. Therefore, we define the PML Descriptor using ℓ levels of the pyramid representation as follows:

$$\ell\text{-PMLD}(f) = \text{COV}(L_1) \parallel \ldots \parallel \text{COV}(L_\ell) \qquad (4)$$

We can observe that the total number of blocks in a pyramid of depth ℓ is $\sum_{i=1}^{\ell} i^2 = \frac{\ell(\ell+1)(2\ell+1)}{6}$. Hence, ℓ-PMLD is composed of $\frac{d(d+1)}{2} \frac{\ell(\ell+1)(2\ell+1)}{6}$ elements, since the number of elements of COV descriptor is $\frac{d(d+1)}{2}$.

4.4 Kinship Verification

Our proposed kinship verification scheme is illustrated in Fig. 3. The modules that needs training are: (i) feature selection, and (ii) binary support vector machine (SVM) classifier. Both can be efficiently learned using a set of positive and negative pairs.

At testing phase, an unseen pair of face images is processed in order to obtain the PML representation of each face. Then,

the obtained two descriptors are merged using the absolute difference giving rise to one single descriptor having the same size as the PML descriptor. Adopting this merging scheme has at least two advantages. First, the order of image presentation of the pair (either in the training phase or in the testing can be arbitrary). This property increases the flexibility of deploying the final algorithm. Second, the size of the final descriptor (associated with the input pair) is not multiplied by two as is the case with a simple vector concatenation. Once the final descriptor is obtained, its components are then filtered out using a trained supervised feature ranking scheme.

4.5 Fisher Score Feature Selection

We use Fisher scoring of the features in order to extract the most relevant and discriminative features of the PML-based descriptors. Fisher scoring is a supervised feature selection method which uses class labels to identify features with best discriminant ability. Let $\mathbf{z} \in \mathbf{R}^D$ denote the PML descriptor associated with a pair of face images. The Fisher score of the rth feature is given by:

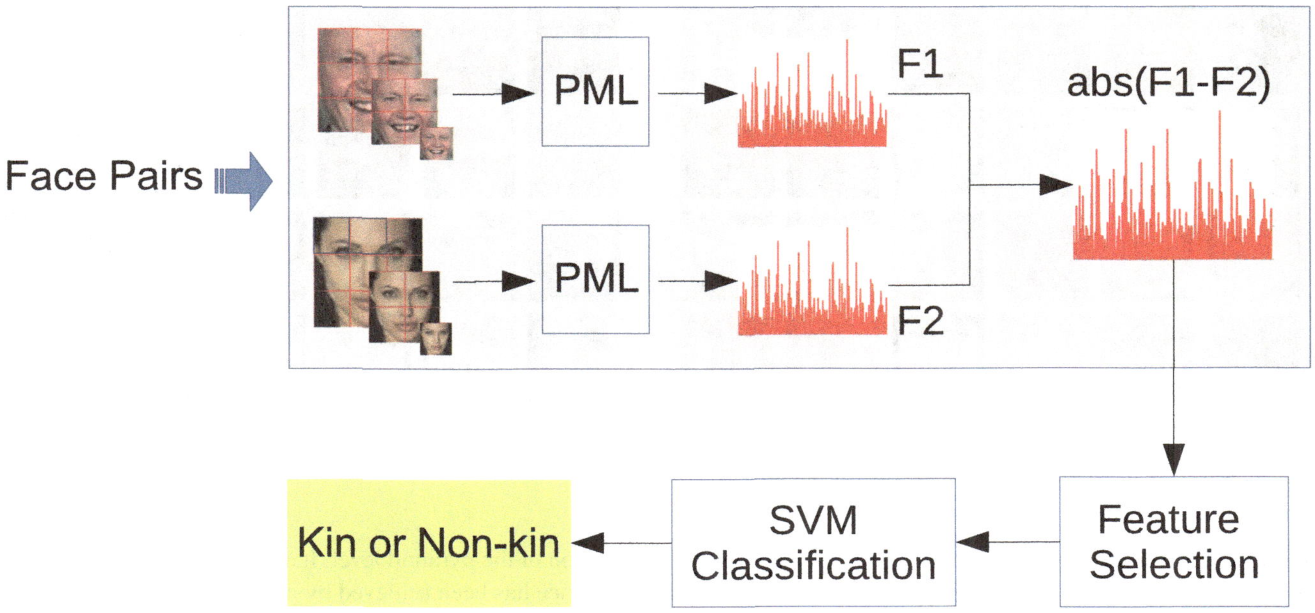

Fig. 3 An illustration of the proposed method for kinface verification using PML representation based on hand-crafted descriptors. Given a pair of images, the PML feature representation is obtained as the absolute difference between the individual PML descriptors. We assume that we are given N training labeled pairs of images. Each pair belongs to either the kinship class (positive class) or the no kinship class (the negative class). The PML feature dimension is reduced by Fisher selection before learning a binary support vector machine (SVM) classifier

$$F_r = \frac{N_1 (\mu_{r,1} - \mu_r)^2 + N_2 (\mu_{r,2} - \mu_r)^2}{N_1 \sigma_{r,1}^2 + N_2 \sigma_{r,2}^2} \quad r = 1, \ldots, D \tag{5}$$

where N_1 and N_2 are respectively the number of positive and negative pairs. $\mu_{r,1}$ and $\sigma_{r,1}^2$ refer to the mean and variance of the rth feature of the positive class, and $\mu_{r,2}$ and $\sigma_{r,2}^2$ refer to the mean and variance of the rth feature of the negative class. μ_r refers to the global mean of the rth feature.

The output of the feature selection is a vector of real scores that can gives a ranking of the attributes composing the PML covariance descriptor. From this obtained ordering, several feature subsets can be chosen by setting a cutoff for the selected features. In this work we have adopted threshold-based criterion. In fact, we have analyzed different cutoff values ranging from 10 to 90% of the relevant features. Once the selection is fixed, it is applied on both the training and test sets.

5   Experimental Results

In this section, we report the kinship verification experiments performed on two benchmark kinship databases, namely KinfaceW-I and KinfaceW-II. These datasets contain face images depicting four classes of relationship: Father-Son (F-S), Father-Daughter (F-D), Mother-Son (M-S), and Mother-Daughter (M-D). KinFaceW-I has respectively 156, 134, 116 and 127 pairs of kinship face images for the aforementioned relationships while KinFaceW-II has 250 pairs for each one. Figure 4 illustrates some pairs in both datasets.

The evaluation protocol followed in this work is the one reported in [18]. All pairs of face images with kinship relation have been considered as positive samples and those without kinship relation as negative samples.

The face images corresponding to each pair are processed according to our proposed kinship verification scheme in order to get the PML-based feature representation for kinship verification (See Fig. 3). In fact, three PML-based hand-crafted descriptors namely, PML-LBP, PML-HOG and PML-COV, have been considered. These PML-based feature vectors characterizing a given pair of face images are obtained as the absolute difference between the individual PML descriptors. We adopt the evaluation protocol described in [18]. We used the pre-specified training/testing splits, which were generated randomly and independently for 5-fold cross validation. As a classifier, we used SVM classifier which has proven to be a good solution when dealing with binary classification.

The different PML-based descriptors have been obtained considering pyramids of different levels ranging from 4 to 7. A summary of the different type of descriptors and their

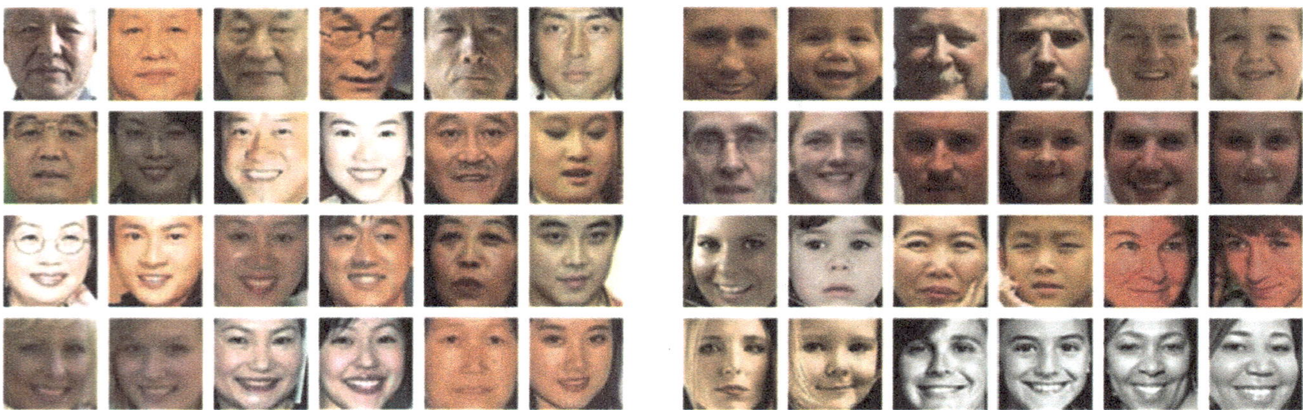

Fig. 4 Some pair samples from KinfaceW-I and KinfaceW-II datasets. From top to bottom are the F-S, F-D, M-S, and M-D kinship relations, and the two neighboring images in each row are with the kinship relation, respectively

dimensions as a function of the pyramid level is disclosed in Table 3. The size of the PML-LBP descriptor can be obtained as the number of blocks times 59 which is the size of the uniform LBP histogram. Similarly, the size of the PML-COV descriptor is given by the number of blocks times 210 which is the covariance feature length (see Sect. 4.1). Firstly, we have analyzed the performance of a binary SVM classifier as a function of the pyramid levels on both kinship databases, and concluded that the optimal configuration corresponds to the face representation based on a pyramid of 7 levels.

Figure 5 gives a graphical illustration of the performance of the different proposed kinship verification algorithms as a

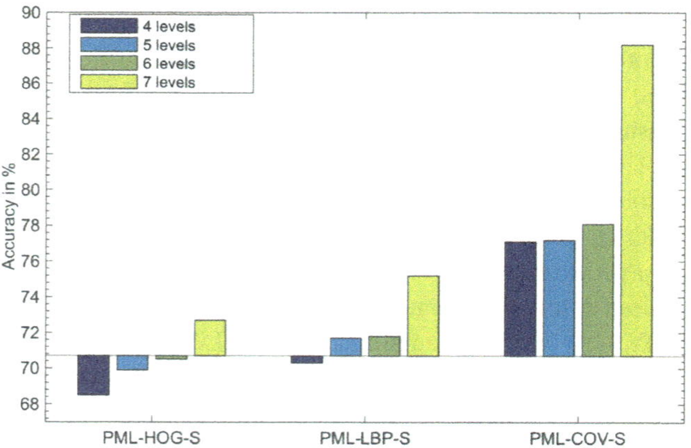

Fig. 5 The performance of the different proposed Kinship verification algorithms on the dataset KinfaceW-I as a function of the number of pyramid levels. We fixed the baseline to the value 70.69% which corresponds to the performance achieved by [12]

function of the pyramid level. It can be seen that the best performance has been achieved by pyramids having high levels.

The classification rates of the different PML-based descriptors on different subsets of the KinfaceW-I and KinfaceW-II datasets are reported in Table 4. In this table, feature selection was not used, i.e.; all original features for the three types of PML are used in training and testing. As can be seen, the PML-COV descriptor achieves kinship verification accuracies of about 84 and 86% for KinfaceW-I and KinfaceW-II, respectively. These results significantly outperform most of the recently proposed methods reported in Tables 1 and 2.

As reported previously, the PML-COV face descriptor is obtained by fusing the information from different texture features, and consequently may contain a lot of redundant and unreliable information. Therefore, performing feature selection can avoid, on one hand, over-fitting problems while improving classification model performance, and on the other hand, to provide efficient and more cost-effective learning models. In this work, we have adopted the feature selection algorithm based on Fisher score method for the automatic weighting of the descriptor attributes (Sect. 4.3). In fact, we have analyzed different cutoff values ranging from 10 to 90% of the relevant features. Once the selection is fixed, it is applied on both the training and test sets. Finally, we evaluate the recognition rate on the test set using the selected features.

Table 5 shows the performance of the SVM classifier on the test sets using the selected features according to Fisher weights. As expected, feature selection has improved the performance of the different algorithms achieving a kinship

Table 3 A summary of the different PML-based features descriptors and their dimensions

Level	Blocks	PML-LBP	PML-HOG	PML-COV
4	30	1770	728	6300
5	55	3245	1560	11,550
6	91	5369	2860	19,110
7	140	8260	4732	29,400

Table 4 Classification accuracy (percent) of different PML-based hand-crafted descriptors on different subsets of the KinfaceW-I and KinfaceW-II data set. Best results are displayed in bold. Feature selection was not used

Kinface-I

	PML-HOG	PML-LBP	PML-COV
F-S	67.1	70.5	**81.7**
F-D	74.0	76.3	**85.9**
M-S	62.9	67.2	**83.6**
M-D	70.5	72.4	**86.3**
Average	68.6	71.6	**84.4**

Kinface-II

	PML-HOG	PML-LBP	PML-COV
F-S	64.6	70.8	**84.2**
F-D	72.2	77.4	**88.6**
M-S	69.4	72.4	**84.0**
M-D	66.8	70.8	**88.6**
Average	68.3	72.9	**86.4**

Table 5 Classification accuracy (percent) of different PML-based hand-crafted descriptors after Fisher score feature selection on different subsets of the KinFaceW-I and KinFaceW-II data set. Best results are displayed in bold

Kinface-I

	PML-HOG-S	PML-LBP-S	PML-COV-S
F-S	71.2	72.4	**84.3**
F-D	76.9	78.9	**91.0**
M-S	69.4	71.5	**87.1**
M-D	73.3	77.9	**90.2**
Average	72.8	75.2	**88.2**

Kinface-II

	PML-HOG-S	PML-LBP-S	PML-COV-S
F-S	66.8	73.6	**85.8**
F-D	74.8	77.6	**88.6**
M-S	72.8	74.8	**87.2**
M-D	68.6	72.8	**91.0**
Average	70.8	74.7	**88.2**

verification accuracy for PML-COV-S around 88% which outperforms the state-of-the-art kinship verification algorithms and schemes that do not exploit external data. In fact, this score improves the performance of deep convolutional neural networks CNN-basic and CNN-Points [48] on KinfaceW-I of about 14 and 11%, respectively. For KinfaceW-II, the performance of our algorithm is comparable with CNN-points and slightly better than CNN-basic.

6 Conclusion

In this paper, a novel and effective framework for Kinship verification is introduced. This framework mainly relies on two components: an efficient and flexible face descriptor for face image analysis, and a pyramid multi level face representation that exploits second order statistics of several texture features. The proposed descriptor and kinship verification scheme, which do not need any external data, outperform state-of-the-art methods on two public datasets KinfaceW-I and KinfaceW-II.

References

[1] T. Ahonen, A. Hadid, and M. Pietikainen. Face description with local binary patterns: Application to face recognition. *IEEE transactions on pattern analysis and machine intelligence*, 28(12):2037–2041, 2006.

[2] P. Alirezazadeh, A. Fathi, and F. Abdali-Mohammadi. A genetic algorithm-based feature selection for kinship verification. *IEEE Signal Processing Letters*, 22(12):2459–2463, 2015.

[3] S. Bekhouche, A. Ouafi, A. Benlamoudi, A. Taleb-Ahmed, and A. Hadid. Automatic age estimation and gender classification in the wild. In *Proceeding of the International Conference on Automatic control, Telecommunications and Signals ICATS'15*, 2015.

[4] S. Bekhouche, A. Ouafi, F. Dornaika, A. Taleb-Ahmed, and A. Hadid. Pyramid multi-level features for facial demographic estimation. *Expert Systems with Applications*, 80(Supplement C):297–310, 2017.

[5] F. Bianconi, R. Bello, P. Napoletano, and F. D. Maria. Improved opponent colour local binary patterns for colour texture classification. In *Workshop Computational Color Imaging Workshop, CCIW*, 2017.

[6] Z. Cao, Q. Yin, X. Tang, and J. Sun. Face recognition with learning-based descriptor. In *2010 IEEE Computer Society Conference on Computer Vision and Pattern Recognition*, pages 2707–2714, June 2010.

[7] N. Dalal and B. Triggs. Histograms of oriented gradients for human detection. In *Computer Vision and Pattern Recognition, 2005. CVPR 2005. IEEE Computer Society Conference on*, volume 1, pages 886–893. IEEE, 2005.

[8] S. H. Davarpanah, F. Khalid, L. Nurliyana Abdullah, and M. Golchin. A texture descriptor: Background local binary pattern (bglbp). *Multimedia Tools Appl.*, 75(11):6549–6568, June 2016.

[9] L. DeBruine, B. Jones, A. Little, and D. Perrett. Social perception of facial resemblance in humans. *Arch. Sexual Behavior*, 37(1):64–77, 2008.

[10] A. Dehghan, O. E.G., and M. Villegas, R.and Shah. Who do i look like? determining parent-offspring resemblance via gated autoencoders. In *IEEE Conference on Computer Vision and Pattern Recognition (CVPR), pp. 1757–1764*, 2014.

[11] F. Dornaika, A. Moujahid, Y. E. Merabet, and Y. Ruichek. Building detection from orthophotos using a machine learning approach: An empirical study on image segmentation and descriptors. *Expert Systems with Applications*, 58:130–142, 2016.

[12] R. Fang, K. D. Tang, N. Snavely, and T. Chen. Towards computational models of kinship verification. In *Image Processing (ICIP), 2010 17th IEEE International Conference on*, pages 1577–1580, 2010.

[13] Y. Fang, Y. Y. S. Chen, H. Wang, and C. Shu. Sparse similarity metric learning for kinship verification. In *Visual Communications and Image Processing (VCIP), 2016*, pages 1–4. IEEE, 2016.

[14] Y. Guo, H. Dibeklioglu, and L. van der Maaten. Graph-based kinship recognition. In *Pattern Recognition (ICPR), 2014 22nd International Conference on*, pages 4287–4292. IEEE, 2014.

[15] J. Hu, J. Lu, J. Yuan, and Y.-P. Tan. Large margin multi-metric learning for face and kinship verification in the wild. In *ACCV (3)*, pages 252–267, 2014.

[16] S. U. Hussain, T. Napoléon, and F. Jurie. Face Recognition using Local Quantized Patterns. In *British Machive Vision Conference*, page 11 pages, Guildford, United Kingdom, Sept. 2012.

[17] J. Kannala and E. Rahtu. Bsif: Binarized statistical image features. In *Pattern Recognition (ICPR), 2012 21st International Conference on*, pages 1363–1366, Nov 2012.

[18] KinFaceW. http://www.kinfacew.com/index.html, 2014.

[19] N. Kohli, M. Vatsa, R. Singh, A. Noore, and A. Majumdar. Hierarchical representation learning for kinship verification. *IEEE Transactions on Image Processing*, 26(1):289–302, 2017.

[20] C. R. Kumar. Harmonic rule for measuring the facial similarities among relatives. *Transactions on Machine Learning and Artificial Intelligence*, 4(6):29, 2017.

[21] Y. Z. R. Lan and Y. Y. Tang. Quaternionic local ranking binary pattern: A local descriptor of color images. *IEEE Transactions on Image Processing*, 25(2):566–579, 2016.

[22] R. Lan and Y. Zhou. Quaternion-michelson descriptor for color image classification. *IEEE Transactions on Image Processing*, 25(11):5281–5292, 2016.

[23] R. Lan, Y. Zhou, and Y. Y. Tang. Quaternionic weber local descriptor of color images. *IEEE Transactions on Circuits and Systems for Video Technology*, 27(2):261–274, 2017.

[24] L. Li, X. Feng, X. Wu, Z. Xia, and A. Hadid. Kinship verification from faces via similarity metric based convolutional neural network. In *International Conference Image Analysis and Recognition*, pages 539–548. Springer, 2016.

[25] Q. Liu, A. Puthenputhussery, and C. Liu. A novel inheritable color space with application to kinship verification. In *Applications of Computer Vision (WACV), 2016 IEEE Winter Conference on*, pages 1–9. IEEE, 2016.

[26] M. B. López, E. Boutellaa, and A. Hadid. Comments on the "kinship face in the wild" data sets. *IEEE Transactions on Pattern Analysis and Machine Intelligence*, 38(11):2342–2344, 2016.

[27] J. Lu, X. Zhou, Y.-P. Tan, Y. Shang, and J. Zhou. Neighborhood repulsed metric learning for kinship verification. *IEEE transactions on pattern analysis and machine intelligence*, 36(2):331–345, 2014.

[28] J. Lu, X. Zhou, Y.-P. Tan, and Y. S. J. Zhou. Neighborhood repulsed metric learning for kinship verification. *IEEE transactions on pattern analysis and machine intelligence*, 36(2):331–345, 2014.

[29] J. Lu, J. Hu, V. E. Liong, X. Zhou, A. Bottino, I. U. Islam, T. F. Vieira, X. Qin, X. Tan, S. Chen, S. Mahpod, Y. Keller, L. Zheng, K. Idrissi, C. Garcia, S. Duffner, A. Baskurt, M. Castrillón-Santana, and J. Lorenzo-Navarro. The fg 2015 kinship verification in the wild evaluation. In *2015 11th IEEE International Conference and Workshops on Automatic Face and Gesture Recognition (FG)*, volume 1, pages 1–7, May 2015.

[30] J. Lu, V. E. Liong, X. Zhou, and J. Zhou. Learning compact binary face descriptor for face recognition. *IEEE transactions on pattern analysis and machine intelligence*, 37(10):2041–2056, 2015.

[31] Mäenpää and M. Pietikainen. Classification with color and texture: jointly or separately? *Pattern Recognition*, 37(8):1629–1640, 2004.

[32] D. T. Nguyen, S. R. Cho, K. Y. Shin, J. W. Bang, and K. R. Park. Comparative study of human age estimation with or without pre-classification of gender and facial expression. *The Scientific World Journal*, 2014:15, 2014.

[33] T. Ojala, M. Pietikainen, and T. Maenpaa. Multiresolution gray-scale and rotation invariant texture classification with local binary

patterns. *Pattern Analysis and Machine Intelligence, IEEE Transactions on*, 24(7):971–987, 2002.

[34] B. Patel, R. Maheshwari, and B. Raman. Evaluation of periocular features for kinship verification in the wild. *Computer Vision and Image Understanding*, 160(Supplement C):24–35, 2017.

[35] A. Puthenputhussery, Q. Liu, and C. Liu. Sift flow based genetic fisher vector feature for kinship verification. In *Image Processing (ICIP), 2016 IEEE International Conference on*, pages 2921–2925. IEEE, 2016.

[36] X. Qin, X. Tan, and S. Chen. Mixed bi-subject kinship verification via multi-view multi-task learning. *Neurocomputing*, 214:350–357, 2016.

[37] C. Silva, T. Bouwmans, and C. Frélicot. An extended center-symmetric local binary pattern for background modeling and subtraction in videos. In *Proceedings of the 10th International Conference on Computer Vision Theory and Applications - Volume 1: VISAPP, (VISIGRAPP 2015)*, pages 395–402, 2015.

[38] R. Szeliski. *Computer vision algorithms and applications.* Springer, London, 2011.

[39] V. Takala, T. Ahonen, and M. Pietik?inen. Block-based methods for image retrieval using local binary patterns. In *Image Analysis, SCIA*, volume LNCS, 3540, 2005.

[40] X. Tan and B. Triggs. Enhanced local texture feature sets for face recognition under difficult lighting conditions. *IEEE Trans. Image Processing*, 19:1635–1650, 2010.

[41] O. Tuzel, F. Porikli, and P. Meer. A fast descriptor for detection and classification. In *European Conf. on Computer Vision*, pages 589–600, 2006.

[42] K. Vinay and B. Shreyas. Face recognition using gabor wavelets. In *Signals, Systems and Computers. Fortieth Asilomar Conference on*, pages 593–597, Oct 2006.

[43] W. Wang, W. Chen, and D. Xu. Pyramid-based multi-scale lbp features for face recognition. In *Multimedia and Signal Processing (CMSP), 2011 International Conference on*, volume 1, pages 151–155, May 2011.

[44] L. Wolf, T. Hassner, and Y. Taigman. Descriptor based methods in the wild. In *Faces in Real-Life Images Workshop in ECCV*, 2008.

[45] S. Xia, M. Shao, J. Luo, and Y. Fu. Understanding kin relationships in a photo. *IEEE Transactions on Multimedia*, 14(4):1046–1056, 2012.

[46] H. Yan. Kinship verification using neighborhood repulsed correlation metric learning. *Image and Vision Computing*, 60:91–97, 2017.

[47] H. Yan, J. Lu, W. Deng, and X. Zhou. Discriminative multimetric learning for kinship verification. *IEEE Transactions on Information forensics and security*, 9(7):1169–1178, 2014.

[48] K. Zhang, Y. Huang, C. Song, H. Wu, and L. Wang. Kinship verification with deep convolutional neural networks. In *Proceedings of the British Machine Vision Conference (BMVC)*, pages 148.1–148.12. BMVA Press, September 2015.

[49] X. Zhou, J. Hu, J. Lu, Y. Shang, and Y. Guan. Kinship verification from facial images under uncontrolled conditions. In *Proceedings of the 19th ACM international conference on Multimedia*, pages 953–956. ACM, 2011.

[50] X. Zhou, Y. Shang, H. Yan, and G. Guo. Ensemble similarity learning for kinship verification from facial images in the wild. *Information Fusion*, 32:40–48, 2016.

[51] X. Zhou, H. Yan, and Y. Shang. Kinship verification from facial images by scalable similarity fusion. *Neurocomputing*, 197:136–142, 2016.

Continuous Wavelet Analysis and Extraction of ECG Features

Mounaim Aqil and Atman Jbari

Abstract

In this chapter, we propose a processing algorithm to measure the features of electrocardiogram records. The continuous wavelet transform is used to analyze the signal in the time-scale domain and evaluate the scalogram for each ECG waves. Thus, we present the literature of wavelet transform and their properties. Next, we propose criteria to choose the mother wavelet more adapted for ECG analysis. Then, the processing algorithm is detailed to extract the features: R-peaks, QRS waves, P waves and T waves. To evaluate the performance, we compute the parameters: sensitivity, predictivity, and error rate for a set of ECG records of the MIT-BIH database. The results of sensitivity $Se = 99.84\%$, positive predictivity $P^+ = 99.53$, and error rate $ER = 0.62\%$ demonstrate the effectiveness of the proposed algorithm and its motivation for implementation to improve the processing quality of health systems.

1 Introduction

Biomedical systems integrate the processing of the biomedical measurements in electronic chips to perform automatically required information. Among these devices, electrocardiography implements analysis and interpretation of the ECG signal to extract features that are not visible by direct visual analysis. Since its clinical information is contained in the different waves of the ECG signal, the development of reliable and robust detection and extraction methods is of great importance. For example, the QRS complex is the most important wave of the ECG signal and can be used as a basis for several other tasks such as automatic heart rate determination, cardiac cycle classification, and ECG data compression.

The development of algorithms for the detection and extraction of the different waves of the ECG signal has been the subject of research for more than 40 years. In the literature, several approaches have been presented and used in electrocardiography systems. The main techniques for ECG feature detection and extraction are given as follows.

- *Algorithms based on the calculation of the derivative*: A calculation is made of the first and second derivatives of the ECG signal with the elaboration of a threshold combined with other treatments such as smoothing, weighted summation, and elimination of the average value [1–3].
- *Algorithms based on digital filtering*: In these algorithms, the ECG signal is filtered by two parallel low pass filters with different cutoff frequencies. The difference between the outputs of the two filters is then squared and smoothed. The coefficients of the two filters, as well as the cutoff frequencies, are calculated on the basis of the ECG signal spectrum [1, 2, 4, 5].
- *Approaches based on neural networks*: Neural networks have been used as nonlinear adaptive predictors. The goal is to predict the value of the current signal from its past values. The principle of detection is based on the prediction error. Indeed, for the different segments of the QRS complex, the neural network converges to a point where the samples are well predicted. While for QRS complex segment samples with abrupt changes, the prediction error becomes important. It follows that this error can be used as a characteristic of the signal for the detection of the QRS complex [6–8].

M. Aqil (✉)
Engineering and Applied Technologies Laboratory, Higher School of Technology, Sultan Moulay Slimane University in Beni Mellal, Beni Mellal, Morocco
e-mail: mounaim.aqil@usms.ac.ma

A. Jbari
Electronic Systems Sensors and Nanobiotechnologies (E2SN), Higher School of Technical Education (ENSET), Mohammed V University in Rabat, Rabat, Morocco
e-mail: atman.jbari@um5.ac.ma

© Springer Nature Switzerland AG 2021
J. Aljaâ am et al. (eds.), *Emerging Technologies in Biomedical Engineering and Sustainable TeleMedicine*, Advances in Science, Technology & Innovation, https://doi.org/10.1007/978-3-030-14647-4_5

- *Algorithms based on the hidden model of Markov*: These algorithms are based on the observation of the sequence of the samples of the signal by a function of probability which varies according to the state of a Markov chain [9–11].
- *Syntactic methods*: In these methods, the signal is divided into short segments of a fixed length. Each segment is then represented by a primitive component and encoded using a predefined alphabet. Because of their computational efficiency, most algorithms use line-shaped segments as primitives for signal representation. The set of linear primitives is extended by peaks, parabolic curves, and additional attributes [12–14].
- *Hilbert-based techniques*: In these approaches, the ideal Hilbert transform is approximated by a pass-band finite impulse response filter (FIR). The Hilbert transform of the ECG signal is used for calculating the signal envelope. In order to eliminate the ripples of the envelope and to avoid ambiguities in the detection of the peak level, the envelope is filtered by a low-pass filter [15–17].
- *Approaches based on wavelet transforms*: The idea of the wavelet transform has been used in many research works to extract the different waves of the ECG signal. In most algorithms, we exploit the Mallat and Hwang approach based on the detection of singularity points and local maxima of the transform coefficients [18–20]. Other algorithms have proposed the use of discrete wavelet transform (DWT) detail coefficients for the detection of the QRS complex [21], while other algorithms exploit the multi-scale resolution to implement bandpass filters to detect the QRS complex [22]. Finally, some approaches are based on the selection of the scale parameters of the coefficients of the DWT [23]. The majority of these techniques use the DWT, whereas few proposed methods exploit the continuous wavelet transform (CWT) [24, 25].

In this chapter, we recall the basis of CWT and its application for the time-scale analysis of ECG signal. Then, we present a new ECG processing technique based on the selection of a scale parameter of CWT coefficients corresponding to each wave of ECG signal. This proposed technique is evaluated and compared with other techniques according to standard performances.

2 Continuous Wavelet Transform and Time-Scale Analysis of ECG Signal

2.1 Limitations of Fourier Frequency Analysis

The Fourier transform of a variable time signal $x(t)$ is a mathematical tool for evaluating its spectrum. This spectrum provides the frequency components and their powers according to the following equation:

$$X(jf) = \int_{-\infty}^{+\infty} x(t)e^{-j2\pi ft}dt \tag{1}$$

The Fourier transform does not give any information about the frequency components of the signal in conjunction with their appearance in time. To do this, one can use the Heisenberg–Gabor inequality which minimizes the product bandwidth and time width of the signal by the factor $\frac{1}{4\pi}$ according to the following expression:

$$\Delta t \cdot \Delta f \geq \frac{1}{4\pi} \tag{2}$$

with:

- Δt is temporal support.
- Δf is the frequency band.

Practically, this implies the impossibility of precisely knowing which components exist in the signal but rather the frequency bands. Because of the absence of any information on the instants of the appearance of the frequency components, the Fourier transform is limited, especially in the case of an analysis of nonstationary signals. Figure 1 illustrates an example of the disadvantage of the Fourier transform. Indeed, we have a signal composed of three waves:

- a sinusoidal wave of 150 Hz,
- a standing wave obtained by superposing two sinusoidal signals of 100 and 50 Hz,
- a sinusoidal wave of 50 Hz.

These three waves appear in this order in the time domain. The spectrum of the signal gives no information on the moment of appearance of the different frequencies constituting the signal.

Thus, the analysis tool of the Fourier transform presents a major limitation. Consequently, this transform cannot locate the singularities in a signal and cannot provide information on some parameters such as the instantaneous frequency. To analyze a nonstationary signal and detect frequency changes with their location in time, the Fourier transform is therefore limited, and it is necessary to use time–frequency analysis tools.

2.2 Continuous Wavelet Transform (CWT)

Definition

In time–frequency transforms, a window is used which is translated throughout the time–frequency domain. Therefore, in the vicinity of a point b, the amplitude of the

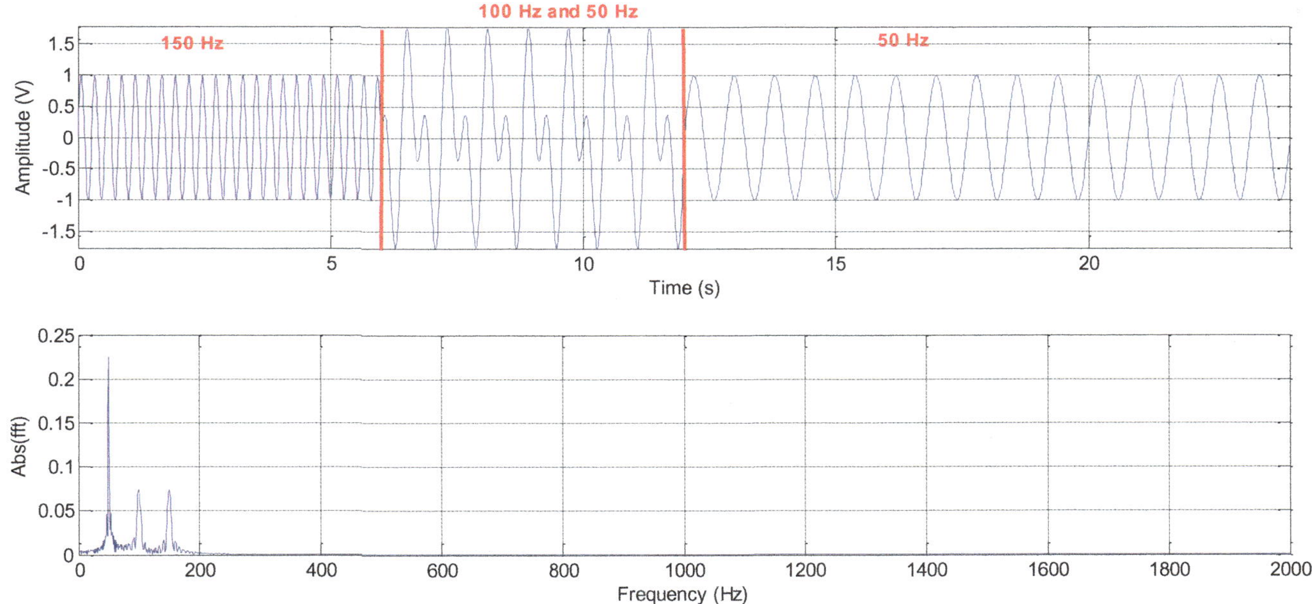

Fig. 1 The spectrum of a composition of sinusoids by Fourier transform

sinusoidal component having a frequency f is measured. The disadvantage of these transforms is the use of a window of the invariant size that covers the time–frequency plane. Now, we look for a window that can analyze the different irregularities of the signal [26–31]. This is the basic principle of wavelet transformation.

A wavelet is a function that has particular properties. In a more general way, the wavelet must satisfy the following conditions:

- It must have a short domain and finite energy in the time domain;
- It must present some oscillations.

From a wavelet function, a family of wavelets can be generated by dilation (or contraction) and translation (along the time axis). Using mathematical notations, this generated family is noted $\{\psi_{a,b}\}$, where ψ is called the analysis wavelet function or the mother wavelet, a is a dilation parameter or scale factor and b is the translation parameter. This set contains all the versions dilated by a and translated by b of the analysis function. In the general context, the continuous wavelet transform (CWT) is defined by the projection of a signal x (t) over all the wavelet functions $\langle f, \psi_{a,b} \rangle$. At each point (a, b) in the time-scale plane, the wavelet transform makes it possible to provide information on the resemblance between the analyzed signal and the scaled version of ψ shifted by b. The CWT analysis of a signal $x(t)$ produces no information in the classical frequency sense but rather coefficients according to scales evaluated according to Eq. (3).

$$C(b,a) = \int_{-\infty}^{+\infty} x(t)\psi_{a,b}^{*}(t)dt \qquad (3)$$

where: $\psi_{a,b}(t) = \frac{1}{\sqrt{a}}\psi\left(\frac{t-b}{a}\right)$ and $\psi_{a,b}^{*}(t)$ is the wavelet conjugate of $\psi_{a,b}(t)$.

Wavelet Properties

The wavelet function must satisfy the following properties:

- *Compact support*: The wavelet must be localized in the domains of time and frequency (or scale).
- *Admissibility condition*: A compact support function is called a wavelet if the following eligibility condition is satisfied:

$$C_{\psi} = \int_{-\infty}^{+\infty} \frac{|\psi(\omega)|^2}{|\omega|^2} d\omega < +\infty \qquad (4)$$

where $\Psi(\omega)$ is the Fourier transform of wavelet function $\psi(t)$.

Two important consequences of this eligibility property are that the mean value of the wavelet function is zero and its spectrum is of the band-pass type. In addition, this property ensures the preservation of the signal energy during the transformation.

- *Frequency selectivity*: A wavelet is said to be frequency-selective when the wavelet frequency band is narrow.
- *Similarity*: The different wavelet functions can be calculated from each other by using a linear combination of the translations and scaling parameters.
- *Symmetry*: To avoid the phase shift during the transformation, it is desirable to have a wavelet which has a temporal symmetry.
- *Regularity* means that there is a rapid decrease in its coefficients. This property leads to the speed of convergence of its coefficients.
- *The number of null moments*: A wavelet has m null moments if it verifies the Eq. (5):

$$\int_{-\infty}^{+\infty} t^k \psi(t)dt = 0 \; avec \; k = 0...m-1 \quad (5)$$

This property makes the wavelet transform more sensitive to the irregularities of a signal.

Main Wavelet Functions

Several wavelet families exist whose most used are:

- *Wavelet of Morlet (Morl)* is defined by the Eq. (6) [32].

$$\psi(t) = e^{-\frac{t^2}{2}} \cdot \cos(5t) \quad (6)$$

- *Wavelet Mexicanhat (Mexh)*: This is the second derivative of Gauss probability density [32]. Its expression is given in Eq. (7).

$$\psi(t) = \frac{2}{\sqrt{3} \cdot \pi^{1/4}} e^{-\frac{t^2}{2}} \cdot (1 - t^2) \quad (7)$$

- *Wavelets of Daubechies of odrer N (dbN)*: For $N = 1$, this wavelet is that of Haar, which is defined by Eq. (8). Except for $db1$, these wavelets do not have an explicit expression. However, these wavelets have been defined so that they have narrow support for a number m of moments. These wavelets are irregular and unsymmetrical.

$$\psi(t) = \begin{cases} 1 \, pour \, 0 \leq t \leq 0.5 \\ -1 \, pour \, 0.5 \leq t \leq 1 \, . \\ \quad 0 \qquad ailleurs \end{cases} \quad (8)$$

- *Wavelets Symmlets of order N (symN)*: This was proposed by Ingrid Daubechies by modification of the construction of dbN so that they are the most symmetrical possible. Apart from symmetry, symmlets wavelets retain the same properties of dbN.

- *Wavelet Coiflet (coifN)*: dbN welets for which the scale function also has zero moments.
- Wavelet of Meyer (meyr): It is an orthogonal wavelet. Even if this wavelet is indefinitely differentiable and with undefined support, it converges rapidly to 0. Moreover, the same fast decay property is preserved for its derivatives [32].

These main mother wavelets are illustrated in Fig. 2.

ECG Analysis and Scalogram

The coefficients of the CWT can be used to evaluate the scalogram $SC(b, a)$ which represents the energy density of the signal for each scale a and position b. The scalogram $SC(b, a)$ is defined by Eq. (9) [33, 34].

$$SC(b, a) = |C(b, a)|^2 \quad (9)$$

An example of the CWT for an ECG signal with a Morlet mother wavelet and a scaling factor from 1 to 32 is shown in Fig. 3.

2.3 Criterion Choice of Mother Wavelet for ECG Analysis

In literature, there is no predefined rule to select a wavelet for a particular application, rather the selection is application-oriented. It is a common practice to select a wavelet function which is having a similar shape as the subject signal as given in Fig. 4.

We have proposed a criterion for choosing the analyzing wavelet published in [35]. The idea of this criterion is to find a method to measure the resemblance between the signal to be analyzed and the wavelet function. This idea comes from the fact that the amplitude of the wavelet transform of a signal provides information on the degree of resemblance of the analyzed signal and the wavelet function.

The proposed method is based on the inequality of Cauchy-Schwartz. Indeed, this inequality is given in Eq. (10) [36, 37].

$$\left| \int_{-\infty}^{+\infty} x(t)\psi_{a,b}^*(t)dt \right|^2 \leq \int_{-\infty}^{+\infty} |x(t)|^2 dt \cdot \int_{-\infty}^{+\infty} \left|\psi_{a,b}^*(t)\right|^2 dt \quad (10)$$

where:

- $\int_{-\infty}^{+\infty} |x(t)|^2 dt$: The energy of the signal
- $\int_{-\infty}^{+\infty} \left|\psi_{a,b}^*(t)\right|^2 dt$: The energy of the wavelet.

The equality of the two members of the inequality implies the collinearity of $x(t)$ and $\psi(t)$. In order to quantify the

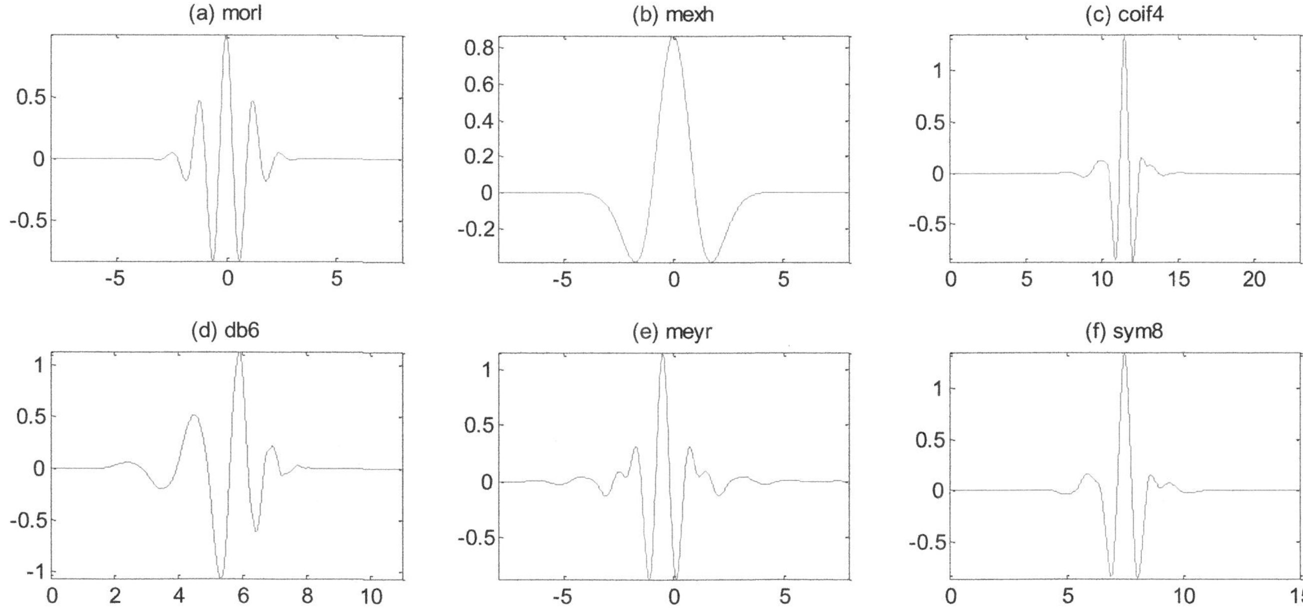

Fig. 2 Examples of mother wavelets

similarity between $x(t)$ and $\psi(t)$, we defined the collinearity ratio L given in Eq. (11).

$$L = \frac{\left| \int_{-\infty}^{+\infty} x(t)\psi_{a,b}^*(t)dt \right|^2}{\int_{-\infty}^{+\infty} |x(t)|^2 dt \int_{-\infty}^{+\infty} \left| \psi_{a,b}^*(t) \right|^2 dt} \qquad (11)$$

The discrete form of Eq. (11) is given in Eq. (12).

$$L = \frac{\sum_{n=1}^{N}\left(\sum_{k=1}^{K} |C_x(n,\sigma_k)|^2\right)}{\sum_{n=1}^{N} |x(n)|^2 \cdot \sum_{n=1}^{N} |\psi(n)|^2} \qquad (12)$$

where

- $C_x(n, \sigma_k)$ are the CWT coefficients.
- N is the number of samples.
- K is the number of scales.
- $x(n)$ is the sample of signal $x(t)$ at time $t_n = nT$; T is the sample period.
- $\psi(n)$ is the sample of the wavelet function ψ.

The criterion choice of mother wavelet consists of computing the collinearity ratio L for each type of mother wavelet and to choose that which gives the best ratio. Table 1 summarizes the result of the method with the following conditions:

- The ECG signal used is the *a01m* record of apnea database [38];
- The scale parameters are $\sigma_k; k = 1,\ldots,32$ and $\sigma_1 = 1$, $\sigma_k = \sigma_{k-1} + 1$.

As shown in Table 1, Morlet's mother wavelet gives the best collinearity ratio L to conserve the maximum of localized energy splint along the acquisition period.

Taking into account this important result, we will use the Morlet's mother wavelet to compute the CWT coefficients of the ECG signal in the following sections.

3 CWT-Based Algorithm for ECG Features

The algorithm is based on CWT coefficients with a selection of scale parameter for each wave of the ECG signal. The process starts with the detection of the R peaks; next a localization of the Q and S points; and then after identification of the P and T waves. The steps of the algorithm are given in Fig. 5 [35].

3.1 R-Peak Detection

The signal is analyzed in a set of scales using the Morlet's wavelet. The wavelet coefficients are exploited to compute the following distributions [39]:

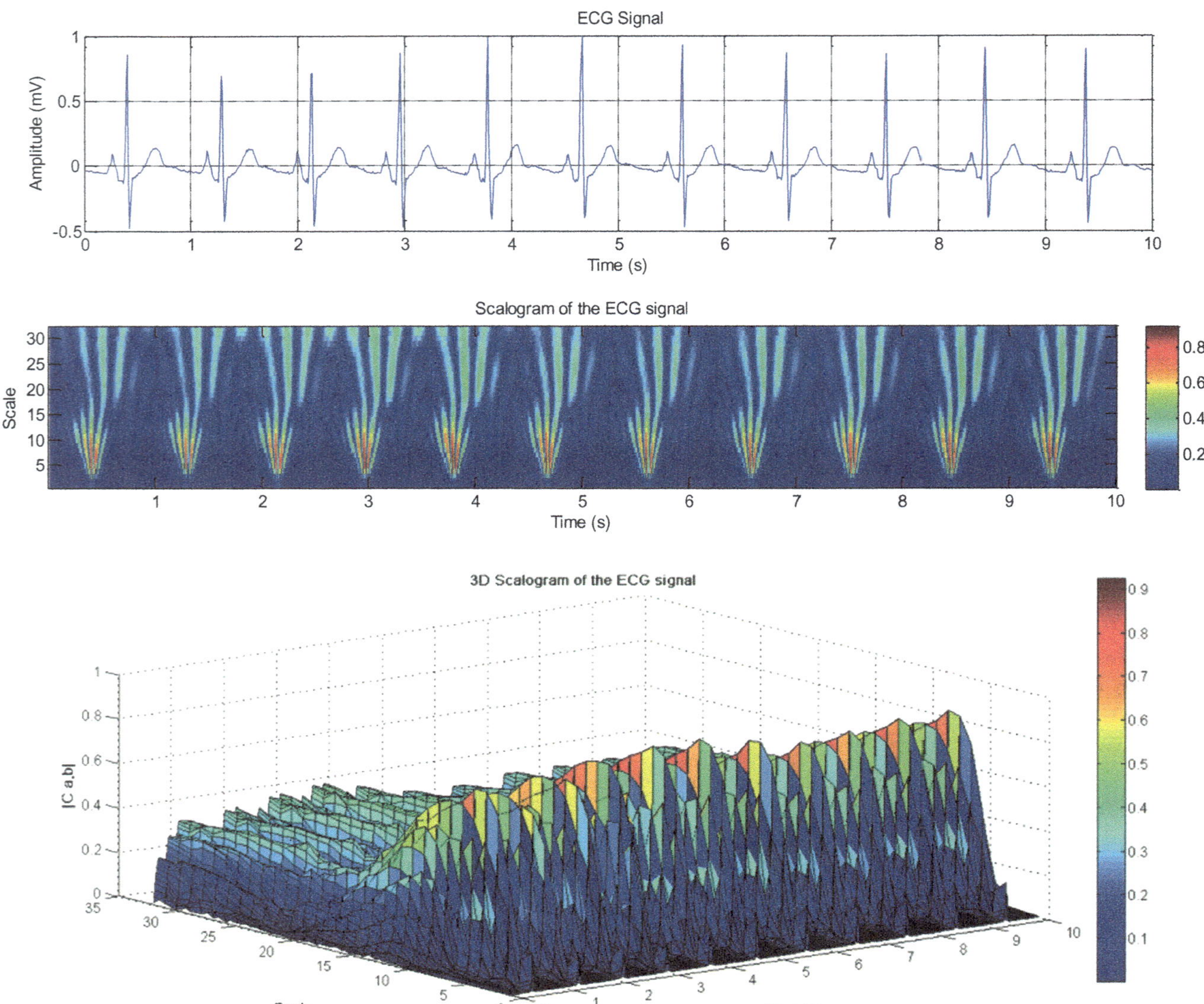

Fig. 3 Scalogramof ECG signal, 2D representation (top), 3D representation (bottom)

- *Time-scale content*: Evaluate the energy $E_x(n)$ of the signal $x(n)$ presented at the time t_n based on the result coefficients $C_x(n, \sigma_k), k = 1, \ldots, K$ of the applied transform. It can be expressed as given in Eq. (13).

$$E_x(n) = \sum_{k=1}^{K} |C_x(n, \sigma_k)|^2 \qquad (13)$$

- *Relative time-scale content*: In order to study the most important contribution at each instant t_n, we propose to evaluate the rate of absolute maximum coefficient and the total energy as given in Eq. (14):

$$RE_x(n) = \frac{max_n\left(|C_x(n, \sigma_k)|^2\right)_{k=1,\ldots,K}}{E_x(n)} \qquad (14)$$

With an aim of automatical:y selecting a scale parameter for R peak detection, we proceed as follows:

- We compute the CWT coefficients $C(n, \sigma_k)$,
- We extract the maximum of the $C(n, \sigma_k)$ at each time point and store them in a vector named y_m,
- We compute the peaks of y_m and looking for all the scales corresponding to these peaks. An averaging of these

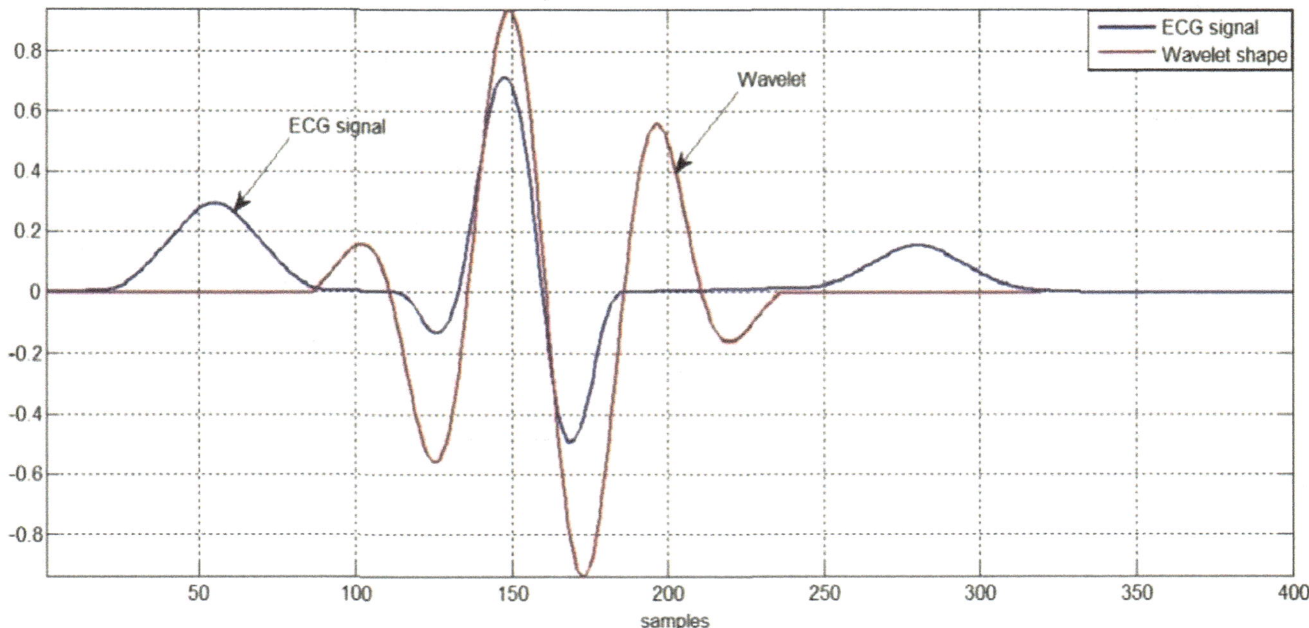

Fig. 4 Representation of ECG's waves and wavelet's shape

Table 1 Collinearity ratio for different mother wavelet

Wavelet	Collinearity ratio
Morl	0.9621
Meyr	0.9508
Mexh	0.8721
Gaus 4	0.5897
Coif 4	0.0606
Sym 4	0.0598
Db 4	0.0598
Haar	0.0549

scales gives us the selected scale called σ_R. The simulation result of this step is illustrated in Fig. 6.

- We analyze the ECG signal with CWT at the selected scale σ_R. This analysis consists of computing the CWT coefficients $C(n, \sigma_R)$. The simulation result of this step is shown in Fig. 7.

In the objective to detect the R-peak starting from the analysis of the signal at the selected scale σ_R, we do as follows:

- We compute the vector M_C containing the mean value $m(k)$ of wavelet coefficients at σ_R along a sliding window w,
- We compute the histogram of vector y_m to determine the distribution of the wavelet coefficients for the different

samples of the ECG signal. The histogram is given in Fig. 8.
- We define a threshold for R detection using the centroid of the histogram method as given in Eq. (15):

$$ECG_{th} = \frac{\sum_{i=1}^{n}(C_i * N_i)}{\sum_{i=1}^{n} N_i} \tag{15}$$

where ECG_{th} is the threshold, C_i is the wavelet coefficient values, N_i is the number of samples and n is the histogram range.

- We detect the peaks in M_C by using the threshold value defined in Eq. (15). These peaks deal with the R peaks of the ECG signal. The results of this step are given in Fig. 9.

3.2 Q and S Points Detection

Once the R peaks are detected, the Q and S points are the next features to locate in order to complete the QRS complex. To select the scale parameter corresponding to Q wave called σ_Q, we follow the given steps:

- We localize the local minima of relative time–frequency content $RE_x(n)$ before each R peak position as given in Fig. 10.

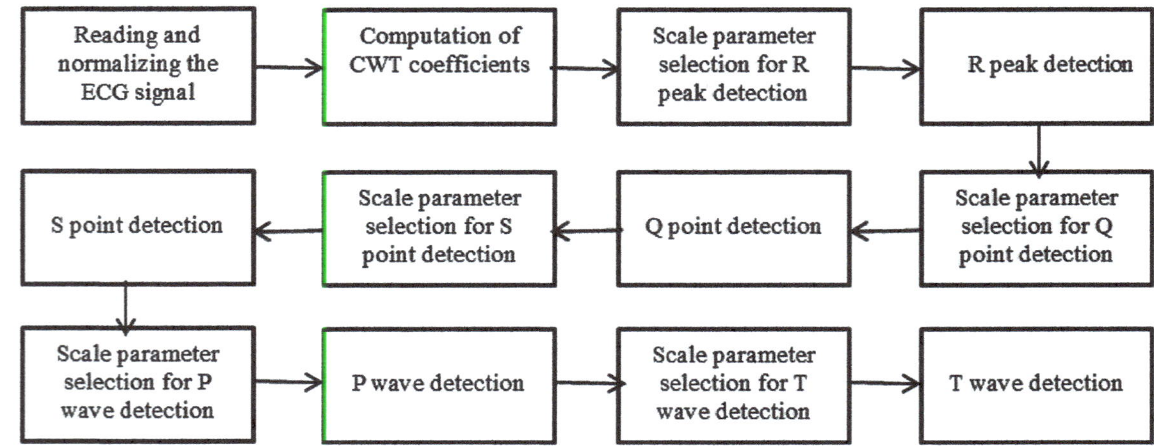

Fig. 5 The steps of the CWT-ECG processing algorithm

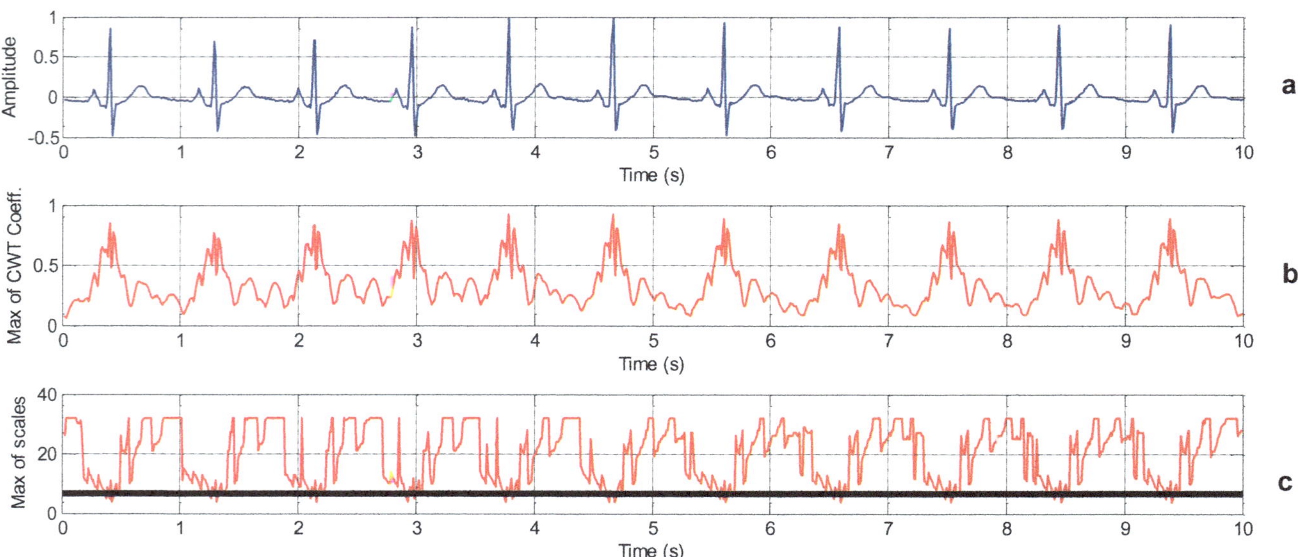

Fig. 6 Scale parameter selection for R peak detection: **a** ECG signal, **b** maximum of CWT coefficients, **c** selection of scale parameter *(the selected scale is plotted in black line)*

- We seek the positions of those local minima in the vector y_m.
- We look for the scales corresponding to those positions.
- An average of obtained scales gives us σ_Q.

To select the scale parameter corresponding to S wave called σ_S, we process as we did for Q wave. The only difference is to localize the local minima after each R peak as given in Fig. 11.

Once the scale parameters σ_Q and σ_S are defined, we compute the CWT coefficients C_{σ_Q} and C_{σ_S}. The plots of those coefficients are given in Fig. 12.

The Q and S points are the inflection points in either side of R peak. So it is thus enough to locate the first zero slope in either side of R peak. For this purpose, we do

differentiation of C_{σ_Q} and C_{σ_S}, then we detect the zero slopes around the position of R peak. The result of this process is given in Fig. 13.

3.3 Detection of P and T Waves

Once the QRS complex is completely localized, we proceed to the next step which consists in locating the P and T waves of ECG signal. In order to select the scale parameter corresponding to P wave called σ_P, the following steps are carried out:

- We compute the energy of the signal locally in a sliding window w according to Eq. (16).

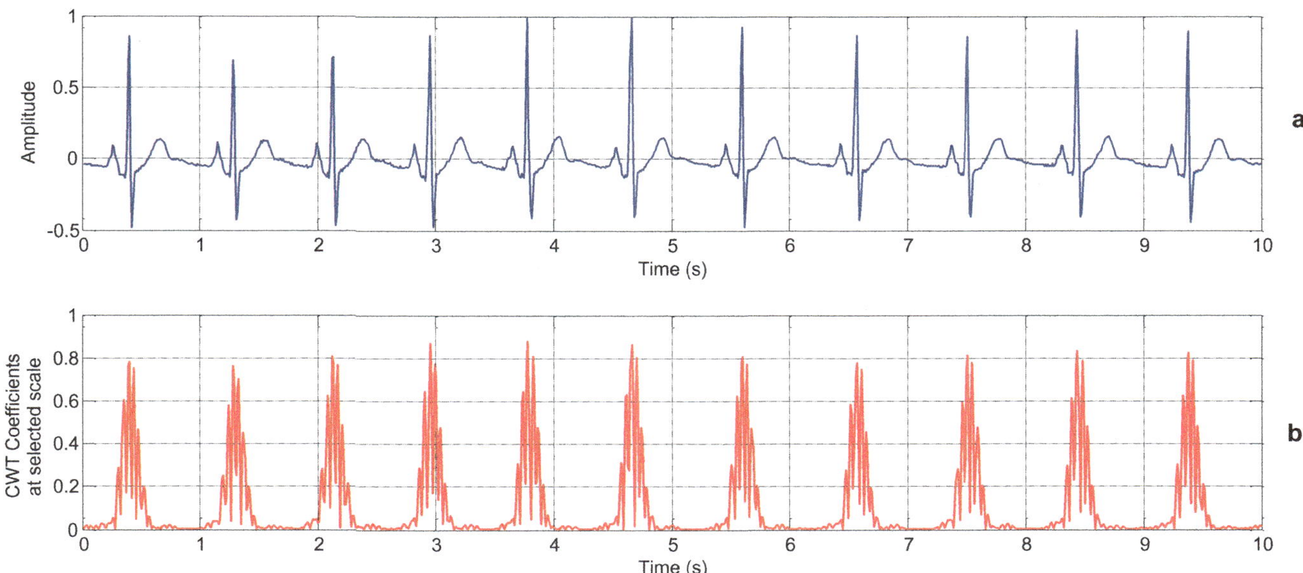

Fig. 7 The CWT coefficients at the selected scale σ_R

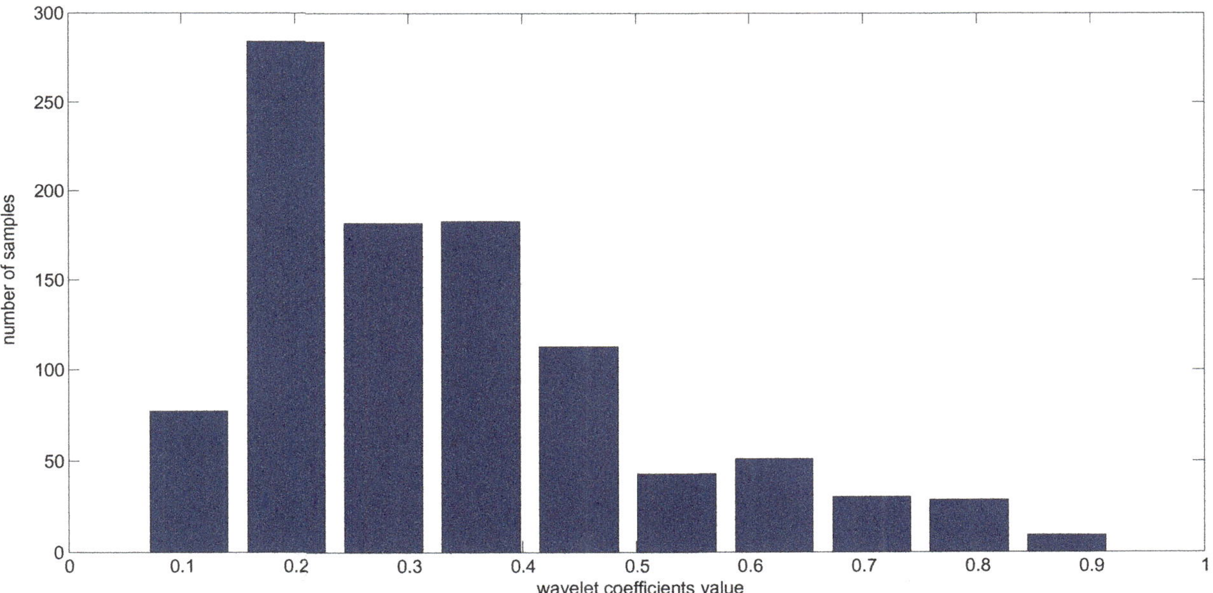

Fig. 8 Distribution of wavelet coefficients at a selected scale

$$E_w = \sum_{new} \sum_{k=1}^{K} |C(n, \sigma_k)|^2 \qquad (16)$$

- We seek the first maxima before each Q point position in E_w. The simulation result of this step is shown in Fig. 14.
- We localize the positions of those maxima in the vector y_m.
- We look for the scales corresponding to those positions.
- An average of obtained scales returns the scale σ_P.

To select the scale parameters corresponding to T wave called σ_T, we follow the same steps given below and we look for the first maxima after the S point positions. The simulation result is shown in Fig. 15.

Once the scale parameters corresponding to P and T waves are selected, we compute the CWT coefficients at these scales. The plot of CWT coefficients C_{σ_P} and C_{σ_T} are given in Fig. 16.

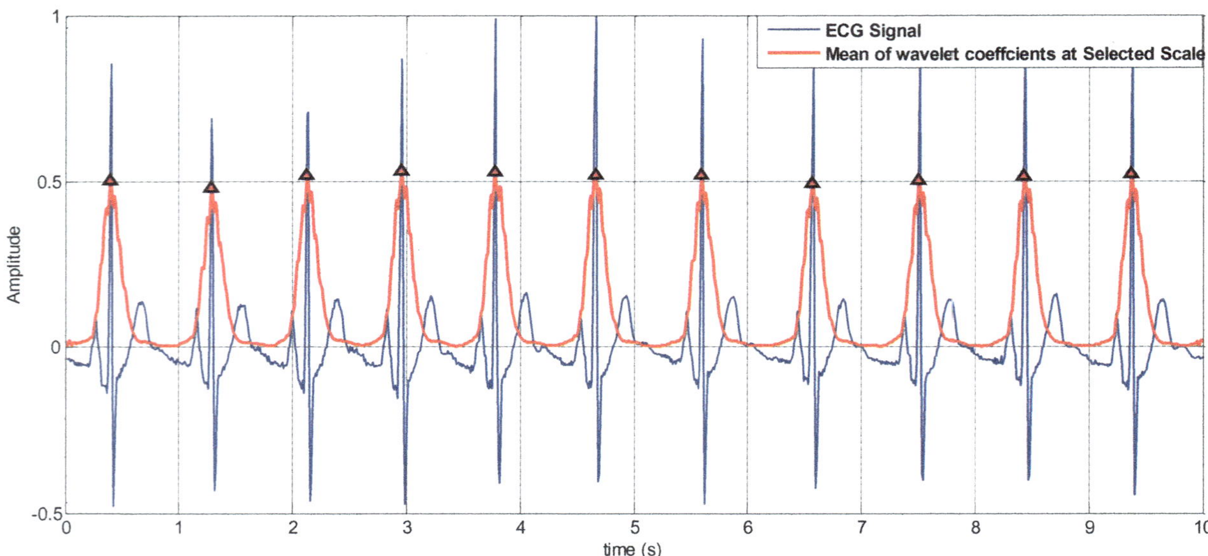

Fig. 9 R-peak detection

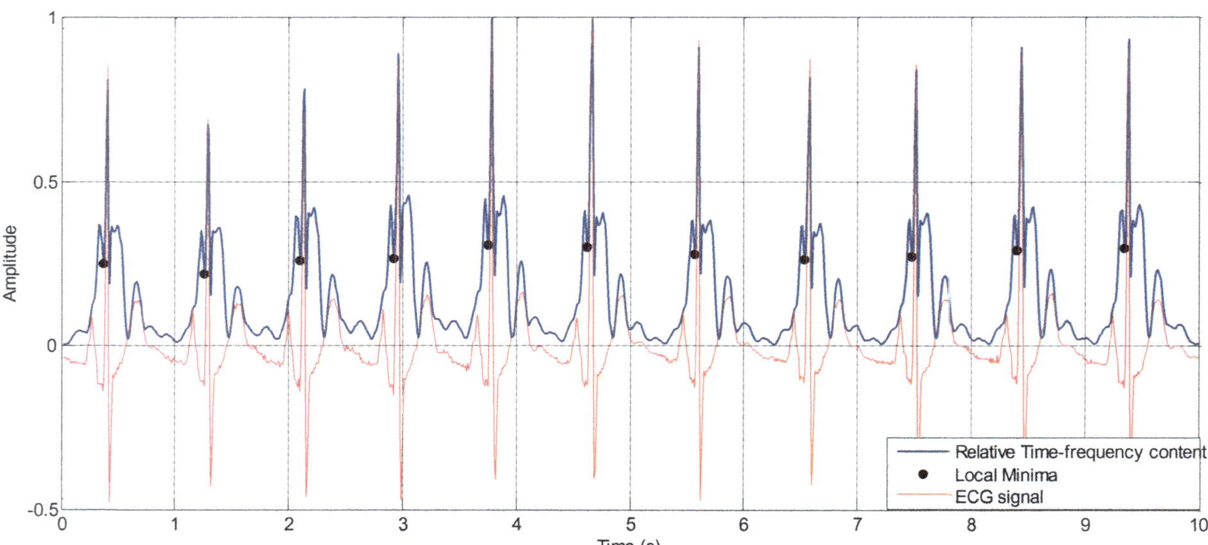

Fig. 10 Local minima before each R peak position in relative time–frequency content

The P wave is identified as the first maxima before each Q point position in the plot of C_{σ_P}. For this goal, we do the derivative of C_{σ_P} named C'_{σ_P}. Then we look for the point P corresponding to the following conditions:

- The point P is before the Q point.
- $C'_{\sigma_P}(P) = 0$.
- C_{σ_P} is increasing before P and decreasing after.

The result of this step is given in Fig. 17.

In order to detect the T wave, we can apply the same method above since the T wave is identified as first maxima after each S point position in the plot of C_{σ_Q}. The result of this detection is shown in Fig. 18.

Finally, the detection of the different waves of the ECG signal is given in Fig. 19.

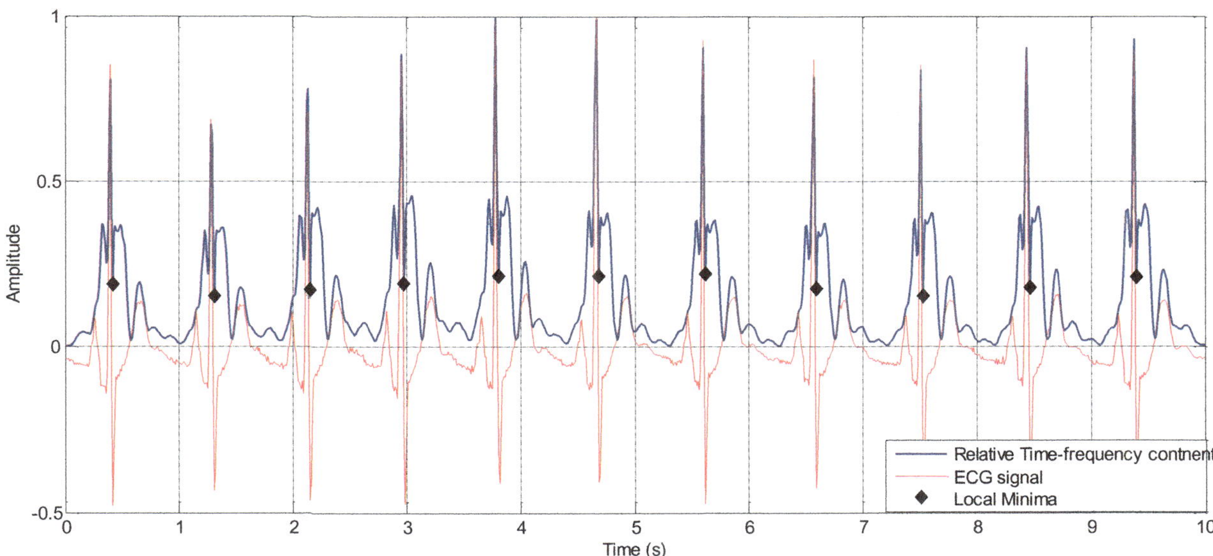

Fig. 11 Local minima after each R peak position in relative time–frequency content

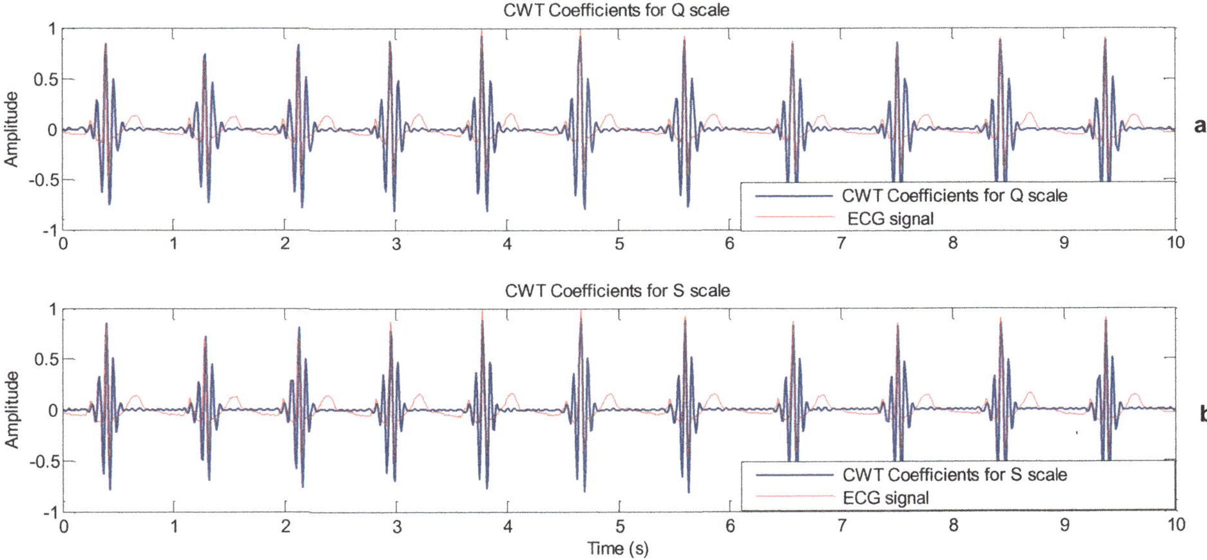

Fig. 12 CWT coefficients: **a** C_{σ_Q}, **b** C_{σ_S}

4   Result and Performances

4.1   MIT-BIH Database Description

In order to evaluate the ECG features extraction and detection algorithm, it should be applied to recordings from MIT-BIH database [40].

This database has been established by scientists to serve as a standard to validate the proposed methods of QRS complex detection. This database contains 48 half-hour recordings. The recordings were digitized at a frequency of 360 Hz with an 11-bit coding.

Each recording contains an annotation made by several cardiologists. Each record of this database is associated with the following files:

- Data file (* .dat): contains digitized samples of the ECG signal.
- Header file (* .hea): contains the interpretation parameters of the data file such as sampling frequency, amplification gain… etc.

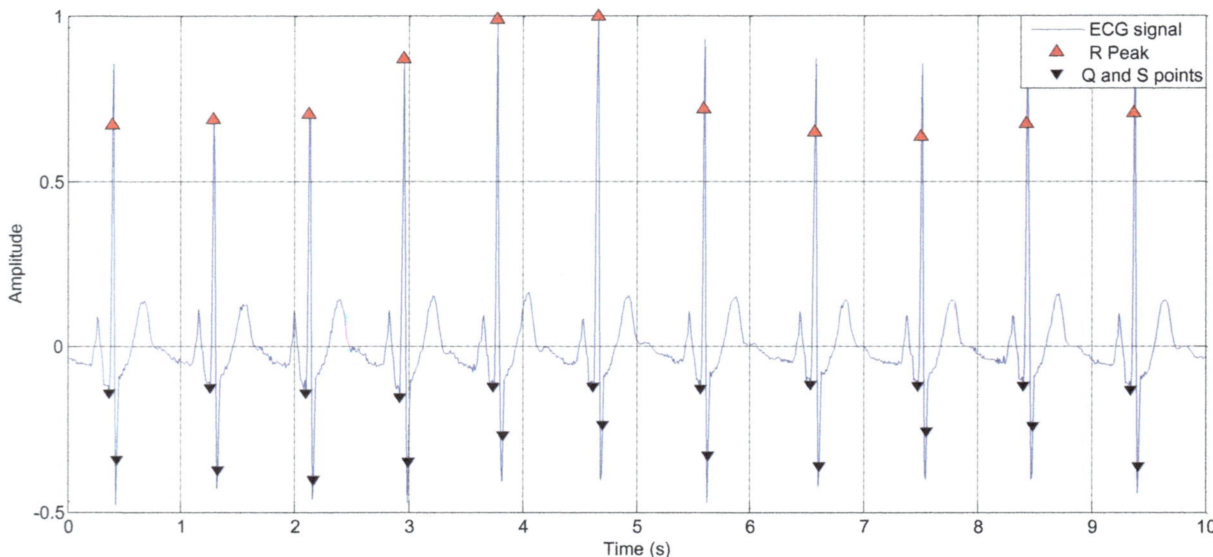

Fig. 13 The detection of Q and S waves

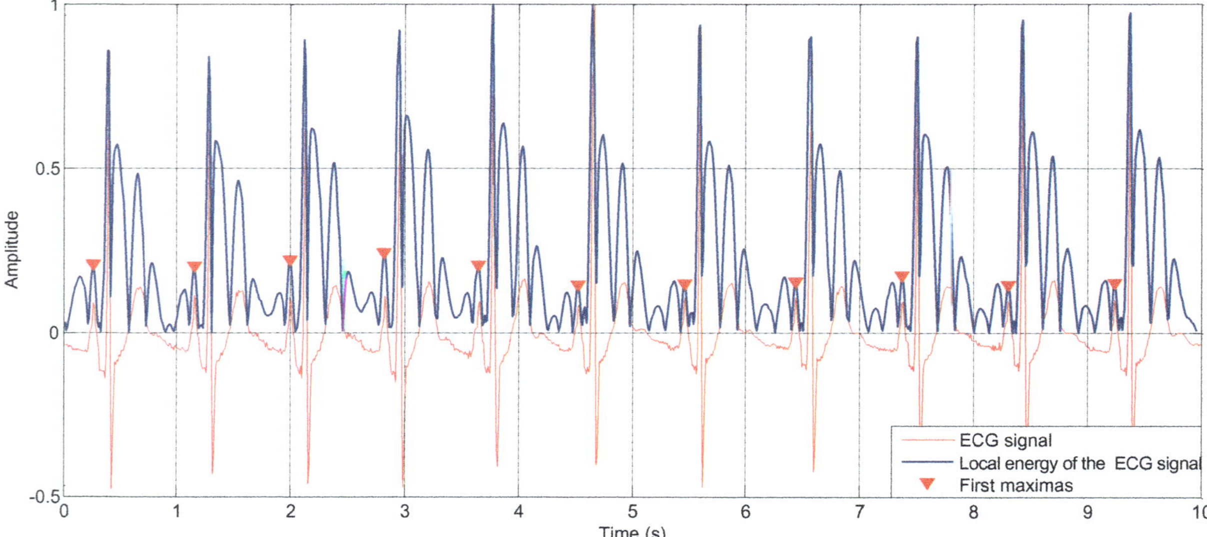

Fig. 14 Local maxima before each Q position

- Annotation file (* .atr): it comprises the positions and instants of the appearance of the peak R of the ECG signal and a mark indicating whether the QRS complex is normal or not.

4.2 Parameters Evaluation

In literature, there are various metrics that are used to evaluate the ECG analysis algorithms. The main measures can be listed as the sensitivity, the positive predictivity, and the error rate.

- Sensitivity (*Se*) can be formalized as follows:

$$Se(\%) = \frac{TP}{TP + FN} \times 100 \qquad (17)$$

- Positive predictivity (P^+) can be defined by the following formula:

$$P^+(\%) = \frac{TP}{TP + FP} \times 100 \qquad (18)$$

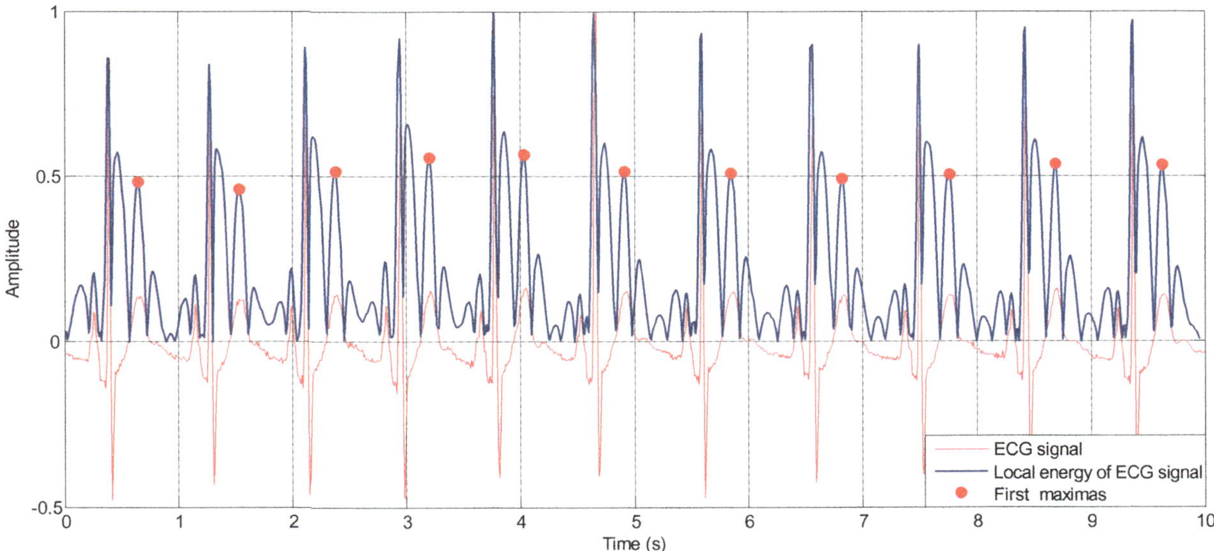

Fig. 15 Local maxima after each S position

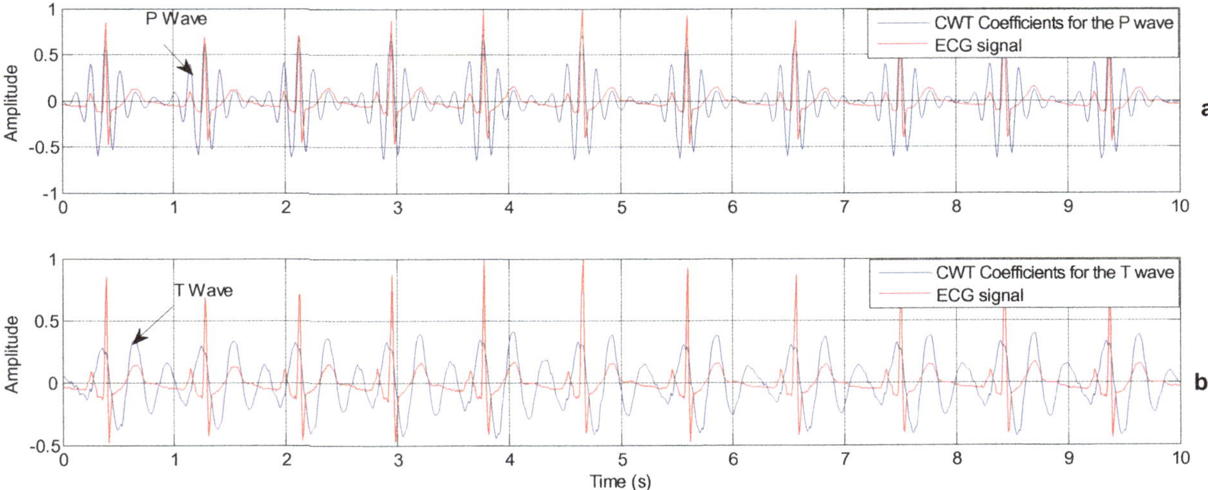

Fig. 16 Wavelet coefficients: **a** C_{σ_P}, **b** C_{σ_T}

- Error rate (*ER*) can be formalized as follows:

$$ER(\%) = \frac{FN + FP}{TB} \times 100 \qquad (19)$$

where

- *TP* is the number of correct predictions for positive samples,
- *TN* is the number of correct predictions for negative samples,
- *FP* is the number of incorrect predictions for positive samples,
- *FN* is the number of incorrect predictions for negative samples,
- *TB* is the total number of beats.

The detection metrics for the proposed method are given in Table 2. The algorithm achieved good performance with the sensitivity of 99.84%, the positive predictivity value of 99.53%, and an error rate of 0.62%.

The comparison of the performance of the proposed method with the other techniques is given in Table 3.

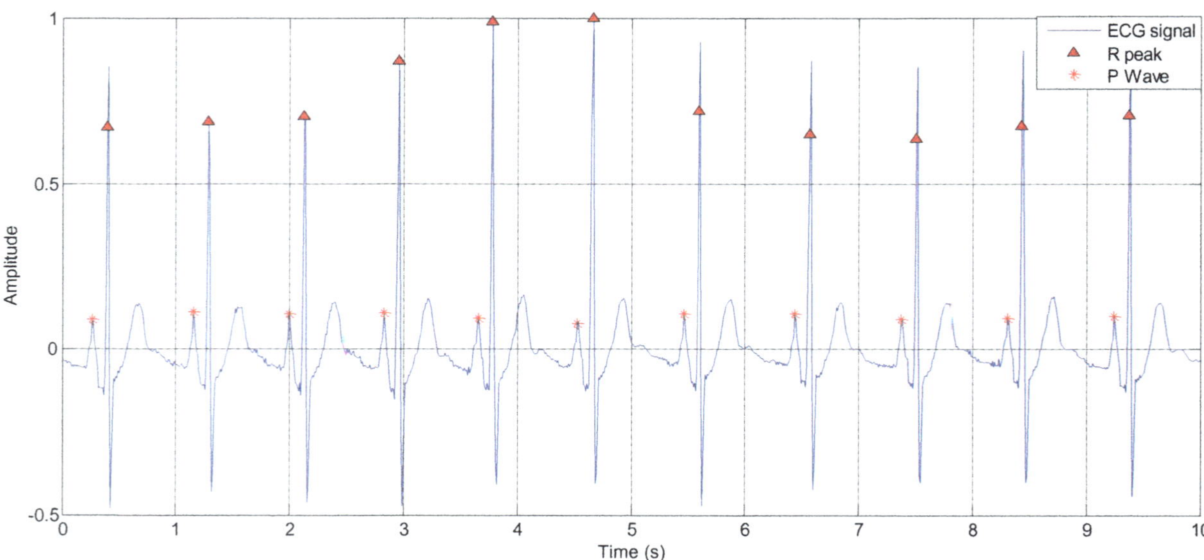

Fig. 17 P wave detection

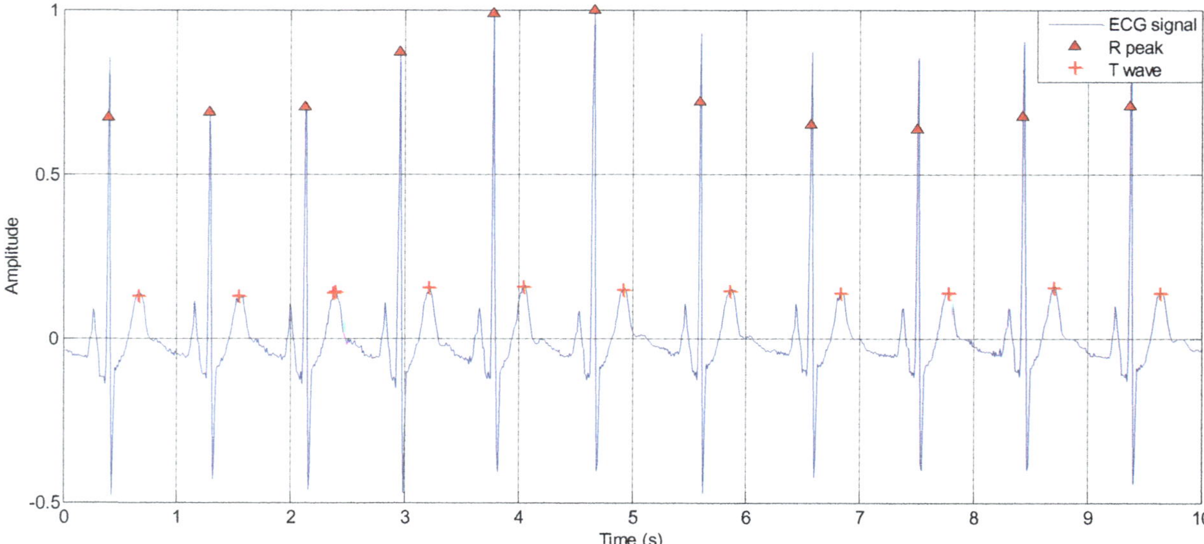

Fig. 18 T wave detection

4.3 Robustness of the Proposed Algorithm

The core of the proposed algorithm is the selection of the scale parameter of the CWT corresponding to each ECG signal wave. This selection can be considered as selective filtering of the wave which will be analyzed. As a result, the features detection of ECG signal can be processed even in the presence of certain noises such as baseline wander (BW) or power line interference (PLI). The denoising of the signal is therefore unnecessary.

To illustrate the robustness of the proposed method, we applied it to an ECG signal separately comprising the following two types of noise:

- **Baseline wander**: a synthetic baseline wander is added to an ECG signal using the sinusoidal model as given below

$$Bw(t) = A_1 \sin(2\pi f_1 t) \tag{20}$$

where the amplitude $A_1 = 0.4$ mV and the frequency $f_1 \in [0 - 0.5 \text{ Hz}]$.

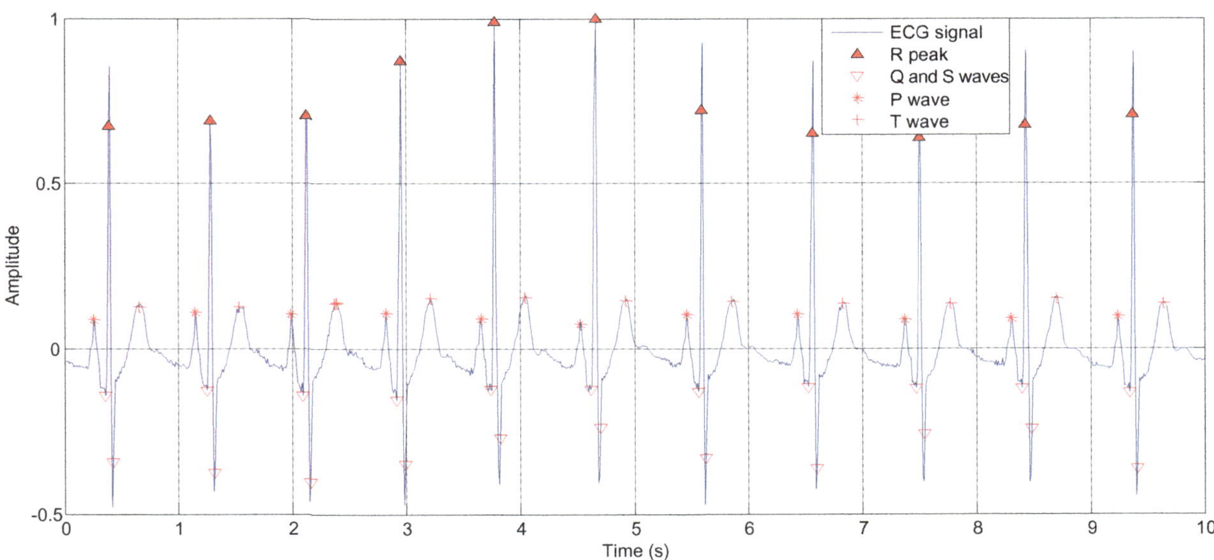

Fig. 19 P, QRS and T waves detection

Table 2 Measures of the QRS detection

Record	TB	TP	FN	FP	Se (%)	P+ (%)	ER (%)
100	2274	2273	1	1	99.95	99.96	0.088
101	1874	1874	0	14	100	99.26	0.747
102	2192	2191	1	15	99.95	99.32	0.729
103	2091	2085	4	2	99.80	99.90	0.286
104	2311	2304	4	16	99.82	99.31	0.865
105	²2691	2682	4	16	99.85	99.41	0.743
106	2098	2094	4	3	99.80	99.86	0.333
107	2140	2137	3	12	99.85	99.44	0.700
108	1824	1819	5	25	99.72	98.64	1.644
109	2535	2534	1	11	99.96	99.57	0.473
111	2133	2126	7	13	99.67	99.39	0.93
112	2550	2547	3	10	99.88	99.61	0.5
113	1796	1795	1	10	99.94	99.45	0.61
114	1890	1879	7	10	99.62	99.47	0.89
115	1962	1951	7	2	99.64	99.90	0.45
116	2421	2410	7	4	99.71	99.83	0.45
117	1539	1539	0	10	100	99.35	0.64
118	2301	2300	1	16	99.95	99.31	0.73
119	2094	2084	5	27	99.76	98.72	1.52
121	1876	1876	0	11	100	99.42	0.58
122	2479	2477	2	0	99.91	100	0.08
123	1519	1519	0	15	100	99.02	0.98
124	1634	1632	2	4	99.87	99.76	0.36
200	2792	2779	5	10	99.82	99.64	0.53
201	2039	1978	8	0	99.59	100	0.39
202	2146	2141	5	4	99.76	99.81	0.41
203	3108	3104	4	10	99.87	99.68	0.45
205	2672	2660	5	0	99.81	100	0.18
Total	60,981	60790	96	271	99.84	99.53	0.62

Table 3 Comparison of QRS detector performance

Algorithm name	Se (%)	P^+ (%)	ER(%)
Karimipour and Homaeinezhad [41]	99.81	99.7	0.49
Pan and Tompkins [5]	99.75	99.53	0.675
Li et al. [20]	99.89	99.94	0.14
Poli et al. [42]	99.6	99.5	0.9
Madeiro et al. [43]	99.15	99.18	1.69
Biel et al. [13]	99.64	99.82	0.54
Yochum et al. [44]	99.85	99.48	0.67
Martinez et al. [45]	99.8	99.86	0.34
Hamilton and Tompkins [46]	99.69	99.77	0.54
The proposed algorithm	99.84	99.53	0.62

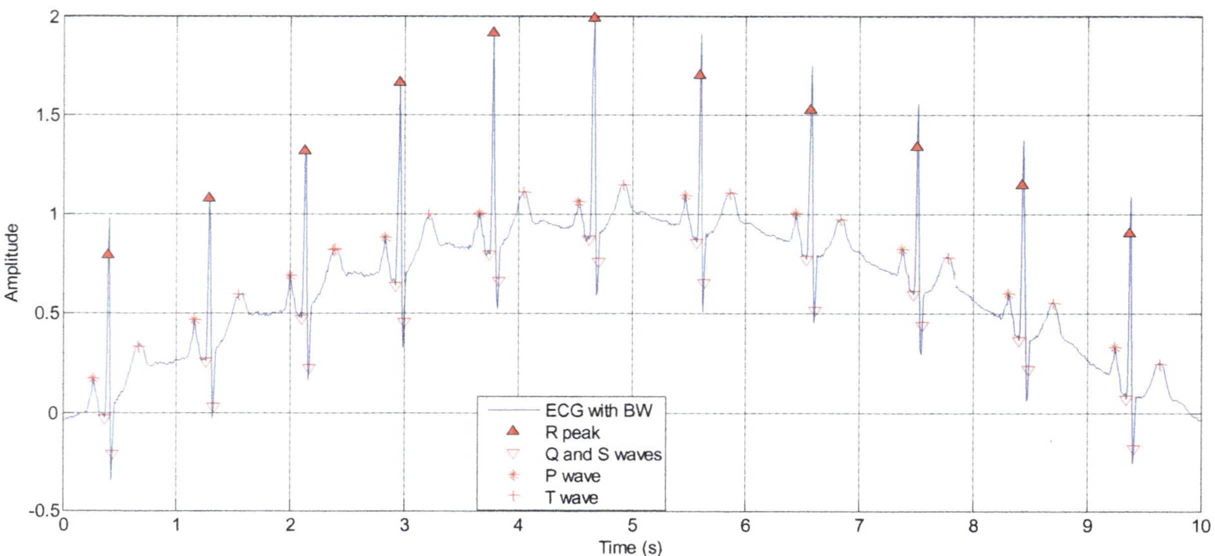

Fig. 20 P, QRS and T waves detection with baseline wander

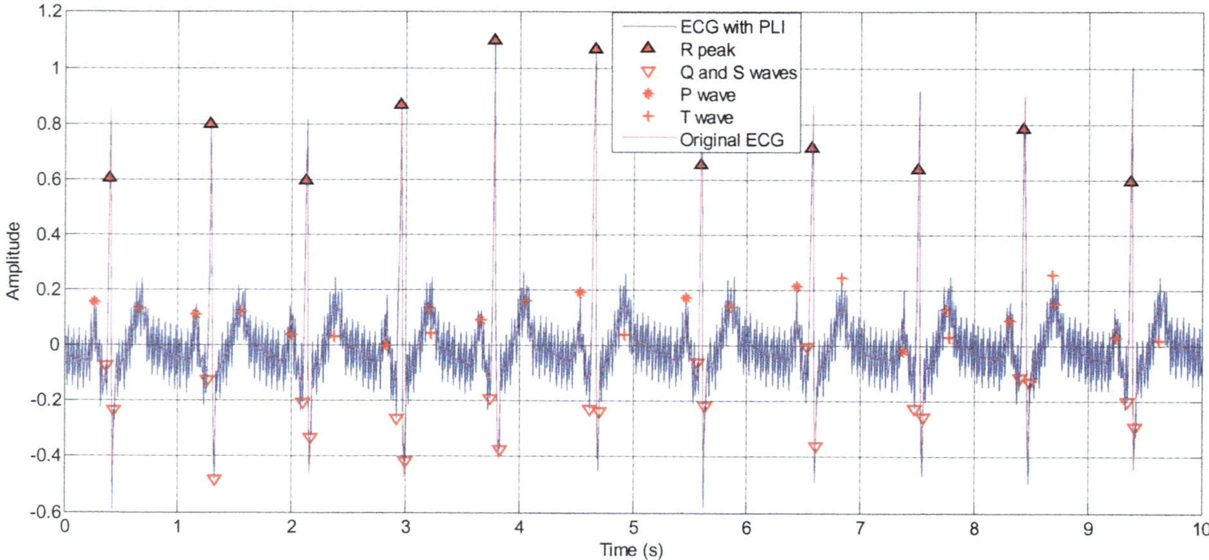

Fig. 21 P, QRS and T waves detection with PLI

The simulation result of the analysis is given in Fig. 20. We note that the ECG features are detected.

– **Power line interference (PLI)**: It is synthesized using the sinusoidal signal formalized as follows:

$$pli(t) = A_2 \sin(2\pi f_2 t) \tag{21}$$

where the amplitude $A_2 = 0.1$ mV and the frequency $f_2 = 50 Hz$.

The result simulation of detection with PLI is given in Fig. 21. It is also clear that the ECG features are extracted without a preprocessing filter. This is an additional benefit of our proposed algorithm based on time-scale analysis of ECG samples.

5 Conclusion

In this chapter, we presented a time-scale analysis and a criterion to choose the mother wavelet for ECG analysis. The idea of this criterion is to find the type of wavelet given the best collinearity with the ECG signal. Indeed, we proved that Mortlet's mother wavelet is best suited to the analysis of the ECG signal since it has the best collinearity ratio.

Also presented in this work a new algorithm based on continuous wavelet transform for detection of QRS, P and T waves of ECG signal. This algorithm exploits a technique of selection of scale parameter for the wavelet coefficients. The algorithm achieved good performance with the sensitivity of 99.84%, the positive predictivity value of 99.53% and an error rate of 0.62%.

The advantages of this selection are multiple, such as the elimination of noise and interference with other parts of the signal while extracting a specific wave as well as a reduced computing time of wavelet coefficients, what makes a reduced duration of the analysis.

The robustness of the algorithm consists in the detection of the P, QRS, and T waves even if the signal is affected by the baseline wander and the power line interference.

References

1. Ahlstrom M. L., Tompkins W. J. (1983) Automated High-Speed Analysis of Holter Tapes with Microcomputers. IEEE Transactions on Biomedical Engineering 30 (110): 651–657. https://doi.org/10.1109/TBME.1983.325067.
2. Fraden J., Neuman M. R. (1980) QRS wave detection. Medical & Biological Engineering & Computing 18 (12): 125–132.https://doi.org/10.1007/BF02443287.
3. Gritzali F., Frangakis G., Papakonstantinou G. (1987) Comparison of the length and energy transformations for the QRS detection. In: IEEE/ Engineering in Medicine and Biology Society Annual Conference.
4. Sun Y., Suppappola S., Wrublewski T. A. (1992) Microcontroller-based real-time QRS detection. Biomedical Instrumentation and Technology 26 (16): 477–484.
5. Pan J., Tompkins W. J. (1985) A Real-Time QRS Detection Algorithm. IEEE Transactions on Biomedical Engineering 32 (13):230–236. https://doi.org/10.1109/TBME.1985.325532.
6. Hu Y. H., Tompkins W. J., Urrusti J. L. et al. (1993) Applications of artificial neural networks for ECG signal detection and classification. Journal of Electrocardiology 26 (Suppl) 6: 66–73.
7. Vijaya G., Kumar V., Verma H. K. (1998) ANN-based QRS-complex analysis of ECG. Journal of medical engineering & technology 22 (14): 160–7. https://doi.org/10.3109/03091909809032534.
8. Xue Q., Hu Y. H., Tompkins W. J. (1992) Neural-Network-Based Adaptive Matched Filtering for QRS Detection. IEEE Transactions on Biomedical Engineering 39 (14): 317–329. https://doi.org/10.1109/10.126604.
9. Andreao R. V., Dorizzi B., Boudy J. (2006) ECG signal analysis through hidden Markov models. IEEE Transactions on Biomedical Engineering 53 (18): 1541–1549. https://doi.org/10.1109/tbme.2006.877103.
10. Pan S.-T., Hong T.-P., Chen H.-C. (2012) ECG signal analysis by using Hidden Markov model. In: International conference on Fuzzy Theory and Its Applications (iFUZZY2012), IEEE, Taichung Taiwan, 16–18 Nov. 2012. https://doi.org/10.1109/ifuzzy.2012.6409718.
11. Hughes N. P., Tarassenko L., Roberts S. J. (2004) Markov models for automated ECG interval analysis. In: 16th International Conference on Advances in Neural Information Processing Systems: 611–618. Whistler, British Columbia, Canada, December 09–11, 2003.
12. Udupa J., Murthy I. (1980) Syntactic approach to ECG rhythm analysis. IEEE Transactions on Biomedical Engineering 27 (17): 370–375. https://doi.org/10.1109/TBME.1980.326650.
13. Biel L., Pettersson O., Philipson L. et al. (2001) ECG analysis: A new approach in human identification. IEEE Transaction on Instrumentation and Measurement 50 (13): 808–812. https://doi.org/10.1109/19.930458.
14. Karpagachelvi S., Arthanari M., Sivakumar M. (2010) ECG Feature Extraction Techniques - A Survey Approach. International Journal of Computer Science and Information Security 8 (1): 76–80.
15. Benitez D. S., Gaydecki P. A., Zaidi A. et al. (2000) A new QRS detection algorithm based on the Hilbert transform. In: Computers in Cardiology, IEEE, Cambridge USA, 24–27 Sept. 2000. https://doi.org/10.1109/CIC.2000.898536.
16. Singh Kohli S., Makwana N., Mishra N. et al. (2012) Hilbert Transform Based Adaptive ECG R-Peak Detection Technique.Int. J. Electr. Comput. Eng. 2 (15): 639–643. http://dx.doi.org/10.11591/ijece.v2i5.1439.
17. Rabbani H., Parsa Mahjoob M., Farahabadi E. et al. (2011) R peak detection in electrocardiogram signal based on an optimal combination of wavelet transform, hilbert transform, and adaptive thresholding. Journal of medical signals and sensors1 (12): 91–98.
18. Bahoura M., Hassani M., Hubin M. (1997) DSP implementation of wavelet transform for real time ECG wave forms detection and heart rate analysis. Computer Methods and Programs in

Biomedicine 52 (11): 35–44. https://doi.org/10.1016/S0169-2607 (97)01780-X.

19. Kadambe S., Murray R., Boudreaux-Bartels G.F. (1999) Wavelet transform-based QRS complex detector. IEEE Transactions on Biomedical Engineering 46 (17): 838–848. https://doi.org/10. 1109/10.771194.

20. Li C., Zheng C., Tai C. (1995) Detection of ECG characteristic points using wavelet transforms. IEEE Transactions on Biomedical Engineering 42 (11): 21–28. https://doi.org/10.1109/10.362922.

21. Zidelmal Z., Amirou A., Adnane M., Belouchrani A. (2012) QRS detection based on wavelet coefficients. Computer Methods and Programs in Biomedicine 107 (13): 490–496. https://doi.org/10. 1016/j.cmpb.2011.12.004.

22. Narayana K., Rao A. (2011) Wavelet based QRS detection in ECG using MATLAB. Innovative Systems Design Engineering 2 (17): 60–70.

23. Rudnicki M., Strumiłło P. (2007) A Real-Time Adaptive Wavelet Transform-Based QRS Complex Detector. In: Beliczynski B., Dzielinski A., Iwanowski M., Ribeiro B. (eds) Adaptive and Natural Computing Algorithms. ICANNGA 2007. Lecture Notes in Computer Science, vol 4432. Springer, Berlin, Heidelberg. https://doi.org/10.1007/978-3-540-71629-7_32.

24. Aqil M., Jbari A., Bourouhou A. (2015) Evaluation of time-frequency and wavelet analysis of ECG signals. In: Third World Conference on Complex Systems (WCCS), Marrakech, Morroco, 23–25 Nov. https://doi.org/10.1109/ICoCS.2015. 7483229.

25. Belkhou A., Jbari A., Belarbi L. (2017) A continuous wavelet based technique for the analysis of electromyography signals. In: International Conference on Electrical and Information Technologies (ICEIT), Rabat, Morroco, 15–18 Nov. DOI:https://doi.org/10. 1109/EITech.2017.8255232.

26. Cohen L. (1994) Time Frequency Analysis: Theory and Applications. Prentice Hall. New Jesey.

27. Boashash B. (2016) Time-frequency signal analysis and processing, 2nd ed. Elsevier Ltd. Amsterdam.

28. Flandrin P. (1998) Time Frequency/ Time-scale Analysis. Elsevier Ltd. Amsterdam.

29. Jbari A.: Séparation Aveugle de Sources par contrastes à références et analyse du contenu temps-échelle. Thesis, University Mohamed V of Rabat (2009).

30. Qian S., Chen D. (1999) Joint time-frequency analysis. IEEE Signal Processing Magazine 16 (12): 52–67. https://doi.org/10. 1109/79.752051.

31. Goswami J. C.,ChanA. K. (2011) Fundamentals of Wavelets. John Wiley & sons Inc. New Jersey.

32. Daubechies I. (1992) Ten Lectures on Wavelets. Society for Industrial and Applied Mathematics. Philadelphia.

33. Semmlow J. (2004) Biosignal and biomedical image processing: MATLAB-based applications. Marcel Dekker Inc.New Jersey.

34. Clifford G. D., Azuaje F., McSharry P. E. (2006) Advanced Methods and Tools for ECG Data Analysis. Artech House. Norwood.

35. Aqil M., Jbari A., Bourouhou A. (2017) ECG-Waves: Analysis and Detection by Continuous Wavelet Transform. J. Telecommun. Electron. Comput. Eng. 9 (13): 45–52.

36. Bernard C.: Wavelets and ill posed problems: optic flow and scattered data. Thesis, University of Paris-Saclay (1999).

37. Mallat S. (2000) Une exploration des signaux en ondelettes. Editions de l'Ecole Polytechnique. Paris.

38. CinC Challenge 2000 data sets (2000) http://www.physionet.org/ Physiobank/database/apnea-ecg. Accessed 25 May 2016.

39. Aqil M., Jbari A., Bourouhou A. (2016) Adaptive ECG Wavelet analysis for R-peaks. In:Proceedings of 2016 International Conference on Electrical and Information Technologies (ICEIT), Tangier. https://doi.org/10.1109/EITech.2016.7519582.

40. MIT-BIH Arrythmia Database (2000) https://www.physionet.org/ physiobank/database/mitdb/. Accessed 20 May 2016.

41. Karimipour A., Homaeinezhad M. R. (2014) Real-time electro-cardiogram P- QRS-T detection-delineation algorithm based on quality-supported analysis of characteristic templates. Computers in Biology and Medicine 52: 153–165. https://doi.org/10.1016/j. compbiomed.2014.07.002.

42. Poli R., Cagnoni S., Valli G. (1995) Genetic Design of Optimum Linear and Nonlinear QRS Detectors. IEEE Transactions on Biomedical Engineering 42 (11): 1137–1141. https://doi.org/10. 1109/10.469381.

43. Madeiro J. P. V., Cortez P. C., Marques J. A. L., et al. (2012) An innovative approach of QRS segmentation based on first-derivative, Hilbert and Wavelet Transforms. Medical Engineering and Physics 34 (19): 1236–1246. https://doi.org/10.1016/j. medengphy/2011.12.011.

44. Yochum M., Renaud C., Jacquir S. (2016) Automatic detection of P, QRS and T patterns in 12 leads ECG signal based on CWT. Biomedical Signal Processing and Control 25: 46–52. https://doi. org/10.1016/j.bspc.2015.10.011.

45. Martinez J. P., Almeida R., Olmos S. et al. (2004) A Wavelet-Based ECG Delineator Evaluation on Standard Databases. IEEE Transactions on Biomedical Engineering 51 (14): 570–581. https://doi.org/10.1109/TBME.2003.821031.

46. Hamilton P., Tompkins W. (1986) Quantitative Investigation of QRS Detection Rules Using the MIT/BIH Arrhythmia Database. IEEE Transactions on Biomedical Engineering 33 (112): 1157–1165. https://doi.org/10.1109/TBME.1986.325695.

e-Health Education Using Automatic Question Generation-Based Natural Language (Case Study: Respiratory Tract Infection)

Wiwin Suwarningsih

Abstract

In the midst of the outbreak, the public is flooded with information that is not necessarily true where hoax messages and fear spread faster than valid information and positive messages. For this reason, it is necessary to have consultation facilities that are accurate, fast and on target. This research creates an educational e-health in the form of a health question and answer system (with an upper respiratory tract infection case study) which can be used to provide answers that are more focused on valid information. Validation of information with answers searched using dynamic neural networks. Documents containing information are extracted to detect the correctness, and document keywords are associated with inquiries from users. The process of clarifying information uses automation of dynamic neural networks which allows the answers given to users to be more focused. The final result of this research is a virtual assistant that provides a corpus in the form of a QA-pair that can be generated automatically to provide accurate information to users working with upper respiratory tract infection with an accuracy of 71.6%.

1 Introduction

Recognition of acute respiratory infections (ARIs) in patients, especially the type of ARI they have, is very important to reduce the risk of spreading the infection. ARI patients may show a variety of clinical symptoms. Some of these diseases have the potential to spread rapidly and could have serious public health consequences. ARIs of potential concern should be identified and reported as early as possible. Infected patients should be provided with appropriate care and services, and infection control measures must be taken immediately to reduce further transmission of the disease. The government in providing accurate information has used a number of various methods. The information provided is in the form of articles such as www.who.int, www.alodokter.com, and www.klikdokter.com and openwho.org. Through this telemedicine service, it is expected that the community can minimize the visits to health facilities and it can make independent isolation and physical distancing more effective. The services in the form of question and answering (QA) or chatbot WhatsApp (WA) are viewed more effective for providing an easy-to-use platform for health consumers to communicate with doctors directly and get the timely personal health consultations [1]. Hence, a knowledge base that can support these consulting services is highly required.

To address these issues, this paper focuses on telemedicine, which provides QA-pairs for natural language-based (i.e. Indonesian) consultations with a deep learning approach. QA-pairs were built using a dynamic neural network approach to facilitate generating sequence responses from valid documents and were always updated with good quality. This approach was used in consideration to the ability of dynamic neural networks to represent the biological nervous systems with a better computational ability as compared to static neural networks [2].

Research and development of natural language-based QA telemedicine with the medical domain has been carried out including research focused on the use of Chinese characters [3, 4], English [5–7] or Spanish [8, 9]. Research conducted by He et al. [3] applied a deep learning method in which the system was made to automatically select the answers of some existing medical records by selecting the most appropriate user questions. Similarly, research conducted by Sinha et al. [4] used a suitable neural network to capture several semantic interactions between words in pairs of questions and answers. Some other studies used a paraphrase

W. Suwarningsih (✉)
Research Center for Informatics, Indonesian Institute of Sciences, Komplek LIPI Gd. 20 Lt. 3 Jl. Cisitu 21, Bandung, Indonesia
e-mail: wiwin.suwarningsih@gmail.com

© Springer Nature Switzerland AG 2021
J. Aljaâam et al. (eds.), *Emerging Technologies in Biomedical Engineering and Sustainable TeleMedicine*, Advances in Science, Technology & Innovation, https://doi.org/10.1007/978-3-030-14647-4_6

">

approach and a summary of test questions [5], machine learning methods [6], the embedment and architectural hyper-parameters of the classifier [7], semi-supervised [8] and statistical data redundancy techniques [9].

Advances in deep learning can replace any complex models created by humans by optimizing processes from beginning to end to demonstrate the potential benefits in various domains such as image and video [10, 11] and image plant classification disease [12] and text processing [2, 13, 14]. Researches that utilize deep learning in the medical domain include [2] presenting a deep learning framework using a multi-level character scale convolutional neural network (CNN). This study conducted a training using Chinese characters for each stage by embedding words and determining the length of the vector of each character. The results showed that deep learning was very optimal in identifying Chinese characters in the form of health consultations for Chinese people. Similar research using Chinese characters was conducted by [3] utilizing a suitable neural network to capture the semantic interactions between words in pairs of question and answer sentences. The results of the matching model carried out by [3] were able to outperform the existing method by increasing the performance of the model to 5.5%. The model used was Match Pyramid with a better performance and as a neural network method with the deepest matching of the latest.

Other research in the online health consultation system was carried out by [9] by introducing a series of unique non-textual features, such as surface linguistic features and new social features for online health QA predicting. This feature supported a multi-modal trust-based learning framework. The semantic representation was studied from the answers to get a classification and to determine the quality of the answers. It is in line with the research conducted by [15] producing BERT language models to evaluate the clinical Why-QA. Deep learning was used to adapt and evaluate the BERT language models. The evaluation in this study was focused on error analysis and compared the benefits of different training data. Researchers [11] introduced deep learning-based early warning score (deep EWS), which adopted a health care system in dealing with emergency response conditions for patient management to minimize the number of false alarm deaths. The deep learning results showed high accuracy to both the response given by medical devices and clinical settings.

The purpose of dynamic neural network used in research was to measure to what extent the effectiveness compared to other methods. The main contributions of this paper are summarized as follows: (i) Interactive question answering using QA-pairs generation-based PICO frame for improving the QA system as a solution for communication during the pandemic; (ii) The availability of corpus in the form of Indonesian QA-pairs for pandemic cases.

The rest of the paper is organized as follows: Sect. 2 describes the proposed method. It is followed by Sect. 3 presenting the implementation of proposed method. Furthermore, Sect. 4 describes the result and discussion. Finally, Sect. 5 presents the conclusion and future work.

2 Materials and Methods

This section explains the proposed method, namely dynamic neural network question generation (DNN-QG). Figure 1 presents the scheme of the method proposed in this study. As shown in Fig. 1, the information retrieval process was taken from Wikipedia, www.klikdokter.com, openwho.org, www. detikhealth.com and www.alodokter.com. Encouraged from the idea [16], we then built a knowledge base providing QA-pairs for the process of information classification and generating a number of sequential questions. Compared to the rule-based question generation systems, it is expected that using dynamic neural network information retrieval processes from social media will be better, selective and optimal.

2.1 Crawling Required Dataset

The information classification carried out in this study was the separation or sorting of objects into classes. In this phase, the dynamic neural network training algorithm attempted to find out a model for class attributes as a function of other variables from the dataset. The classification process automatically assigned text into predefined categories and classified the information categories based on some features extracted from training datasets.

Data were collected from some health website, the types of data crawled were the sentences containing medical elements and other key words related to the disease. The data generated were in the form of semi-structured data such as

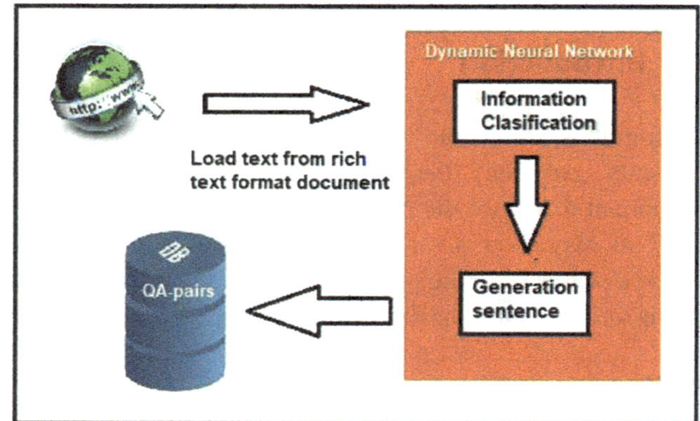

Fig. 1 Schematic proposed method DNN-QG

Table 1 DNNQG dataset

Dataset (train/test)	Wikipedia.id	openwho.org	www.detikhealth.com	www.alodokter.com
Problem	1152/230	1109/322	992/218	967/113
Population	997/319	867/213	993/219	881/116
Intervention	1.120/224	890/118	1.101/320	976/105
Compare	889/318	879/116	1.116/323	874/115
Control	1.109/422	997/119	987/117	983/117
Outcome	898/220	789/118	789/118	872/114
Organs	975/315	980/116	890/119	965/113

JSON or XML files. Table 1 shows the amount of data (27.037 statement sentences) used for training and testing data based on both social media sources and PICO base classification [17].

The network built consisted of a large number of interdependent processing elements for cooperation in solving any problems. A connection between two neurons determined the authority of one neuron to another one, while the weight on the connection determined the power of authority between the two neurons. The learning method used was a neural network trained with the help of a series of inputs and the required output patterns.

2.2 Information Classification

A research conducted by [18] focused on the enhancing features at the attention-based lexical level to increase the addition of exploration at the sentence level. The approach used was the dynamic feature creation network (DFGN) to produce features in sentence representation. This feature was automatically designed for dynamic feature extraction and selection at the sentence level. Other studies such as [19] proposed a multi-view fusion neural network where each component produced a QA-pair. The fusion recurrent neural network (RNN) function was used to integrate the results to form a more holistic representation and gate filters were used to collect important information from the input. However, the residual network was used to add the output as a result of the QA-pair representation process.

Research [20] applied a dynamic neural network for the classification of input data as a basis for basic decision making. The developed application was used for learning during real-time operations and as input data in the form of labeled actions. Similarly, research conducted by [21] used neural networks for text classification as the input vectors of words with several variable dimensions without any loss of information. The learning process was used for Hebrew by combining neural network learning rules with the supervised or semi-supervised modes. Whereas [22] proposed a new technique for text classification, namely recurrent neural networks as a combination of recurrent neural networks and convolution neural networks.

However, [23] classified a number of questions as the facts or opinion base with a deep neural network-based approach. The proposed model was made to capture the representative features of the questions through the semantic analysis of the questions, compared to the features extracted from the questions, and determined whether the new questions raised were fact or opinion. This classification could then be used as the input for further systems, where the aim was to determine whether answers to questions could be provided with the existing resources.

Although the five studies above have used neural networks for sentence classification with several different approaches, there has never been filtering information (hoax or fact) and classification using frames such as problem, intervention, control and outcome (PICO) [23]. PICO is used to form more specific classes to make the information extraction process faster and more precise and handled correctly for words out of vocabulary.

The general structure proposed for our information classification systems (adapting from [16]) based on dynamic neural networks is presented as follows:

1. Extracting a set of core features of language $f_1, \ldots, f_k$ relevant to predict the hoax information or not and create a PICO class based on output pair
2. For each interesting feature f_i, taking the corresponding vector $v (f_i)$.
3. Merging vectors (either by combining, adding or by combining both) into x input vectors.
4. Entering x into the nonlinear classifier (neural feed-forward network).

The feature extraction stage carried out in the classification of information using dynamic neural networks was only done by extracting the core features. This was to make it simpler to find the indicative feature combinations so as to reduce the need for engineered feature combinations, compared to the traditional NLP systems based on linear models, which must determine the core features manually by creating combination features. This was to obtain the dimensions to the input. We thus needed a large combination of space to make an effective set of combinations. Different from when we used DNN, feature extraction was found more effective because it only defined and focused on the core features without having to manually create other features.

2.3 Question Generation

Understanding exactly how data is digested, analyzed and returned to end users can have a large impact on the expectations for good accuracy and reliability by tracing neural network algorithms for sequence generation. Research conducted by [17] used a neural network to take answers with a sequence-to-sequence model according to the input context to produce some relevant questions as the output. The main problem discussed was in handling a number of interrogative words that did not match the type of answer and managing words that were irrelevant to the answer. Similarly, research conducted by [24] developed an online feedback for web-based users by expressing questions and answers on system service satisfaction. But handling feedback using a combination of neural networks and dynamic processes of the question and answer system has not been implemented. It aims to achieve the increased training in high-quality and sustainable samples.

Another use of neural networks is [14, 25] for sequence-to-sequence systems. A research [14] proposed a transformer-based neural network for the choice of answers in combining both global information and sequential features of a sentence. Experiments were carried out comprehensively to verify the effectiveness of the proposed model on a public dataset in well-known metrics. Research [25] created a knowledge-based chat model based on a sequence-to-sequence neural network for more natural questioning to overcome the same words being repeated during decoding. As the proposed distribution mechanism of the generation of words produced previously did not produce a significant generation, we then needed a dynamic generation method using DNN.

The proposed dynamic neural network question generation (as a modification of [19]s) is a neural network consisting of four layers:

(1) Input layer. It contains a single neuron receiving as input a text represented as a sentence of variable dimension m. This layer is connected directly to the learning layer.
(2) Learning layer-1.
   - The number of learning neurons Z is identical to the predefined sentences categories.
   - Each neuron Z represents a category defined by a dictionary and x_k represents a possible question.
   - A dictionary dicZ is denoted as an unordered set of unique tuples (x_k, z, w_k, z) of a token (x_k, z) and its weight (w_k, z).
   - Each token is associated to a weight, which indicates its membership of the corresponding category and relationship with others tokens in the same category.
(3) Learning layer-2.
   - Reviewing generated question (x_k).
   - Ranking the hardness of each question and removing the incorrect questions.
   - The learning process involves restructuring of the neuron, adding new words and updating the weights of the words associated to the dictionaries. dicZ = $\{(x_1, z, w_1, z), \ldots, (x_k, z, w_k, z)\}$.
(4) Output layer. It is an affine layer with the learning layer. The number of output neurons corresponds to the pre-defined categories QA-pairs. In this layer, question is generated as a probability vector. It represents the membership of the input vector into each category.

Figure 2 depicts the architecture of the DNN-QG.

Our model training are: (i) Number of features mapped for each layer, 100 features, (ii) pretrained word embedding using 100 dimensions, (iii) using three convolutional layers of 5×100, 4×1 and 2×1 size and using three-layer pooling with sizes 4×100, 3×1 and 3×1. Figure 3 presents the scheme of learnt QA-pairs representation

3 Result and Discussion

3.1 Baseline Model

We established two baselines, such as recurrent neural network (RNN) and long short-term memory (LSTM) for information classification and question generation without any multi-task trainings. The RNN model was trained to produce the classifications derived from social media as the alternative form of answer [19]. Conventionally, the results of this classification were then trained to generate the pairs of question and answer sentences. The embodiment was carried out by inputting data from the generation of questions and answers to the model alternately. The alternative representations are like this; to make it clear that there is only one RNN module (Fig. 4).

All RNNs have feedback loops in the repeating layer. This allows them to retain information in 'memory' over time. However, it may be difficult to train standard RNN to solve problems that require long-term temporal dependency

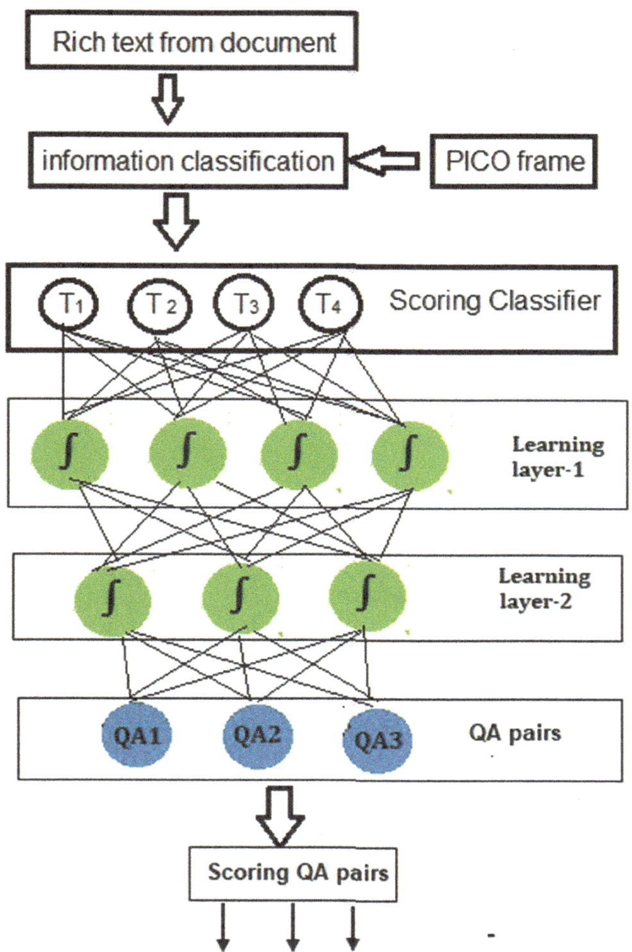

Fig. 2 Dynamic neural network question generation (DNN-QG)

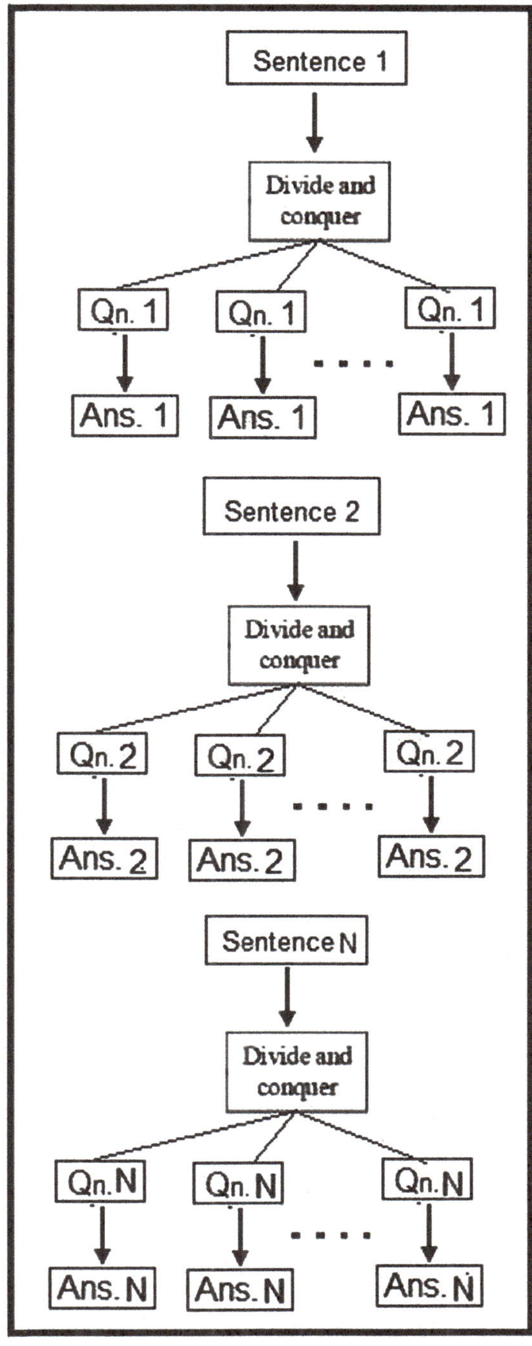

Fig. 3 Learning QA-pairs representation

learning. This is because the gradient of the loss function decays exponentially with time (called the missing gradient problem).

In addition to the information classification process, we compared the question generation performance with the LSTM model variant [24]. This was to predict the sequence of information positions as the answer. LSTM can store information for a long duration with the system parameters that can be trained in a reasonable amount of time (Fig. 5).

LSTM network is a type of RNN that uses special units other than standard units. LSTM units include 'memory cells' which can store information in memory for long periods of time. A series of gates is used to control when information enters memory, when it is released and when it is forgotten. This architecture allows them to study long-term dependencies. GRU is similar to LSTM, but use a simplified structure.

3.2 Result

Our evaluation method was to measure the performance by measuring the accuracy of each model. The baseline method used for classification and question generation could only do a few PICO frames including problem, compare and

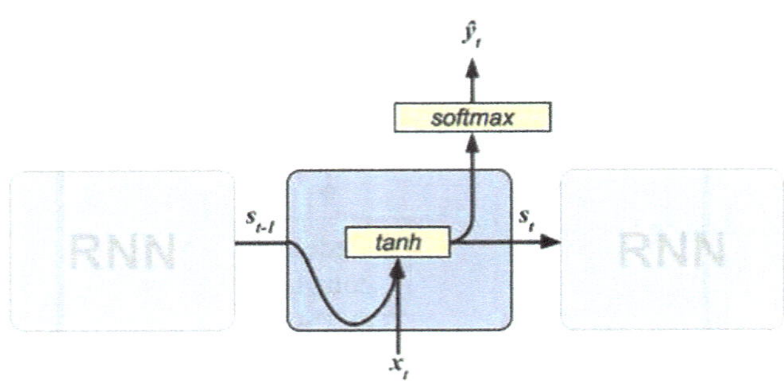

Fig. 4 RNN representation [28]

Fig. 5 LSTM representation [29]

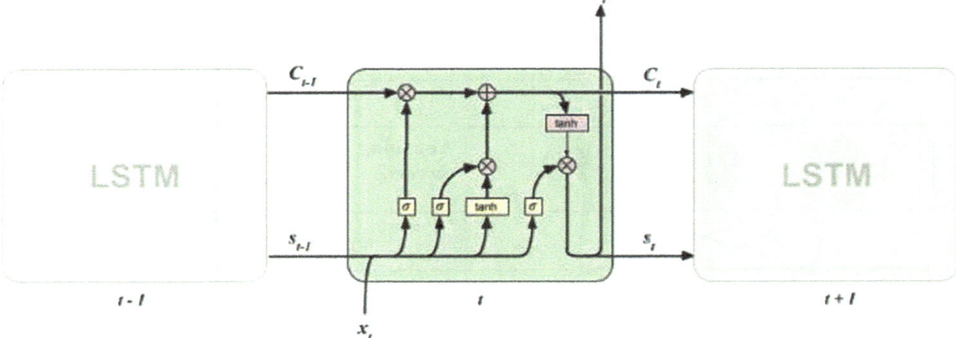

language absorption) cannot be classified. Classification results based on input sentences can only fit into some of these classifications, which cause the QA-pairs model built to be overfitting.

As seen in Table 4, if the input data in the form of information was detected as hoax news, then the data would be discarded and information in the form of facts would be processed for classification and question generation. The sequence generation process was conducted by raising questions coming from the important words based on the weight calculation of each word. Then, the sequence gen-

outcome for RNN models with a maximum accuracy of 71.2%. However, the LSTM model was only in the population, intervention and control categories with a maximum accuracy of 71.4%. The results of performance measurements from the baseline model with the method we proposed can be seen in Table 2.

Because the baseline model could only classify some PICO frames, we only conducted question generation experiments on the definable PICO frames, whereas in the proposed model the question generation testing process was carried out on all PICO frames even though the amount of information classification for each element in the PICO frame was uneven. (The results of definable PICO-based classification can be seen in Table 3.)

As seen in Table 3, DNNQG was able to surpass the baseline method. The results varied greatly because the input data obtained could be more than one sentence (the examples can be seen in Table 4). The types of sentences can be classified properly if the sentence is a simple sentence with the standard language. Any sentences containing words out of vocabulary (such as slang, local languages or foreign

eration process continued until the words with high weight were completely finished to generate the question. There were some words without any weight and unable to be defined for containing some sentences out of vocabulary, such as the affix words (such as '*kok*', '*lho*' or '*deh*') and other slang languages such as 'hatija' (stand for *hati-hati di jalan*, in English: be careful), uptake of the local language that is Sundanese language 'hanupis' (stand for *hatur nuhun pisan*, in English: thank you very much).

The training conducted in this study used a number of sentence variations such as active sentences, passive sentences, speech sentences and solicitation sentences. The types of sentences classified as the non-standard sentences are those as a combination of regional languages and English written according to the pronunciation of the word '*donlot*' (in English: download), the word '*lola*' = '*loding lama*' (in English: long loading), the word '*mager*' = '*males gerak*' (in English: lazy) and so on. The model that is produced from this training process continued to be studied to produce an optimal model for handling various types of sentences from input data.

Table 2 The results of performance measurements from the baseline model

Task	RNN (%)	LSTM (%)	DNNQG (%)
Classification information	71.5	71.9	72.1
Question generation	70.9	70.9	71.1
Average	71.2	71.4	71.6

Table 3 The results of definable PICO-based classification

Classification class	RNN	LSTM	DNNQG
Problem	212	112	230
Population	112	370	356
Intervention	102	325	320
Compare	250	89	233
Control	115	323	345
Outcome	356	102	318
Organs	103	108	114

3.3 Discussion

A number of phrases in the source language were mapped to phrases in the target language. In this task, the facts nouns, which constituted intervention classifications, were mapped into natural language questions. Then, it was continued by limiting the tasks to a set of valid and limited outputs. Two tasks were very limited, e.g., limited valid output set. This applied especially to short phrases, such as one sentence question with answer pairs yes or no. Most valid outputs were paraphrased with a series of words interconnected with each other based on the vectors defined during the information classification.

The proposed model may not recognize certain paraphrases, especially the entity paraphrases. We therefore optimized the log possibilities by using Adam's first-order gradient-based optimization algorithm [26] and automatic evaluation metrics [27]. This evaluation metric used the word similarity score in which in our experiment it was the similarity and non-exclusive harmony between words in two QA-pairs, maximizing a similarity between words in harmony. Then, it was followed by calculating the similarity of sentences as the average of aligned words.

Adam's First-Order Gradient
Our experiments used a separate dataset including QA-pairs with Yes/No answers. QA-pairs with simple questions with short answers consisted of 2–3 words (see Table 5). We used these two types of sentences into training, validation and testing data. The DNN model we set using a learning rate of 0.00015 and a gradient parameter greater than 0.1. We continued to improve these dimensions to produce some optimal dimensions (the Adam algorithm for stochastic optimization [26] can be seen below):

```
for t in range(num_iterations):
    g = compute_gradient(x, y)
    m = beta_1 * m + (1 - beta_1) * g
    v = beta_2 * v + (1 - beta_2) * np.power(g, 2)
    v_hat = np.maximum(v, v_hat)
    w = w - step_size * m / (np.sqrt(v_hat) + epsilon)
```

where t = initialize timestep, m = initialize 1st moment vector, v = initialize 2nd moment vector, g = gradient, and w = weights.

Table 5 presents the calculation results for the dataset Yes/No answer, short answer (2–3 words) and definition answer classification, which shows Yes/No answer is superior and optimal for its accuracy value followed by short answer and definition answer has the lowest accuracy than the two other types of QA. The average convergence time is 2.4 h but Yes/No answer has a convergence time for the most optimal compared to short answer and definition answer. When viewed as a whole dataset type definition answer has the least performance. This happens because the experiments conducted confirm performance optimization very much depending on the type and size of the dataset, with each optimizer exhibiting different levels of accuracy and loss in the three datasets.

Referring to the result of Adam's algorithm analysis of our dataset testing, there are a number of things that can be concluded, namely: (i) The actual step size in each iteration is limited to the property size parameter. This property is used to add intuitive understanding to hyperparameter learning levels that were not intuitive before, (ii). Adam is designed to combine the advantages possessed by DNNQG which works well in online data management.

Automation Evaluation Metrix
DNNQG was trained end-to-end with QA-pair models limited to the answer to questions with short Yes/No answers or answers consisting of a maximum of four words. Our model proposed a performance failure on the question with some answers in the form of definitions or exposures that required a reasoning. In this paper, the IMeQG dataset was also used to evaluate all models. The IMeQG dataset was taken from several social media with very general information. Thus, there were some strange results on using natural datasets.

Evaluation matrix is used to evaluate the performance of the algorithm that we use. The evaluation carried out is to calculate accuracy, precision and recall with the formula defined as follows:

Table 4 Example of the results of the formation process of classification and QA generation

Data input	Sentence generate	Classification	Question answer generation	
			Question	Answer
WHO telah menetapkan ISPA sebagai pandemi yg artinya penyebarannya sudah global. Tidak perlu takut ya. Yuk, kenali bagaimana penyebaran dan langkah-langkah pencegahannya! (In English: WHO has established ARI as a pandemic which means its spread is global. You don't need to be afraid. Come on, recognize how the spread and preventive measures!)	**Sentence-1**: *WHO telah menetapkan ISPA sebagai pandemi yg artinya penyebarannya sudah global.* (In English: WHO has designated ARI as a pandemic which means its spread is global.)	Problem, Population	*Siapa yang menetapkan ARI sebagai pandemi?* (In English: Who established ARI as a pandemic?) *Apa yang menjadi pademi?* (in English: What becomes pademic?) *Mengapa menjadi pandemic?* (In English: Why become a pandemic?)	WHO ISPA (In English: ARI) *penyebarannya sudah global* (In English: the distribution is global)
	Sentence-2: *Tidak perlu takut ya.* (In English: No need to be afraid.)	Not classified	No generate	No generate
	Sentence-3: *Yuk, kenali bagaimana penyebaran dan langkah-langkah pencegahannya!* (In English: Come on, recognize how the spread and preventive measures!)	Intervention	*Bagaimana penyebaran dan langkah-langkah pencegahannya?* (In English: How is the spread and prevention steps?)	No Answer
Bantu lawan virus ISPA dengan diam dirumah. Sayangi keluarga kita dengan diam saja dirumah, bila harus keluar gunakan masker, ya cinta!!!! Serius lho ISPA bahaya banget.... seremmm dehhh. (In English: Help the ARI virus opponent by staying quietly at home. Love our family quietly at home, if you have to go out using a mask, yes love!!!! Seriously, ARI is very dangerous.... so scary.)	**Sentence-1**: *Bantu lawan virus ISPA dengan diam dirumah.* (In English: Help the ARI virus opponent by staying quietly at home.)	Problem, Intervention, Outcome	*Apa yang bantu?* (In English: What help?) *Bagaimana bantu lawan* (In English: How to help opponents?) *Dimana bantu lawan ISPA?* (In English: Where can you help ARI opponents?)	*Lawan virus ISPA* (In English: ARI virus opponents) *Diam di rumah* (In English: stay at home) *Diam di rumah* (In English: stay at home)
	Sentence-2: *Sayangi keluarga kita dengan diam saja dirumah, bila harus keluar gunakan masker, ya cinta!!!!* (In English: Love our family quietly at home, if you have to go out using a mask, yes love!!!!)	Outcome, Intervention	*Siapa yang disayang?* (In English: Who is loved?) *Bagaimana keluarga disayang?* (In English: How is the family loved?) *Bagaimana bila harus keluar?* (In English: What if I have to get out?) *Apa yang digunakan bila keluar?* (In English: What is used when leaving?)	*Keluarga* (In English: family) *Diam di rumah* (In English: stay at home) *Gunakan masker* (In English: wear a mask) *Masker* (In English: face mask)
	Sentence-3: *Serius lho ISPA bahaya banget ......* (In English: Seriously, ARI is very dangerous......)	Problem, Outcome	*Apa yang bahaya banget?* (In English: What is so dangerous?) *Apa ISPA bahaya?* (In English: What corona danger?) *Apa yang serius?* (In English: What's serious?)	ISPA (In English: ARI) Ya (in English: yes) ISPA (In English: ARI)
	Sentence-4: *seremmm deh*	Not classified	No generate	No generate

Table 5 Result of Adams first-order gradient

Type of QA	Convergence time (h)	Accuracy	Loss
Yes/No answer	2.125	0.848	0.429
Short answer	2.425	0.829	0.400
Definition answer	2.725	0.624	0.687

Table 6 Evaluation matrix

Type of QA	Method	RNN (%)	LSTM (%)	DNN (%)
Yes/No answer	Accuracy	70.5	71.4	**74.5**
	Precision	67.9	68.5	71.4
	Recall	62.3	63.4	64.3
Short answer	Accuracy	71.9	72.9	**73.6**
	Precision	67.2	68.2	69.3
	Recall	60.3	61.6	62.2
Definition	Accuracy	67.2	66.8	**65.6**
	Precision	63.4	62.3	61.3
	Recall	57.2	58.6	57.8

$$Precision = \frac{TP}{TP + FP} \qquad (1)$$

$$Recall = \frac{TP}{TP + FN} \qquad (2)$$

$$Accuracy = \frac{(TP + TN)}{TP + TN + FP + FN} \qquad (3)$$

where TP is true positive and TN is true negative, while FP is false positive and FN is false negative (Table 6).

The accuracy of the model tests on dataset using a modified DNN showed the improved performance compared to the baseline. A dramatic increase achieved by DNNQG was related to the fact that DNN could store information and created the QA-pairs. In matrix evaluation, it was observed that DNNQG experienced some errors during the training data because some words were not recognized, especially for the non-standardized words or out of vocabulary. To overcome this, DNN's ability needs to be improved by the introduction of all types of words or phrases included in the OOV.

Based on the results of the calculation of the optimization of the model that we proposed, it can be concluded that the weakness of DNN-QG in this study was that the training process was quite time-consuming, coupled with the variations of words that were not uniform, the learning process that was difficult to be interrupted and the difficulties faced by the users to interpret it, and the users often constrained by overfitting. However, there were several advantages we obtained by using this DNN, including the excellent results

with varied and complex types of data in accordance with our dataset with a variety of discrete and continuous data. Another advantage is that the testing process was relatively very fast compared to the training process.

4 Conclusions

This paper presents the DNN approach to classify the questions into PICO frames and automatic question generation for early information on the type of pandemic disease. The proposed model was compared with the Indonesian language dataset collected from social media containing a number of labeled statement sentences, called the IMeQG dataset, used for the evaluation experiments. Two deep learning techniques, RNN and LSTM, were trained for the classification resulting from the statement sentences in the dataset. The RNN model achieved a maximum accuracy of 71.2% for the problem, compare and outcome dataset categories, but it experienced some overfitting problems, while using LSTM for the population, intervention and control categories achieved an accuracy of 71.4%. The DNN model fitted the data well and outperformed the RNN and LSTM with a significant difference by achieving an accuracy of 71.6% for the electronic dataset category.

For future research, in identifying the words or phrases that are out of vocabulary by establishing a series of formulas for classification of the model, the system is expected to be able to produce and find appropriate and up-to-date answers to new knowledge.

Acknowledgements The author would like to thank all the facilities provided by Indonesian Institute of Sciences (LIPI) particular Research Center for Informatics and, during the process of making this manuscript.

Declaration

Funding Statement

This research did not receive any specific grant from funding agencies in the public, commercial or not-for-profit sectors.

Conflict of Interest The author declares no conflict or interest.

References

1. Y. Sharma and S. Gupta, "Deep Learning Approaches for Question Answering System," *Procedia Comput. Sci.*, vol. 132, pp. 785–794, 2018, https://doi.org/10._016/j.procs.2018.05.090.

2. S. Zhang, X. Zhang, H. Wang, J. Cheng, P. Li, and Z. Ding, "Chinese medical question answer matching using end-to-end character-level multi-scale CNNs," *Appl. Sci.*, vol. 7, no. 8, pp. 1–17, 2017, https://doi.org/10.3390/app7080767.

3. J. He, M. Fu, and M. Tu, "Applying deep matching networks to Chinese medical question answering: A study and a dataset," *BMC Med. Inform. Decis. Mak.*, vol. 19, no Suppl 2, 2019, https://doi.org/10.1186/s12911-019-0761-8.

4. N. K. Sinha, M. M. Gupta, and D. H. Rao, "Dynamic neural networks: An overview," *Proc. IEEE Int. Conf. Ind. Technol.*, vol. 1, pp. 491–496, 2000, https://doi.org/10.1109/icit.2000.854201.

5. A. Ben Abacha and D. Demner-Fushman, "On the Role of Question Summarization and Information Source Restriction in Consumer Health Question Answering.," *AMIA Jt. Summits Transl. Sci. proceedings. AMIA Jt. Summits Transl. Sci.*, vol. 2019, no. September, pp. 117–126, 2019, [Online]. Available: http://www.ncbi.nlm.nih.gov/pubmed/31258963%0Ahttp://www.pubmedcentral.nih.gov/articlerender.fcgi?artid=PMC6568117.

6. A. Ben Abacha and P. Zweigenbaum, "MEANS: A medical question-answering system combining NLP techniques and semantic Web technologies," *Inf. Process. Manag.*, vol. 51, no. 5, pp. 570–594, 2015, https://doi.org/10.1016/j.ipm.2015.04.006.

7. A. Pérez, R. Weegar, A. Casillas, K. Gojenola, M. Oronoz, and H. Dalianis, "Semi-supervised medical entity recognition: A study on Spanish and Swedish clinical corpora." *J. Biomed. Inform.*, vol. 71, pp. 16–30, 2017, https://doi.org/10.1016/j.jbi.2017.05.009.

8. J. L. Vicedo, R. Izquierdo, F. Llopis, and R. Muñoz, "Question answering in Spanish," *CEUR Workshop Proc.*, vol. 1169, no. May 2014, 2003, https://doi.org/10.1007/978-3-540-30222-3.

9. Z. Hu, Z. Zhang, H. Yang, Q. Chen, and D. Zuo, "A deep learning approach for predicting the quality of online health expert question-answering services," *J. Biomed. Inform.*, vol. 71, pp. 241–253, 2017, https://doi.org/10.1016/j.jbi.2017.06.012.

10. I. Hachchane, A. Badri, A. Sahel, and Y. Ruichek, "Large-scale image-to-video face retrieval with convolutional neural network features," *IAES Int. J. Artif. Intell.*, vol 9, no. 1, pp. 40–45, 2020, https://doi.org/10.11591/ijai.v9.i1.pp40-45.

11. Y. Lee, J. myoung Kwon, Y. Lee, H. Park, H. Cho, and J. Park, "Deep learning in the medical domain: Predicting cardiac arrest using deep learning," *Acute Crit. Care*, vol. 33, no. 3, pp. 117–120, 2018, https://doi.org/10.4266/acc.2018.00290.

12. S. B. Jadhav, V. R. Udupi, and S. B. Patil, "Convolutional neural networks for leaf image-based plant disease classification," *IAES Int. J. Artif. Intell.*, vol. 8, no. 4, pp. 328–341, 2019, https://doi.org/10.11591/ijai.v8.i4.pp328-341.

13. S. Deshmukh, R. Balani, V. Rohane, and A. Singh, "Sia: An interactive medical assistant using natural language processing," *Proc. - Int. Conf. Glob. Trends Signal Process. Inf. Comput. Commun. ICGTSPICC 2016*, pp. 584–586, 2017, https://doi.org/10.1109/icgtspicc.2016.7955368.

14. T. Shao, Y. Guo, H. Chen, and Z. Hao, "Transformer-Based Neural Network for Answer Selection in Question Answering," *IEEE Access*, vol. 7, pp. 26146–26156, 2019, https://doi.org/10.1109/access.2019.2900753.

15. A. Wen, M. Y. Elwazir, S. Moon, and J. Fan, "Adapting and evaluating a deep learning language model for clinical why-question answering," *JAMIA Open*, vol. 0, no. 0, pp. 1–5, 2020, https://doi.org/10.1093/jamiaopen/ooz072.

16. Y. Goldberg, "A primer on neural network models for natural language processing," *J. Artif. Intell. Res.*, vol. 57, pp. 345–420, 2016, https://doi.org/10.1613/jair.4992.

17. X. Sun, J. Liu, Y. Lyu, W. He, Y. Ma, and S. Wang, "Answer-focused and Position-aware Neural Question Generation Xingwu," pp. 3930–3939, 2018.

18. L. Ma, P. Wang, and L. Zhang, "Dynamic Feature Generation Network for Answer Selection," 2018, [Online]. Available: http://arxiv.org/abs/1812.05366.

19. L. Sha, X. Zhang, F. Qian, B. Chang, and Z. Sui, "A multi-view fusion neural network for answer selection," *32nd AAAI Conf. Artif. Intell. AAAI 2018*, pp. 5422–5429, 2018.

20. A. K. Yadav and A. K. Sachan, "Research and application of dynamic neural network based on reinforcement learning," *Adv. Intell. Soft Comput.*, vol. 132 AISC, pp. 931–942, 2012, https://doi.org/10.1007/978-3-642-27443-5-107.

21. L. Vega and A. Mendez-Vazquez, "Dynamic neural networks for text classification," *Proc. - 2016 Int. Conf. Comput. Intell. Appl. ICCIA 2016*, pp. 6–11, 2016, https://doi.org/10.1109/iccia.2016.15 .

22. A. Bharathi and E. Deepankumar, "Natural object classification using artificial neural network," *Int. J. Appl. Eng. Res.*, vol. 10, no. 20, pp. 16359–16363, 2015, https://doi.org/10.1109/ijcnn.2000.861294.

23. B. A. Upadhya, S. Udupa, and S. S. Kamath, "Deep Neural Network Models for Question Classification in Community Question-Answering Forums," *2019 10th Int. Conf. Comput. Commun. Netw. Technol. ICCCNT 2019*, pp. 1–6, 2019, https://doi.org/10.1109/icccnt45670.2019.8944861.

24. B. Kratzwald and S. Feuerriegel, "Learning from on-line user feedback in neural question answering on the web," *Web Conf. 2019 - Proc. World Wide Web Conf. WWW 2019*, pp. 906–916, 2019, https://doi.org/10.1145/3308558.3313661.

25. S. Kim, H. Kim, O. W. Kwon, and Y. G. Kim, "Improving Response Quality in a Knowledge-Grounded Chat System Based on a Sequence-to-Sequence Neural Network," *2019 IEEE Int. Conf. Big Data Smart Comput. BigComp 2019 - Proc.*, pp. 1–4, 2019, https://doi.org/10.1109/bigcomp.2019.8679339.

26. D. P. Kingma and J. L. Ba, "Adam: A method for stochastic optimization," *3rd Int. Conf. Learn. Represent. ICLR 2015 - Conf. Track Proc.*, pp. 1–15, 2015.

27. I. V. Serban *et al.*, "Generating factoid questions with recurrent neural networks: The 30 M factoid question-answer corpus," *54th Annu. Meet. Assoc. Comput. Linguist. ACL 2016 - Long Pap.*, vol. 1, pp. 588–598, 2016.

28. T. Mikolov, M. Karafiát, L. Burget, C. Jan, and S. Khudanpur, "Recurrent neural network based language model," *Proc. 11th Annu. Conf. Int. Speech Commun. Assoc. INTERSPEECH 2010*, no. September, pp. 1045–1048, 2010.

29. S. Hochreiter and J. Schmidhuber, "Long Short-Term Memory," *Neural Comput.*, vol. 9, no. 8, pp. 1735–1780, 1997, https://doi.org/10.1162/neco.1997.9.8.1735.

A Novel Machine Learning Model for Adaptive Tracking and Real-Time Forecasting COVID-19 Dynamic Propagation

Daiana Caroline dos Santos Gomes
and Ginalber Luiz de Oliveira Serra

Abstract

This chapter presents a computational model with intelligent machine learning for the analysis of epidemiological data. The innovations of adopted methodology consist of an interval type-2 fuzzy clustering algorithm based on adaptive similarity distance mechanism for defining specific operation regions associated with the behavior and uncertainty inherited to epidemiological data, and an interval type-2 fuzzy version of Observer/Kalman Filter Identification (OKID) algorithm for adaptive tracking and real-time forecasting according to unobservable components computed by recursive spectral decomposition of experimental epidemiological data. Experimental results and comparative analysis illustrate the efficiency and applicability of the proposed methodology for adaptive tracking and real-time forecasting the dynamic propagation behavior of novel coronavirus 2019 (COVID-19) outbreak in Brazil.

1 Introduction

In sciences and engineering is very common the solution of problems with stochastic nature such as prediction, separation, and detection of signals in the presence of random noise [1–4]. Kalman filter (KF) is the most well-known and used mathematical tool for stochastic estimation from noisy and uncertain measurements. It was proposed by Rudolph E. Kalman in 1960, who published his famous paper "A New Approach to Linear Filtering and Prediction Problem" [5], describing a recursive solution to discrete-time linear filtering problem, and becoming a standard approach for optimal estimation. Since the time of its introduction, the Kalman filter has been the subject of extensive research and applications in the fields of orbit calculation, target tracking, integrated navigation, dynamic positioning, sensor data fusion, microeconomics, control, modeling, digital image processing, pattern recognition, image segmentation and image edge detection, and others. This broad interest in KF is due to its optimality, convenient form for online real-time processing, easy formulation, and implementation [6].

Fuzzy systems have been widely used for modeling [7–10], and also for health area [11,12]. The successful applications of fuzzy systems are due to its structure based on rules, where the antecedent propositions of the rules define fuzzy operation regions and the consequent describes a corresponding physical behavior in those regions, and its capability of approximate functions as well as treat nonlinearities and uncertainties [13]. Recently, type-2 fuzzy systems have been highlighted in several applications due to their better ability to deal with uncertain information [14,15]. A special case within the study of type-2 fuzzy logic is the interval type-2 fuzzy sets that, by simplifying the membership functions assigned to the sets, define a Footprint of Uncertainty (FoU) in data processing, which is limited by upper and lower membership functions [16].

With the emergence caused by COVID-19 and its rapid spread to several countries, authorities around the world have been implemented plans for fighting the transmission of the virus based on guidelines provided by the World Health Organization (WHO) [17–19]. The impacts caused by COVID-19 pandemic have affected health, social, economic, political, and cultural spheres, unprecedented in the recent worldwide history of epidemics [20]. In view to the problems faced to COVID-19 crisis, researchers from all scientific areas has proposed new studies and contributions as an effort to fight and understand the coronavirus disease [21–26]. In these contexts, computational modeling applied to analysis of epidemiolog-

D. C. dos Santos Gomes (✉)
Federal University of Maranhão, Av. dos Portugueses, 1966, Bacanga, São Luís 65080-805, Brazil
e-mail: daianagomes159@gmail.com

G. L. de Oliveira Serra
Federal Institute of Education, Science and Technology of Maranhão, Av. Getúlio Vargas, 04, Monte Castelo, São Luís 65030-005, Brazil
e-mail: ginalber@ifma.edu.br

© Springer Nature Switzerland AG 2021
J. Alja'am et al. (eds.), *Emerging Technologies in Biomedical Engineering and Sustainable TeleMedicine*, Advances in Science, Technology & Innovation, https://doi.org/10.1007/978-3-030-14647-4_7

ical data has received increasing interest from the scientific community, aiming to characterize the dynamic evolution of infectious diseases outbreak, and also helping in its control and prevention [27–34].

Associated to epidemiological data analysis, the proposal for adaptive and real-time modeling methodologies which take into account the processing of uncertainties inherited to these types of experimental data (underreportings, lack of information, incubation period of the virus, time to seek care, and diagnosis), is still open. The proposed methodology, based on interval type-2 fuzzy Kalman filter, is useful for adaptive and real-time forecasting of uncertain experimental data. A new formulation of type-2 fuzzy version of Observer/Kalman Filter Identification (OKID) algorithm, is proposed, for updating, recursively, the consequent proposition of type-2 fuzzy Kalman filter using spectral components extracted from the experimental data. Interval fuzzy sets characterizing the antecedent of type-2 fuzzy Kalman filter inference system are estimated by, also proposed, a formulation of interval type-2 fuzzy version of Gustafson–Kessel clustering algorithm. The applicability of the proposed methodology is illustrated through experimental results from adaptive tracking and real-time forecasting of the COVID-19 dynamic propagation in Brazil.

1.1 Related Works

In the last years, studies involving the integration of fuzzy systems and Kalman filters have been proposed in the literature [35–39]. In [40], fuzzy sets are combined with an optimization method based on an extended Kalman filter with probabilistic–numerical linguistic information applied for tracking a maneuvering target. According to limited and uncertain information from different sensors, the methodology is able to merge this information and be applied to the problem of trace optimization in an unknown maneuvering target in Sichuan province in China. In [41], an optimization methodology of adaptive Unscented Kalman Filter (UKF) is presented by an evolutionary fuzzy algorithm named Fuzzy Adaptive Grasshopper Optimization Algorithm, and it is efficiently applied to different benchmark functions, such as robotic manipulator and servo-hydraulic system, whose performance is better compared to previous versions of UKF. In [42], a reformulation in the uncertainty representation in fuzzy Kalman filters (FKF) is proposed to solve problems related to uncertainty propagation, where trapezoidal possibility distributions are used to represent fuzzy variables, defining regions of possibility and impossibility of asymmetric sets for modeling sensor's uncertainty. In [43], a strategy based on fuzzy logic control to treat pathological symptoms of movement-disorder with higher performance is presented. A slowly varying hidden variable in a neural network is estimated using an

unscented Kalman filter and is used as a feedback variable to enhance control performance. The presented design has significant potential for clinical treatment of movement disorders and opens a new perspective for the applications in the fields of neural control engineering and brain-machine interfaces. Despite the extensive literature in this context, there are still many fields to be explored regarding the association of Kalman filters and fuzzy logic.

Several mathematical, computational, and statistical methods have already been proposed and widely applied in the prediction of infectious diseases worldwide [44–47]. In [48], a seasonal autoregressive integrated moving average (SARIMA) model was used to predict the incidence of Chlamydia Trachomatis (CT) infection in Shenzhen city, China. The proposed model breaks down the time series data corresponding to monthly cases of CT infection into behavioral patterns such as trend, seasonal and random, in order to understand the epidemiological behavior of the disease and obtain more accurate predictions. In [49], negative binomial regression models were developed to forecast human infections by the Ross River virus (RRV), which is Australia's most epidemiologically important mosquito-borne disease. The model uses data from climatic, environmental, and oceanographic variables in order to understand the factors associated with RRV transmission in epidemiologically important regions in the state of Victoria and to establish an early warning forecasting system. In [50], ensemble niche models to predict spatiotemporally varying bat birthing to examine how birthing cycles of African fruit bats, molossid bats, and non-molossid microbats inform the spatiotemporal occurrence of Ebola Virus Disease (EVD) spillover. The model uses pool sparse data and predicted the risk of EVD spillover at locations of the two 2018 EVD outbreaks in the Democratic Republic of the Congo. In [34], an ensemble model was introduced for sequential forecasting that weights a set of plausible models and use a frequentist computational bootstrap approach to evaluate its uncertainty. The feasibility of the approach was demonstrated using simple dynamic differential-equation models and the trajectory of outbreak scenarios of the Ebola Forecasting Challenge, providing forecasting horizon of 1–4 weeks. In [51], a novel multi-layered dynamic transmission model is presented for hepatitis-C virus (HCV) transmission within a people who inject drugs (PWID) population. The approach based on this model is able to estimate the number of undiagnosed PWIDs, the true incidence, the average time until diagnosis, the reproduction numbers, and associated uncertainties, using routine surveillance data.

Recently, with the beginning of the Covid-19 epidemic outbreak, several researchers have proposed model-based data analysis approaches applied to novel Coronavirus 2019 [52–57]. The objective of these studies is to characterize the evolution of a pandemic in certain regions and, thus, to contribute to the requirements adopted to contain the contamination by virus and allocation of resources. In [58], a mathematical model based on the SEIR (Susceptible–Exposed–Infectious–Recovered) model for forecasting the transmission dynamics of Covid-19 in Korea, is proposed. This study is able to predict the final size and the timing of the end of epidemic, as well as the maximum number of isolated individuals using daily, confirmed cases comparing epidemiological parameters between the national level and the Daegu/Gyeongbuk area. In [59], the role of asymptomatic carriers in transmission poses challenges for control of the Covid-19 pandemic, is addressed. This methodology models the viral propagation using a renewal equation framework, which allows modeling of the current incidence of infected individuals in the function of the previous incidence, and how infectiousness of an infected individual varies over the course of their infection. In [60], an SEIR model is developed for predicting the 2019 Novel Coronavirus outbreak at the early stage in India and helping to take active measures prior to propagation of 2019-nCoV disease, based on reproduction number (R_0) criterion. In [61], several supervised machine learning models are compared to predict the number of patients affected by Covid-19. The four standard forecast models were used: linear regression (LR), least absolute shrinkage and selection operator (LASSO), support vector machine (SVM), and exponential smoothing (ES). Three types of predictions are made by each of the models, such as the number of newly infected cases, the number of deaths, and the number of recoveries in the next 10 days.

Differently from the aforementioned approaches and other ones found in literature, the scope of this chapter outlines the integration of the Kalman filter and interval type-2 fuzzy systems for tracking and forecasting the COVID-19 dynamic spread behavior. The design of interval type-2 fuzzy Kalman filter, according to the proposed methodology, is based on spectral unobservable components and uncertainty regions extracted from experimental data.

1.2 Motivation and Contributions of the Proposed Methodology

The impacts caused by novel coronavirus pandemic has motivated the analysis of epidemiological data, for support of political/health authorities and decision-making [25,60]. In this context, several modeling methodologies has been proposed in literature for solving epidemiological problems [62–65]. However, the uncertainties inherent to experimental epidemiological data (underreporting, lack of information, incubation period of the virus, time to seek care, and diagnosis) have opened a new research field, to which

the proposed methodology belongs. The originality of the proposed methodology is outlined by the following main contributions:

- A new machine learning computational tool based on the successful integration of Kalman filters and type-2 fuzzy systems for adaptive tracking and real-time forecasting of experimental epidemiological data, which is useful for analysis of COVID-19 dynamic propagation;
- Formulation of new interval type-2 fuzzy clustering algorithm based on adaptive similarity distance mechanism ables to define specific operation regions in the epidemiological data associated to the behavior and uncertainty inherent to COVID-19 dynamic propagation;
- Formulation of a new computational model with intelligent machine learning based on interval type-2 fuzzy Kalman filter, for adaptive tracking and real-time forecasting the behavior and uncertainty inherent to COVID-19 dynamic propagation, from the specific operation regions in the epidemiological data.

2 Interval Type-2 Fuzzy Computational Model

In this section, the proposed methodology for designing the interval type-2 fuzzy Kalman filter computational model from experimental data is presented. Formulations for preprocessing the experimental dataset by spectral analysis, parametric estimation of interval type-2 fuzzy Kalman filter antecedent proposition, parametric estimation of interval type-2 fuzzy Kalman filter consequent proposition, and its recursive updating mechanism, are addressed.

2.1 Pre-processing by Singular Spectral Analysis

The Singular Spectral Analysis technique is a mathematical tool for analyzing and decomposing complex time series into simpler components within the original data [66].

Training Step

Let the initial experimental dataset referring to p time series under analysis, with N_b samples, given by

$$\mathbf{y} = [\mathbf{y}_1 \quad \mathbf{y}_2 \quad \cdots \quad \mathbf{y}_{N_b}], \quad \mathbf{y} \in \mathbb{R}^{p \times N_b} \tag{1}$$

where $\mathbf{y}_k \in \mathbb{R}^p$, with $k = 1, \ldots, N_b$, is the time series vector at instant of time k. From this initial dataset, a trajectory matrix $\mathbf{H}$ is defined, for each of the dimensions of $\mathbf{y}$, considering a set of ρ delayed vectors with dimension δ, which is an integer number defined by user with $2 \leq \delta \leq N_b - 1$ and $\rho = N_b - \delta + 1$, given by

$$\mathbf{H} = \begin{bmatrix} y_1 & y_2 & y_3 & \cdots & y_\rho \\ y_2 & y_3 & y_4 & \cdots & y_{\rho+1} \\ \vdots & \vdots & \vdots & \ddots & \vdots \\ y_\delta & y_{\delta+1} & y_{\delta+2} & \cdots & y_{N_b} \end{bmatrix}, \quad \mathbf{H} \in \mathbb{R}^{\delta \times \rho} \quad (2)$$

and the covariance matrix $\mathbf{S}$ is obtained as follows:

$$\mathbf{S} = \mathbf{H}\mathbf{H}^T, \quad \mathbf{S} \in \mathbb{R}^{\delta \times \delta} \quad (3)$$

Applying the Singular Value Decomposition (SVD) procedure to matrix $\mathbf{S}$, is obtained a set of eigenvalues in decreasing order such that $\sigma^1 \geq \sigma^2 \geq \cdots \geq \sigma^\delta \geq 0$ with their respective eigenvectors $\boldsymbol{\phi}^1, \boldsymbol{\phi}^2, \ldots, \boldsymbol{\phi}^\delta$. Considering $d = max \, \{\varsigma, \text{ such that } \sigma^\varsigma > 0\}$, and $\mathbf{V}^\varsigma = \mathbf{H}^T \boldsymbol{\phi}^\varsigma / \sqrt{\sigma^\varsigma}$ with $\varsigma = 1, \ldots, d$, the singular value decomposition of the trajectory matrix $\mathbf{H}$, can be rewritten as follows:

$$\mathbf{H} = \mathbf{H}^1 + \mathbf{H}^2 + \cdots + \mathbf{H}^d \quad (4)$$

where the matrix $\mathbf{H}^\varsigma|^{\varsigma=1,\ldots,d}$ is elementary (it has rank equal to 1), and is given by

$$\mathbf{H}^\varsigma = \sqrt{\sigma^\varsigma}\boldsymbol{\phi}^\varsigma \mathbf{V}^{\varsigma T}, \quad \mathbf{H}^\varsigma \in \mathbb{R}^{\delta \times \rho} \quad (5)$$

The regrouping of $\mathbf{H}^\varsigma|^{\varsigma=1,\ldots,d}$ into ξ linearly independent matrices terms $\mathbf{I}^j|^{j=1,\ldots,\xi}$, such that $\xi \leq d$, results in

$$\mathbf{H} = \mathbf{I}^1 + \mathbf{I}^2 + \cdots + \mathbf{I}^\xi \quad (6)$$

where ξ is the number of unobservable components extracted from experimental dataset. The unobservable spectral components $\alpha^j|^{j=1,\ldots,\xi}$ obtained from matrices $\mathbf{I}^j|^{j=1,\ldots,\xi}$, are given by

$$\alpha_k^j = \begin{cases} \dfrac{1}{k}\displaystyle\sum_{v=1}^{k+1} I_{v,k-v+1}^j & 1 \leq k \leq \delta^* \\[2ex] \dfrac{1}{\delta^*}\displaystyle\sum_{v=1}^{\delta^*} I_{v,k-v+1}^j & \delta^* \leq k \leq \rho^* \\[2ex] \dfrac{1}{N_b-k+1}\displaystyle\sum_{v=k-\rho^*+1}^{N_b-\rho^*+1} I_{v,k-v+1}^j & \rho^* < k \leq N_b \end{cases} \quad (7)$$

where $\delta^* = \min(\delta, \rho)$, $\rho^* = \max(\delta, \rho)$, such that δ and ρ are associated to number of rows and columns of the trajectory matrix $\mathbf{H}$, respectively, and $N_b = \delta + \rho - 1$ is the length of initial experimental dataset.

Recursive Step

After the initialization of spectral analysis algorithm in the training step, the next steps will be repeated for each time instant $k = N_b + 1, N_b + 2, \ldots$, as formulated in sequel. The value of ρ is increased by $\rho = k - \delta + 1$ and the covariance matrix is updated, recursively, as follows:

$$\mathbf{S}_k = \mathbf{S}_{k-1} + \Upsilon_k, \quad \mathbf{S}_k \in \mathbb{R}^{\delta \times \delta} \quad (8)$$

where $\Upsilon_k = \boldsymbol{\psi}_k \boldsymbol{\psi}_k^T \in \mathbb{R}^{\delta \times \delta}$ with $\boldsymbol{\psi}_k = \left[y_\rho, y_{\rho+1}, \ldots, y_k\right]^T \in \mathbb{R}^{\delta \times 1}$. Applying SVD procedure to covariance matrix $\mathbf{S}_k$, the set of eigenvalues $\sigma_k^1, \sigma_k^2, \ldots, \sigma_k^\delta$ and their respective eigenvectors $\boldsymbol{\phi}_k^1, \boldsymbol{\phi}_k^2, \ldots, \boldsymbol{\phi}_k^\delta$ are updated at time instant k so that y_k can be rewritten by

$$y_k = h_k^1 + h_k^{\hat{2}} + \cdots + h_k^d \quad (9)$$

where $h_k^\varsigma = \kappa_k^\varsigma \boldsymbol{\psi}_k^T \boldsymbol{\phi}_k^\varsigma$, with $\varsigma = 1, \ldots, d$, such that κ_k^ς corresponds to the last element of the eigenvector $\boldsymbol{\phi}_k^\varsigma$. Finally, the regrouping of the terms $h_k^\varsigma|^{\varsigma=1,\ldots,d}$ in ξ disjoint terms $I_k^j|^{j=1,\ldots,\xi}$, results in

$$y_k = I_k^1 + I_k^{\hat{2}} + \cdots + I_k^\xi \quad (10)$$

such that $I_k^j = \alpha_k^j$, with $j = 1, \ldots, \xi$ and $k = N_b + 1, N_b + 2, \ldots$, represents the samples of extracted unobservable components at instant k. The Recursive Singular Spectral Analysis, according to proposed methodology, is implemented as described in Algorithm 1.

2.2   Parametric Estimation of Interval Type-2 Fuzzy Kalman Filter

The adopted structure of interval type-2 fuzzy Kalman filter presents the $i|^{[i=1,2,\ldots,c]}$th fuzzy rule, given by

$$R^{(i)}: \quad \text{IF } \mathbf{Z}_k \text{ IS } \widetilde{W}^i$$
$$\text{THEN } \begin{cases} \widetilde{\widetilde{\mathbf{x}}}_{k+1}^i = \widetilde{\mathbf{A}}_k^i \widetilde{\widetilde{\mathbf{x}}}_k^i + \widetilde{\mathbf{B}}_k^i \mathbf{u}_k + \widetilde{\mathbf{K}}_k^i \widetilde{\boldsymbol{\epsilon}}_k^i \\ \widetilde{\widetilde{\mathbf{y}}}_k^i = \widetilde{\mathbf{C}}_k^i \widetilde{\widetilde{\mathbf{x}}}_k^i + \widetilde{\mathbf{D}}_k^i \mathbf{u}_k \end{cases} \quad (11)$$

with nth order, m inputs, p outputs, where $\mathbf{Z}_k$ is the linguistic variable of the antecedent; $\widetilde{W}^i$ is the interval type-2 fuzzy set; $\widetilde{\widetilde{\mathbf{x}}}_k^i \in \mathbb{R}^n$ is the estimated interval states vector; $\widetilde{\widetilde{\mathbf{y}}}_k^i \in \mathbb{R}^p$ is the estimated interval output vector and $\mathbf{u}_k \in \mathbb{R}^m$ is the input signal. The matrices $\widetilde{\mathbf{A}}_k^i \in \mathbb{R}^{n \times n}$, $\widetilde{\mathbf{B}}_k^i \in \mathbb{R}^{n \times m}$, $\widetilde{\mathbf{C}}_k^i \in \mathbb{R}^{p \times n}$, $\widetilde{\mathbf{D}}_k^i \in \mathbb{R}^{p \times m}$ and $\widetilde{\mathbf{K}}_k^i \in \mathbb{R}^{n \times p}$ are, respectively, state matrix, input matrix, output matrix, direct transmission matrix and Kalman gain matrix, which are uncertain parameters that

<table>
<tr><td>

Algorithm 1: Recursive Singular Spectral Analysis

input : $\mathbf{y}, \delta, \xi$

output: $\alpha_k^j |^{j=1,\dots,\xi}$

:

%Training step;

Step 1: Compute $\rho = N_b - \delta + 1$;

Step 2: Construct the trajectory matrix $\mathbf{H}$ - Eq. (2);

Step 3: Compute the covariance matrix $\mathbf{S}$ - Eq. (3);

Step 4: Apply the SVD method in the covariance matrix $\mathbf{S}$ and obtain the set of eigenvalues $\sigma^1 \geq \sigma^2 \geq \cdots \geq \sigma^\delta \geq 0$ with their respective eigenvectors $\boldsymbol{\phi}^1, \boldsymbol{\phi}^2, \dots, \boldsymbol{\phi}^\delta$;

Step 5: Rewrite the SVD of the matrix $\mathbf{S}$ in the form of Eq. (4);

Step 6: Regroup the matrices $\mathbf{H}^\varsigma |^{\varsigma=1,\dots,d}$ in ξ linearly independent matrix terms $\mathbf{I}^j |^{j=1,\dots,\xi}$ - Eq. (6);

Step 7: Compute the unobservable components $\alpha_k^j |^{j=1,\dots,\xi}$ - Eq. (7);

%Recursive step;

while $k \geq N_b + 1$ **do**

    Step 1: Update ρ;

    Step 2: Update the covariance matrix $\mathbf{S}_k$ - Eq. (8);

    Step 3: Update the set of eigenvalues with their respective eigenvectors applying the SVD method in $\mathbf{S}_k$;

    Step 4: Rewrite the sample y_k in the form of Eq. (9);

    Step 5: Regroup the terms $h_k^\varsigma |^{\varsigma=1,\dots,d}$ in ξ disjoint terms $I_k^j |^{j=1,\dots,\xi}$, such that $I_k^j = \alpha_k^j$ - Eq. (10);

end

</td></tr>
</table>

describe the dynamics of experimental dataset within a region of uncertainty. The residual error $\widetilde{\epsilon}_k^i$ for ith rule is defined as $\widetilde{\epsilon}_k^i = \mathbf{y}_k - \widetilde{\widehat{\mathbf{y}}}_k^i$, where $\mathbf{y}_k \in \mathbb{R}^p$ is the real-time series and $\widetilde{\widehat{\mathbf{y}}}_k^i$ is the interval estimated time series by ith interval Kalman filter.

The interval type-2 fuzzy Kalman filter approximates the dynamic behavior inherited to experimental dataset through the weighted sum of Kalman filters defined in the consequent proposition of type-2 fuzzy Kalman filter rules, according to normalized interval activation degrees $\widetilde{\mu}_{\widetilde{W}^i}^i(\mathbf{Z}_k)$, of each ith rule, as follows:

$$\widetilde{\widehat{\mathbf{x}}}_{k+1} = \sum_{i=1}^{c} \widetilde{\mu}_{\widetilde{W}^i}^i(\mathbf{Z}_k)\widetilde{\mathbf{A}}_k^i\widetilde{\widehat{\mathbf{x}}}_k + \sum_{i=1}^{c} \widetilde{\mu}_{\widetilde{W}^i}^i(\mathbf{Z}_k)\widetilde{\mathbf{B}}_k^i\mathbf{u}_k + \sum_{i=1}^{c} \widetilde{\mu}_{\widetilde{W}^i}^i(\mathbf{Z}_k)\widetilde{\mathbf{K}}_k^i\widetilde{\epsilon}_k^i$$

$$\widetilde{\widehat{\mathbf{y}}}_k = \sum_{i=1}^{c} \widetilde{\mu}_{\widetilde{W}^i}^i(\mathbf{Z}_k)\widetilde{\mathbf{C}}_k^i\widetilde{\widehat{\mathbf{x}}}_k + \sum_{i=1}^{c} \widetilde{\mu}_{\widetilde{W}^i}^i(\mathbf{Z}_k)\widetilde{\mathbf{D}}_k^i\mathbf{u}_k \qquad (12)$$

with $\widetilde{\mu}_{\widetilde{W}^i}^i(\mathbf{Z}_k) = \left[\underline{\mu}_{\widetilde{W}^i}^i(\mathbf{Z}_k), \overline{\mu}_{\widetilde{W}^i}^i(\mathbf{Z}_k) \right]$, where $\underline{\mu}_{\widetilde{W}^i}^i(\mathbf{Z}_k)$ and $\overline{\mu}_{\widetilde{W}^i}^i(\mathbf{Z}_k)$ corresponds to lower and upper activation degrees in ith rule, respectively, and c is the number of rules of interval type-2 fuzzy Kalman filter, such that

$$\sum_{i=1}^{c} \widetilde{\mu}_{\widetilde{W}^i}^i(\mathbf{Z}_k) = 1, \qquad \widetilde{\mu}_{\widetilde{W}^i}^i(\mathbf{Z}_k) \geq 0 \qquad (13)$$

Parametric Estimation of Antecedent

The interval type-2 fuzzy version of Gustafson–Kessel clustering algorithm [67], is proposed, as formulated in the sequel. Given the experimental dataset $\mathbf{Z} \in \mathbb{R}^{p \times N_b}$, previously collected, choose the number of clusters c such that $1 < c < N_b$; the random initial interval partition matrix $\widetilde{\mathbf{U}}^{(0)} \in \mathbb{R}^{c \times N_b}$, the termination tolerance $\mathcal{E} > 0$ and the interval weighting exponent $\widetilde{m} = \left[\underline{m}, \overline{m} \right]$, where $\underline{m}$ and $\overline{m}$ correspond to, respectively, weighting exponent of upper and lower membership functions of the interval type-2 fuzzy set $\widetilde{W}^i$.

Repeat for $l = 1, 2, \dots$

Step 1—Compute the centers of the clusters $\widetilde{\mathbf{v}}^{i(l)}$:

$$\widetilde{\mathbf{v}}^{i(l)} = \frac{\sum_{k=1}^{N_b} \left(\widetilde{\mu}_{\widetilde{W}^i}^i(\mathbf{Z}_k)^{i(l-1)} \right)^{\widetilde{m}} \mathbf{Z}_k}{\sum_{k=1}^{N_b} \left(\widetilde{\mu}_{\widetilde{W}^i}^i(\mathbf{Z}_k)^{(l-1)} \right)^{\widetilde{m}}}, \quad 1 \leq i \leq c \qquad (14)$$

where $\mathbf{Z}_k$ is the data at sample k and $\widetilde{\mu}_{\widetilde{W}^i}^i(\mathbf{Z}_k)$ is the interval membership degree of $\mathbf{Z}_k$ in the ith cluster.

Step 2—Compute the covariance matrices $\widetilde{\mathbf{F}}^i$ of the clusters:

$$\widetilde{\mathbf{F}}^i = \frac{\sum_{k=1}^{N_b} \left(\widetilde{\mu}_{\widetilde{W}^i}^i(\mathbf{Z}_k)^{(l-1)} \right)^{\widetilde{m}} \left(\mathbf{Z}_k - \widetilde{\mathbf{v}}^{i(l)} \right) \left(\mathbf{Z}_k - \widetilde{\mathbf{v}}^{i(l)} \right)^T}{\sum_{k=1}^{N} \left(\widetilde{\mu}_{\widetilde{W}^i}^i(\mathbf{Z}_k)^{(l-1)} \right)^{\widetilde{m}}},$$

$$1 \leq i \leq c, \quad 1 \leq k \leq N_b \qquad (15)$$

Step 3—Compute the distances $\widetilde{D}_{k\widetilde{\mathbf{F}}^i}^i$ between the sample $\mathbf{Z}_k$ and the center $\widetilde{\mathbf{v}}^{i(l)}$ of the ith cluster:

$$\widetilde{D}_{k\widetilde{\mathbf{F}}^i}^i = \sqrt{\left(\mathbf{Z}_k - \widetilde{\mathbf{v}}^{i(l)} \right)^T \left[\det\left(\widetilde{\mathbf{F}}^i \right)^{1/n} \left(\widetilde{\mathbf{F}}^i \right)^{-1} \right] \left(\mathbf{Z}_k - \widetilde{\mathbf{v}}^{i(l)} \right)}$$

$$(16)$$

Step 4—Update the interval partition matrix $\widetilde{\mathbf{U}}^{(l)}$:
If $\widetilde{D}_{k\widetilde{\mathbf{F}}^i}^i > 0$ for $1 \leq i \leq c, 1 \leq k \leq N_b$

$$\widetilde{\mu}_{\widetilde{W}^i}^{i(l)}(\mathbf{Z}_k) = \left[\underline{\mu}_{\widetilde{W}^i}^i(\mathbf{Z}_k), \overline{\mu}_{\widetilde{W}^i}^i(\mathbf{Z}_k) \right] \qquad (17)$$

where

$$\underline{\mu}_{\widetilde{W}^i}^{i(l)}(\mathbf{Z}_k) = \min \left[\frac{1}{\sum_{j=1}^{c} \left(\underline{D}_{k\mathbf{F}^i}^i / \underline{D}_{k\mathbf{F}^i}^i \right)^{2/(\underline{m}-1)}} \; , \; \frac{1}{\sum_{j=1}^{c} \left(\overline{D}_{k\overline{\mathbf{F}}^i}^i / \overline{D}_{k\overline{\mathbf{F}}^i}^i \right)^{2/(\overline{m}-1)}} \right] \tag{18}$$

$$\overline{\mu}_{\widetilde{W}^i}^{i(l)}(\mathbf{Z}_k) = \max \left[\frac{1}{\sum_{j=1}^{c} \left(\underline{D}_{k\mathbf{F}^i}^i / \underline{D}_{k\mathbf{F}^i}^i \right)^{2/(\underline{m}-1)}} \; , \; \frac{1}{\sum_{j=1}^{c} \left(\overline{D}_{k\overline{\mathbf{F}}^i}^i / \overline{D}_{k\overline{\mathbf{F}}^i}^i \right)^{2/(\overline{m}-1)}} \right] \tag{19}$$

otherwise

$$\widetilde{\mu}_{\widetilde{W}^i}^{i(l)}(\mathbf{Z}_k) = [0, \; 0] \text{ with } \underline{\mu}_{\widetilde{W}^i}^{i(l)}(\mathbf{Z}_k) \in [0, 1] \text{ e } \overline{\mu}_{\widetilde{W}^i}^{i(l)}(\mathbf{Z}_k) \in [0, 1]$$

Until $\left\| \widetilde{\mathbf{U}}^{(l)} - \widetilde{\mathbf{U}}^{(l-1)} \right\| < \mathcal{E}$

The interval type-2 fuzzy Gustafson–Kessel clustering algorithm, according to the proposed methodology, is implemented as described in Algorithm 2.

Algorithm 2: Interval Type-2 Fuzzy Gustafson-Kessel Clustering Algorithm

  input : $\mathbf{Z}, \widetilde{m}, \mathcal{E}, \widetilde{\mathbf{U}}^{(0)}$

  output: $\widetilde{\mathbf{U}}$
:

  $l = 0$;

  repeat

    $l = l + 1$;

    for $i = 1$ **to** c **do**

      Step 1: Compute the centers of the clusters $\widetilde{\mathbf{v}}^{i(l)}$ - Eq. (14);

      Step 2: Compute the covariance matrices of the clusters $\widetilde{\mathbf{F}}^i$ - Eq. (15);

      Step 3 - Compute the distances $\widetilde{D}_{k\widetilde{\mathbf{F}}^i}^i$ - Eq. (16);

      Step 4: Update the interval partition matrix $\widetilde{\mathbf{U}}^{(l)}$ - Eq. (17)–(19);

    end

  until $\left\| \widetilde{\mathbf{U}}^{(l)} - \widetilde{\mathbf{U}}^{(l-1)} \right\| < \mathcal{E}$;

Parametric Estimation of Consequent

Once the interval type-2 fuzzy Kalman filter is obtained by the black-box modeling approach, it is necessary the estimation, from experimental data, of matrices that compose the interval type-2 fuzzy Kalman filter inference system consequent proposition, as formulated in Eq. (11). In this sense, an interval type-2 fuzzy OKID (Observer/Kalman Filter Identification) algorithm [68], is proposed. The interval type-2 membership values from partitions defined on experimental data, which were estimated by interval type-2 Gustafson–Kessel clustering algorithm, have been considered as weighting criteria for computing the consequent proposition of interval type-2 fuzzy Kalman filter inference system. The interval type-2 fuzzy OKID algorithm is formulated in the sequel.

Let the experimental dataset $\mathbf{Z}$, such that $\mathbf{Z}_k = \begin{bmatrix} \mathbf{u}_k & \boldsymbol{\alpha}_k^* \end{bmatrix}^T$, where $\boldsymbol{\alpha}_k^*$ corresponds to spectral components extracted from the experimental dataset that presents higher eigenvalue and are more significant to represent the dynamics of experimental dataset. Choose an appropriate number of Markov parameters q, through the following steps:

Step 1—Compute the matrix of regressors Λ, given by

$$\Lambda = \begin{bmatrix} \mathbf{u}_q & \mathbf{u}_{q+1} & \cdots & \mathbf{u}_{N_b-1} \\ \mathbf{Z}_{q-1} & \mathbf{Z}_q & \cdots & \mathbf{Z}_{N_b-2} \\ \mathbf{Z}_{q-2} & \mathbf{Z}_{q-1} & \cdots & \mathbf{Z}_{N_b-3} \\ \vdots & \vdots & \ddots & \vdots \\ \mathbf{Z}_0 & \mathbf{Z}_1 & \cdots & \mathbf{Z}_{N_b-q-1} \end{bmatrix} \tag{20}$$

Step 2—Compute the interval Observer Markov Parameters $\widetilde{\overline{\mathbf{Y}}}^i$:

$$\widetilde{\hat{\mathbf{y}}}^T = \sum_{i=1}^{c} \widetilde{\Gamma}^i \Lambda^T \widetilde{\overline{\mathbf{Y}}}^{i^T} \tag{21}$$

where

$$\widetilde{\Gamma}^i = \begin{bmatrix} \widetilde{\mu}_{\widetilde{W}^i}^i(\mathbf{Z}_q) & 0 & \ldots & 0 \\ 0 & \widetilde{\mu}_{\widetilde{W}^i}^i(\mathbf{Z}_{q+1}) & \ldots & 0 \\ 0 & 0 & \ldots & 0 \\ \vdots & \vdots & \ddots & \vdots \\ 0 & 0 & \ldots & \widetilde{\mu}_{\widetilde{W}^i}^i(\mathbf{Z}_{N_b-1}) \end{bmatrix} \tag{22}$$

is the diagonal weighting matrix of the ith fuzzy rule obtained from the interval type-2 Gustafson–Kessel fuzzy clustering algorithm and

$$\begin{aligned} \widetilde{\overline{\mathbf{Y}}}^i &= \begin{bmatrix} \widetilde{\mathbf{D}}_k^i & \widetilde{\mathbf{C}}_k^i \widetilde{\overline{\mathbf{B}}}_k^i & \widetilde{\mathbf{C}}_k^i \widetilde{\overline{\mathbf{A}}}_k^i \widetilde{\overline{\mathbf{B}}}_k^i & \cdots & \widetilde{\mathbf{C}}_k^i \widetilde{\overline{\mathbf{A}}}_k^{i(q-1)} \widetilde{\overline{\mathbf{B}}}_k^i \end{bmatrix} \\ &= \begin{bmatrix} \widetilde{\overline{\mathbf{Y}}}_0^i & \widetilde{\overline{\mathbf{Y}}}_1^i & \widetilde{\overline{\mathbf{Y}}}_2^i & \cdots \widetilde{\overline{\mathbf{Y}}}_q^i \end{bmatrix} \end{aligned} \tag{23}$$

are the interval observer Markov parameters of ith rule such that $\widetilde{\overline{\mathbf{A}}}_k^i = \begin{bmatrix} \widetilde{\mathbf{A}}_k^i + \widetilde{\mathbf{K}}_k^i \widetilde{\mathbf{C}}_k^i \end{bmatrix}$ and $\widetilde{\overline{\mathbf{B}}}_k^i = \begin{bmatrix} \widetilde{\mathbf{B}}_k^i + \widetilde{\mathbf{K}}_k^i \widetilde{\mathbf{D}}_k^i, & -\widetilde{\mathbf{K}}_k^i \end{bmatrix}$. Manipulating the Eq. (21):

$$\Lambda \widetilde{\Gamma}^i \mathbf{y}^T = \Lambda \widetilde{\Gamma}^i \Lambda^T \widetilde{\overline{\mathbf{Y}}}^{i^T} \tag{24}$$

where $\mathbf{y} = \begin{bmatrix} \mathbf{y}_1 & \mathbf{y}_2 & \cdots & \mathbf{y}_{N_b} \end{bmatrix} \in \mathbb{R}^{p \times N_b}$ corresponds to experimental dataset. Assuming $\widetilde{\mathfrak{U}}^i = \Lambda \widetilde{\Gamma}^i \Lambda^T$ and $\widetilde{\mathbf{S}}^i = \Lambda \widetilde{\Gamma}^i \mathbf{y}^T$,

Eq. (24) is rewriting as:

$$\widetilde{\mathfrak{U}}^i \, \widetilde{\mathbf{Y}}^{i^T} = \widetilde{\mathbf{s}}^i \tag{25}$$

The Eq. (25) is solved by QR factorization method, which is numerically robust since it avoids matrix inverse operations. Applying QR factorization to the term $\widetilde{\mathfrak{U}}^i$ on the right side of the Eq. (25), it has:

$$\widetilde{\mathbf{Q}}^i \widetilde{\mathbf{R}}^i \widetilde{\mathbf{Y}}^{i^T} = \widetilde{\mathbf{s}}^i \tag{26}$$

where $\widetilde{\mathbf{Q}}^i$ is an orthogonal matrix, such that $\left(\widetilde{\mathbf{Q}}^i\right)^{-1} = \left(\widetilde{\mathbf{Q}}^i\right)^T$ and $\widetilde{\mathbf{R}}^i$ is an upper triangular matrix. Because the matrix $\widetilde{\mathbf{R}}^i$ is upper triangular, Eq. (26) can be solved by backward replacement, obtaining the observer's Markov parameter vector $\widetilde{\mathbf{Y}}^i$.

Step 3—Compute the observer gain and system Markov parameters:

$$\widetilde{\mathbf{Y}}_0^i = \widetilde{\mathbf{D}}_k^i \tag{27}$$

$$\widetilde{\mathbf{Y}}_j^i = \widetilde{\mathbf{C}}_k^i \widetilde{\mathbf{A}}^{i^{(j-1)}} \widetilde{\mathbf{B}}_k^i \tag{28}$$

$$= \left[\widetilde{\mathbf{C}}_k^i \left(\widetilde{\mathbf{A}}_k^i + \widetilde{\mathbf{K}}_k^i \widetilde{\mathbf{C}}_k^i \right)^{(j-1)} \left(\widetilde{\mathbf{B}}_k^i + \widetilde{\mathbf{K}}_k^i \widetilde{\mathbf{D}}_k^i \right), \, -\widetilde{\mathbf{C}}_k^i \left(\widetilde{\mathbf{A}}_k^i + \widetilde{\mathbf{K}}_k^i \widetilde{\mathbf{C}}_k^i \right)^{(j-1)} \widetilde{\mathbf{K}}_k^i \right] \tag{29}$$

$$= \left[\widetilde{\mathbf{Y}}_j^{i^{(1)}}, \, -\widetilde{\mathbf{Y}}_j^{i^{(2)}} \right], \quad j = 1, 2, 3, \ldots \tag{30}$$

where $\widetilde{\mathbf{Y}}_j^i$ are the interval observer Markov parameters obtained from Step 2 for ith cluster. Thus, the system Markov parameters $\widetilde{\mathbf{Y}}_j^i$ are obtained as follows:

$$\widetilde{\mathbf{Y}}_0^i = \widetilde{\mathbf{Y}}_0^i = \widetilde{\mathbf{D}}_k^i \tag{31}$$

$$\widetilde{\mathbf{Y}}_j^i = \widetilde{\mathbf{Y}}_j^{i^{(1)}} - \sum_{\iota=1}^{j} \widetilde{\mathbf{Y}}_j^{i^{(2)}} \widetilde{\mathbf{Y}}_{j-\iota}^i, \quad \text{for } j = 1, \ldots, q \tag{32}$$

$$\widetilde{\mathbf{Y}}_j^i = -\sum_{\iota=1}^{q} \widetilde{\mathbf{Y}}_j^{i^{(2)}} \widetilde{\mathbf{Y}}_{j-\iota}^i, \quad \text{for } j = q+1, \ldots, \infty \tag{33}$$

and the observer gain Markov parameters $\widetilde{\mathbf{Y}}_j^{i^o}$ are obtained by

$$\widetilde{\mathbf{Y}}_1^{i^o} = \widetilde{\mathbf{Y}}_1^{i^{(2)}} = \widetilde{\mathbf{C}}_k^i \widetilde{\mathbf{K}}_k^i \tag{34}$$

$$\widetilde{\mathbf{Y}}_j^{i^o} = \widetilde{\mathbf{Y}}_j^{i^{(2)}} - \sum_{\iota=1}^{j-1} \widetilde{\mathbf{Y}}_j^{i^{(2)}} \widetilde{\mathbf{Y}}_{j-\iota}^{i^o}, \quad \text{for } j = 2, \ldots, q \tag{35}$$

$$\widetilde{\mathbf{Y}}_j^{i^o} = -\sum_{\iota=1}^{q} \widetilde{\mathbf{Y}}_j^{i^{(2)}} \widetilde{\mathbf{Y}}_{j-\iota}^{i^o}, \quad \text{for } j = q+1, \ldots, \infty \tag{36}$$

Step 4—Construct the Hankel matrix $\widetilde{\mathbf{H}}^i (j-1) \in \mathbb{R}^{\gamma p \times \beta m}$:

$$\widetilde{\mathbf{H}}^i (j-1) = \begin{bmatrix} \widetilde{\mathbf{Y}}_j^i & \widetilde{\mathbf{Y}}_{j+1}^i & \cdots & \widetilde{\mathbf{Y}}_{j+\beta-1}^i \\ \widetilde{\mathbf{Y}}_{j+1}^i & \widetilde{\mathbf{Y}}_{j+2}^i & \cdots & \widetilde{\mathbf{Y}}_{j+\beta}^i \\ \vdots & \vdots & \ddots & \vdots \\ \widetilde{\mathbf{Y}}_{j+\gamma-1}^i & \widetilde{\mathbf{Y}}_{j+\gamma}^i & \cdots & \widetilde{\mathbf{Y}}_{j+\gamma+\beta-2}^i \end{bmatrix} \tag{37}$$

where γ and β are sufficiently large arbitrary integers defined by user.

Step 5—For $j = 1$, decompose the Hankel matrix $\widetilde{\mathbf{H}}^i (0)$ using Singular Value Decomposition:

$$\widetilde{\mathbf{H}}^i (0) = \widetilde{\Xi}^i \widetilde{\Sigma}^i \widetilde{\Psi}^{i^T} \tag{38}$$

where $\widetilde{\Xi}^i \in \mathbb{R}^{\gamma p \times \gamma p}$ and $\widetilde{\Psi}^i \in \mathbb{R}^{\beta m \times \beta m}$ are orthogonal matrices and $\widetilde{\Sigma}^i \in \mathbb{R}^{\gamma p \times \beta m}$ is the diagonal matrix of singular values defined as follows:

$$\widetilde{\Sigma}^i = \begin{bmatrix} \widetilde{\Sigma}_n^i & 0 \\ 0 & 0 \end{bmatrix} \tag{39}$$

such that n is the number of significant singular values and determines the minimum order of the type-2 fuzzy Kalman filter. Thus, the size of matrices in Eq. (38) is reduced to the minimum order, as follows:

$$\widetilde{\mathbf{H}}_n^i (0) = \widetilde{\Xi}_n^i \widetilde{\Sigma}_n^i \widetilde{\Psi}_n^{i^T} \tag{40}$$

where $\widetilde{\Xi}_n^i \in \mathbb{R}^{\gamma p \times n}$, $\widetilde{\Psi}_n^i \in \mathbb{R}^{n \times \beta m}$, $\widetilde{\Sigma}_n^i \in \mathbb{R}^{n \times n}$ are the resulting matrices after the reduction to minimum order.

Step 6—Compute the observability and controllability matrices:

$$\widetilde{\mathcal{P}}_\gamma^i = \widetilde{\Xi}_n^i \left(\widetilde{\Sigma}_n^i \right)^{1/2} \tag{41}$$

$$\widetilde{\mathcal{Q}}_\beta^i = \left(\widetilde{\Sigma}_n^i \right)^{1/2} \widetilde{\Psi}_n^{i^T} \tag{42}$$

where

$$\widetilde{\mathcal{P}}_\gamma^i = \begin{bmatrix} \widetilde{\mathbf{C}}_k^i \\ \widetilde{\mathbf{C}}_k^i \widetilde{\mathbf{A}}_k^i \\ \widetilde{\mathbf{C}}_k^i \widetilde{\mathbf{A}}_k^{i^2} \\ \vdots \\ \widetilde{\mathbf{C}}_k^i \widetilde{\mathbf{A}}_k^{i^{\gamma-1}} \end{bmatrix} \tag{43}$$

is the observability matrix and

$$\widetilde{\mathcal{Q}}_\beta^i = \begin{bmatrix} \widetilde{\mathbf{B}}_k^i & \widetilde{\mathbf{A}}_k^i \widetilde{\mathbf{B}}_k^i & \widetilde{\mathbf{A}}_k^{i\,2} \widetilde{\mathbf{B}}_k^i & \cdots & \widetilde{\mathbf{A}}_k^{i\,\beta-1} \widetilde{\mathbf{B}}_k^i \end{bmatrix} \tag{44}$$

is the controllability matrix.

Step 7—Compute the matrices that make up the consequent proposition of interval type-2 fuzzy Kalman filter:

$$\widetilde{\mathbf{A}}_k^i = \left(\widetilde{\Sigma}_n^i \right)^{-1/2} \widetilde{\Xi}_n^{i\,T} \widetilde{\mathbf{H}}_n^i (1) \widetilde{\Psi}_n^{i\,T} \left(\widetilde{\Sigma}_n^i \right)^{-1/2} \tag{45}$$

$$\widetilde{\mathbf{B}}_k^i = \text{first } m \text{ collumns of } \widetilde{\mathcal{Q}}_\beta^i \tag{46}$$

$$\widetilde{\mathbf{C}}_k^i = \text{first } p \text{ rows of } \widetilde{\mathcal{P}}_\gamma^i \tag{47}$$

$$\widetilde{\mathbf{D}}_k^i = \widetilde{\mathbf{Y}}_0^i \tag{48}$$

Step 8—Compute the interval Kalman gain matrix $\widetilde{\mathbf{K}}_k^i$:

$$\widetilde{\mathbf{Y}}_j^{i\,o} = -\widetilde{\mathcal{P}}_\gamma^i \widetilde{\mathbf{K}}_k^i \tag{49}$$

where $\widetilde{\mathbf{Y}}_j^{i\,o}$ are the observer gain Markov parameters computed in Step 3, $\widetilde{\mathcal{P}}_\gamma^i$ is the observability matrix computed in Step 6 and $\widetilde{\mathbf{K}}_k^i$ is the interval Kalman gain matrix. Manipulating the Eq. (49):

$$\widetilde{\mathcal{P}}_\gamma^{i\,T} \widetilde{\Gamma}^i \widetilde{\mathbf{Y}}_j^{i\,o} = -\widetilde{\mathcal{P}}_\gamma^{i\,T} \widetilde{\Gamma}^i \widetilde{\mathcal{P}}_\gamma^i \widetilde{\mathbf{K}}_k^i \tag{50}$$

Assuming $\widetilde{\mathfrak{A}}^i = -\widetilde{\mathcal{P}}_\gamma^{i\,T} \widetilde{\Gamma}^i \widetilde{\mathcal{P}}_\gamma^i$ and $\widetilde{\mathfrak{N}}^i = \widetilde{\mathcal{P}}_\gamma^{i\,T} \widetilde{\Gamma}^i \widetilde{\mathbf{Y}}_j^{i\,o}$, Eq. (50) is rewriting as follows:

$$\widetilde{\mathfrak{A}}^i \widetilde{\mathbf{K}}_k^i = \widetilde{\mathfrak{N}}^i \tag{51}$$

The Eq. (51) is solved by QR factorization method being applied to $\widetilde{\mathfrak{A}}^i$ and obtaining the interval Kalman gain matrix $\widetilde{\mathbf{K}}_k^i$ in the same way as done in Step 2 for determining interval observer Markov parameters.

Recursive Updating of Interval Type-2 Fuzzy Kalman Filter Inference System After the initial estimation of interval type-2 fuzzy Kalman filter, the Kalman filters, into consequent proposition of interval type-2 fuzzy Kalman filter inference system, are updated recursively at instants of time $k = N_b + 1, k = N_b + 2, \ldots$, to each new sample from experimental dataset. Considering the regressors vector λ_k, at instant k, given by

$$\lambda_k = \begin{bmatrix} \mathbf{u}_{k+1} \\ \mathbf{Z}_k \\ \mathbf{Z}_{k-1} \\ \vdots \\ \mathbf{Z}_{k-q} \end{bmatrix} \tag{52}$$

the interval observer Markov parameters $\widetilde{\mathbf{Y}}_k^i$ are obtained by recursive updating of Eq. (25), as follows:

$$\widetilde{\mathfrak{U}}_k^i = \widetilde{\mathfrak{U}}_{k-1}^i + \widetilde{\mu}_{\widetilde{W}^i}^i (\mathbf{Z}_k) \lambda_k \lambda_k^T \tag{53}$$

$$\widetilde{\mathbf{S}}_k^i = \widetilde{\mathbf{S}}_{k-1}^i + \widetilde{\mu}_{\widetilde{W}^i}^i (\mathbf{Z}_k) \lambda_k \mathbf{y}_k^T \tag{54}$$

Once $\widetilde{\mathfrak{U}}_k^i$ and $\widetilde{\mathbf{S}}_k^i$ have been updated, and applying the QR factorization in $\widetilde{\mathfrak{U}}_k^i$, the observer Markov parameters for ith cluster at sample k, $\widetilde{\mathbf{Y}}_k^i$, are updated. The consequent proposition of the type-2 fuzzy Kalman filter is updated recursively by repeating the Step 3–Step 7. Similarly, the interval type-2 fuzzy Kalman gain matrix $\widetilde{\mathbf{K}}_k^i$ is obtained by recursive updating of Eq. (51), as follows:

$$\widetilde{\mathfrak{A}}_k^i = \widetilde{\mathfrak{A}}_{k-1}^i + \widetilde{\mu}_{\widetilde{W}^i}^i (\mathbf{Z}_k) \lambda_k \lambda_k^T \tag{55}$$

$$\widetilde{\mathfrak{N}}_k^i = \widetilde{\mathfrak{N}}_{k-1}^i + \widetilde{\mu}_{\widetilde{W}^i}^i (\mathbf{Z}_k) \lambda_k \lambda_k^T \tag{56}$$

Once $\widetilde{\mathfrak{A}}_k^i$ and $\widetilde{\mathfrak{N}}_k^i$ have been updated, and applying the QR factorization method in $\widetilde{\mathfrak{A}}_k^i$, the interval type-2 fuzzy Kalman gain matrix is updated.

The interval type-2 fuzzy Observer/Kalman Filter Identification algorithm, according to the proposed methodology, is implemented as described in Algorithm 3.

In the sense to illustrate the sequential steps of the computational aspects for interval type-2 fuzzy Kalman filter design, for better understanding from readers, a flowchart of the proposed methodology is shown in Fig. 1.

3 Experimental Results

In this section, experimental results for forecasting analysis the COVID-19 dynamic propagation, including comparative analysis with the approaches in [69–73] and with the machine learning models Least Absolute Shrinkage and Selection Operator (LASSO), Autoregressive Integrated Moving Aver-

---

Algorithm 3: Interval Type-2 Fuzzy Observer/Kalman Filter Identification Algorithm

input : $\mathbf{Z}, \gamma, \beta, q, \widetilde{\Gamma}^i$

output: $\widetilde{\mathbf{A}}_k^i, \widetilde{\mathbf{B}}_k^i, \widetilde{\mathbf{C}}_k^i, \widetilde{\mathbf{D}}_k^i, \widetilde{\mathbf{K}}_k^i$

:

%Training step;

Step 1: Construct the matrix of regressors Λ - Eq. (20);

for $i = 1$ **to** c **do**

    Step 2: Compute the interval observer Markov parameters $\widetilde{\widetilde{\mathbf{Y}}}^i$ - Eq. (24)-(26);

    Step 3: Compute the interval system Markov parameters $\widetilde{\mathbf{Y}}^i$ - Eq. (31)–(33) and the interval observer gain Markov parameters $\widetilde{\mathbf{Y}}^{i^o}$ - Eq. (34)–(36) ;

    Step 4: Construct the Hankel matrices $\widetilde{\mathbf{H}}^i(0)$ and $\widetilde{\mathbf{H}}^i(1)$ - Eq. (37);

    Step 5: Decompose $\widetilde{\mathbf{H}}^i(0)$ using SVD method - Eq. (38) and determine the minimum order n of type-2 fuzzy Kalman filter - Eq. (39);

    Step 6: Compute the observability matrix $\widetilde{\mathcal{P}}_\gamma^i$ - Eq. (41) and the controlability matrix $\widetilde{\mathcal{Q}}_\beta^i$ - Eq. (42);

    Step 7: Compute the matrices $\widetilde{\mathbf{A}}_k^i, \widetilde{\mathbf{B}}_k^i, \widetilde{\mathbf{C}}_k^i, \widetilde{\mathbf{D}}_k^i$ - Eq. (45)–(48);

    Step 8: Compute the interval Kalman gain matrix $\widetilde{\mathbf{K}}_k^i$ - Eq. (49)-(51);

end

%Recursive update of interval type-2 fuzzy Kalman filter;

while $k \geq N_b + 1$ **do**

    Construct the regressors vector λ_k - Eq. (52);

    for $i = 1$ **to** c **do**

        Update the interval observer Markov parameters $\widetilde{\widetilde{\mathbf{Y}}}_k^i$ through Eq. (53)–(54);

        Repeat **Step 3** to **Step 7** as described in training step;

        Update the interval Kalman gain matrix through Eq. (55)–(56)

    end

end

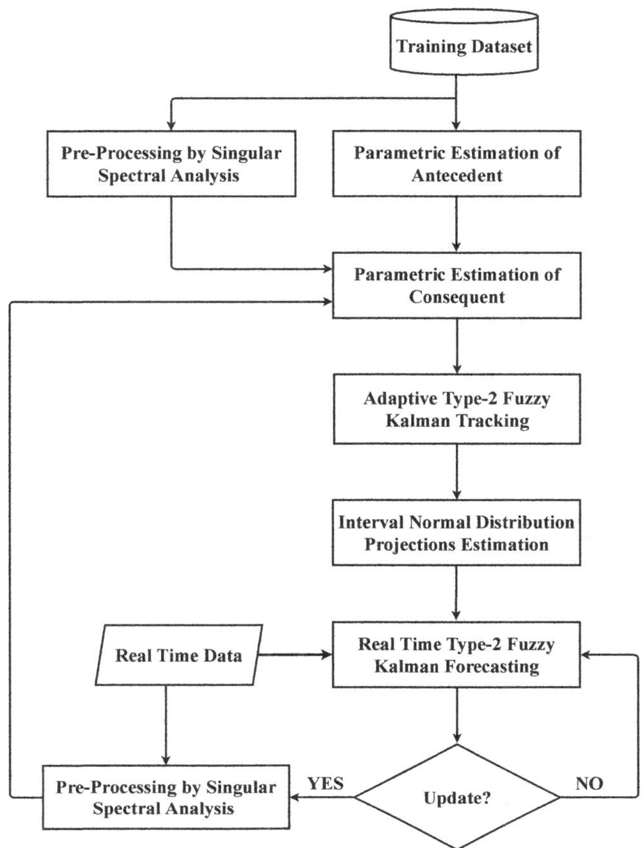

Fig. 1 The flowchart of the proposed methodology corresponding to computational aspects for designing the interval type-2 fuzzy Kalman filter

age (ARIMA), and Recurrent Neural Network (RNN), taking into account the experimental dataset of daily deaths reports caused by coronavirus disease in Brazil, are presented.

3.1   Interval Type-2 Fuzzy Kalman Filtering and Forecasting Analysis of COVID-19 Dynamic Propagation in Brazil

The experimental dataset corresponding to daily deaths reports within the period ranging from 29 February 2020 to 18 May 2020, in Brazil, is shown in Fig. 2, which were extracted from the official report by the Ministry of Health

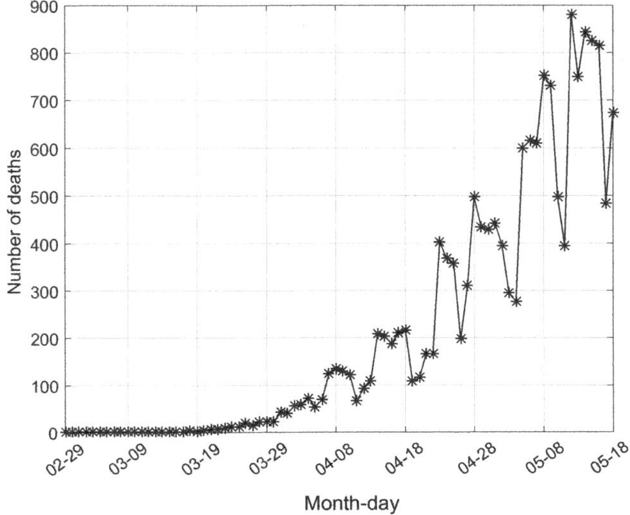

Fig. 2 The experimental dataset of daily deaths reports within the period from 29 February 2020 to 18 May 2020, in Brazil

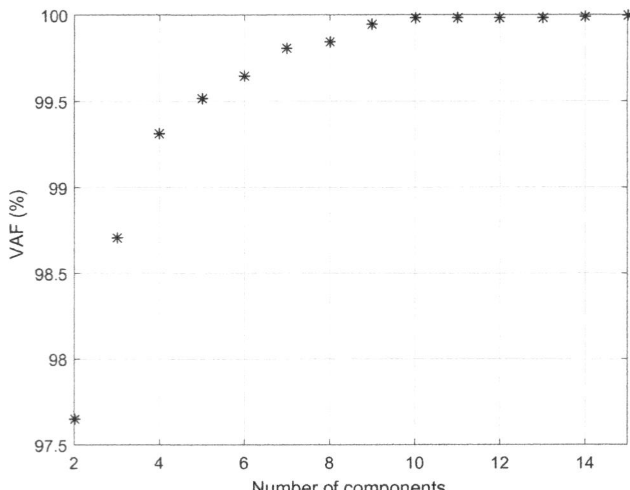

Fig. 3 The efficiency of unobservable components, according to VAF criterion, for representing the experimental dataset of the reports of the daily deaths, in Brazil

of Brazil.[1] Once that the problem of interest, in this chapter, is based on the time series related to daily deaths reports in Brazil, the variable $\mathbf{u}_k$, in Eq. (11), is considered as white noise signal with low amplitude.

The pre-processing of experimental dataset by singular spectral analysis was able for extracting the unobservable components associated with daily death reports. The Variance Accounted For (VAF) was considered for evaluating the appropriate number of these components, within a range from 2 to 15 ones, for the best representation of experimental dataset, as shown in Fig. 3. As it can be seen, considering the cost-benefit balance for computational practical application of the proposed methodology, the appropriated number of unobservable components was $\xi = 10$, with a VAF value of 99.98% in efficiency to represent as accurately as possible the experimental dataset and, at the same time, reducing the computational load of interval type-2 fuzzy Kalman filter algorithm. These spectral unobservable components are shown in Fig. 4. The partitions of experimental dataset related to daily deaths reports were defined by interval type-2 fuzzy Gustafson–Kessel clustering algorithm, as shown in Fig. 5, so the antecedent proposition, the rules number, and consequent proposition, of the type-2 fuzzy Kalman filter, could be

estimated successfully. For implementing the proposed type-2 fuzzy clustering algorithm, the following parameters were adopted: number of clusters $c = 3$, interval weighting exponent $\widetilde{m} = [1.5, 2.3]$ and termination tolerance $\mathcal{E} = 10^{-5}$. The implementation of interval type-2 fuzzy OKID algorithm, for parametric estimation of the consequent proposition in the type-2 fuzzy Kalman filter inference system, in Eq. (11), took into account the partitions on daily deaths reports, in Fig. 5, as weighting criterion, and the parameter values: $q = 1$ (associated to number of Markov parameters), $\gamma = 15$ (associated to number of rows of Hankel matrix) e $\beta = 15$ (associated to number of columns of Hankel matrix). According to the experimental dataset of daily deaths reports in Brazil shown in Fig. 2, the pre-processed unobservable components are shown in Fig. 4, the interval type-2 fuzzy normalized membership values shown in Fig. 5, the initial parametric estimation of the type-2 fuzzy Kalman filter was computed by training step. The confidence region, as shown in Fig. 6, created by initial estimation of interval type-2 fuzzy Kalman filter taking into account uncertainties estimated by interval type-2 membership functions shown in Fig. 5, inherited to experimental dataset ranging from 29 February 2020 to 18 May 2020, illustrates its efficiency for tracking the experimental dataset of daily death reports in Brazil. From this confidence region, shown in Fig. 6, an interval normal distribution projections were estimated, delimiting upper and lower limits for forecasting the further daily deaths reports in Brazil. The efficiency of interval type-2 fuzzy Kalman filter based on its initial estimation by training step from the experimental dataset of daily deaths reports ranging from 29 February 2020 to 18 May 2020, for forecasting the further (validation) experimental dataset of daily death reports, is shown in Fig. 7a. Interval normal distributions are adopted for modeling the COVID-19 dynamic propagation related to the daily death reports. This interval normal distribution model is computed as projections that are estimated from the recursive parameterization of interval type-2 fuzzy Kalman filter for adaptive tracking and real-time forecasting the experimental epidemiological dataset of COVID-19. The efficiency of the interval normal distribution model is measured in the sense that if the estimated projections are no longer sufficient to represent the experimental epidemiological dataset, an updating of interval type-2 fuzzy Kalman filter is necessary for new tracking and

---

[1] Available at: https://covid.saude.gov.br/.

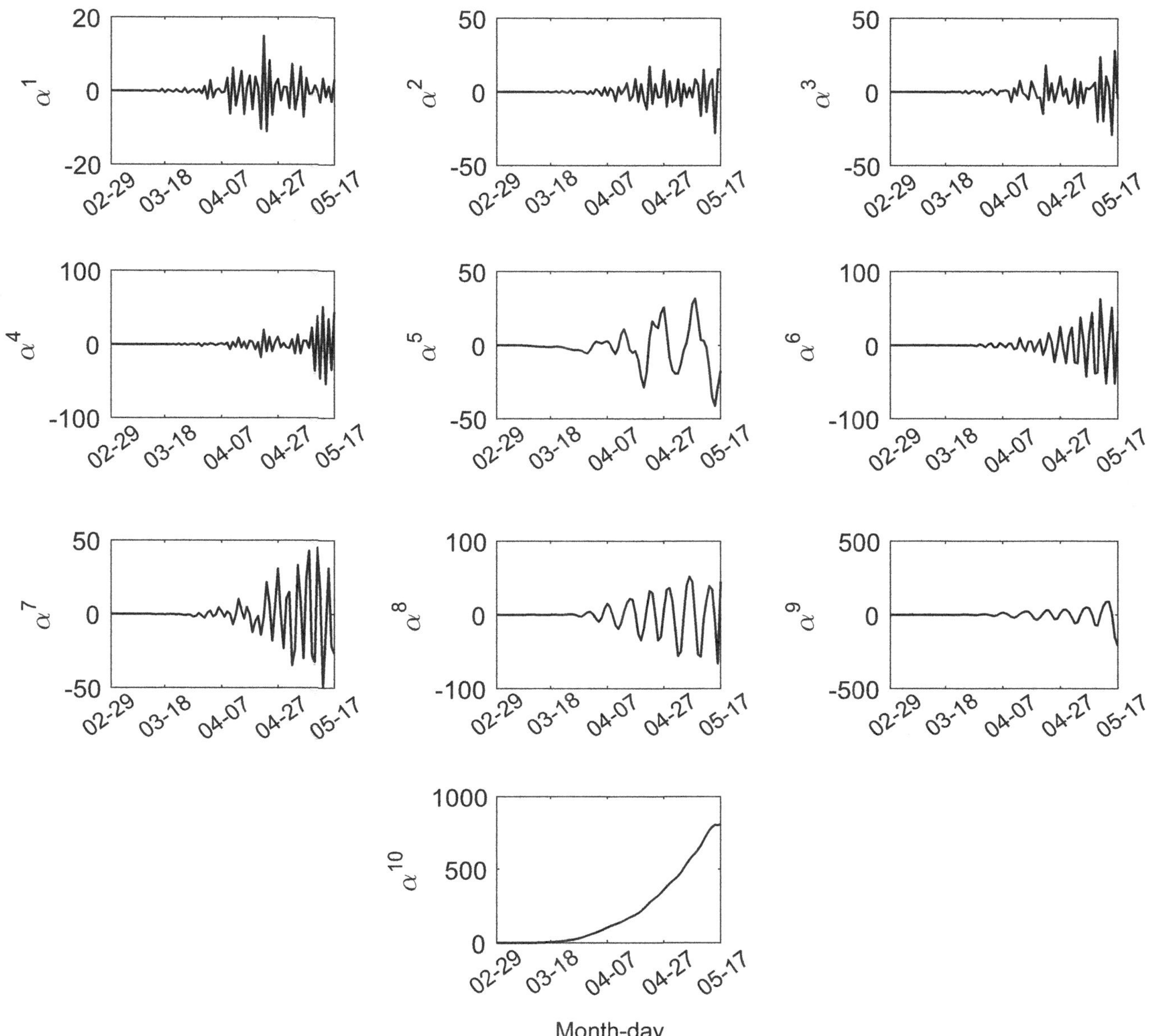

Fig. 4 The temporal behavior of spectral unobservable components $\alpha^j\,|^{j=1,\ldots,10}$, which were extracted from experimental dataset of daily deaths, in Brazil

forecasting the COVID-19 dynamic propagation related to the further daily deaths reports. According to this criterion, the results of updating of interval type-2 fuzzy Kalman filter for tracking and forecasting the COVID-19 dynamic propagation related to the daily death reports, are shown in Fig. 7b–f. It can be seen an efficiency in the adaptability of estimated projections defined by interval type-2 fuzzy Kalman filter, which illustrates its applicability for adaptive tracking and real-time forecasting the COVID-19 dynamic propagation.

The estimation of interval type-2 fuzzy Kalman gain matrices $\widetilde{\mathbf{K}}^i\,|^{i=1,\ldots,3}$, during recursive updating of interval type-2 fuzzy Kalman filter, is shown in Fig. 8. The recursive estimation of the interval type-2 fuzzy matrices $\widetilde{\mathbf{A}}^i$, $\widetilde{\mathbf{B}}^i$, $\widetilde{\mathbf{C}}^i$ and $\widetilde{\mathbf{D}}^i$,

with $i = 1, \ldots, 3$, in the consequent proposition of the interval type-2 fuzzy Kalman filter inference system, during recursive updating of interval type-2 fuzzy Kalman filter, are shown in Figs. 9, 10, 11 and 12. The upper and lower instantaneous activation degrees related to interval type-2 fuzzy Kalman filter inference system, during the training and recursive steps, are shown in Fig. 13. The efficiency of interval type-2 fuzzy Kalman filter, during its recursive updating for tracking and forecasting the COVID-19 dynamic propagation related to daily death reports in Brazil, was validated through the Variance Accounted For (VAF) criterion, as shown in Fig. 14.

According to results from adaptive tracking and real-time forecasting COVID-19 dynamic propagation related daily

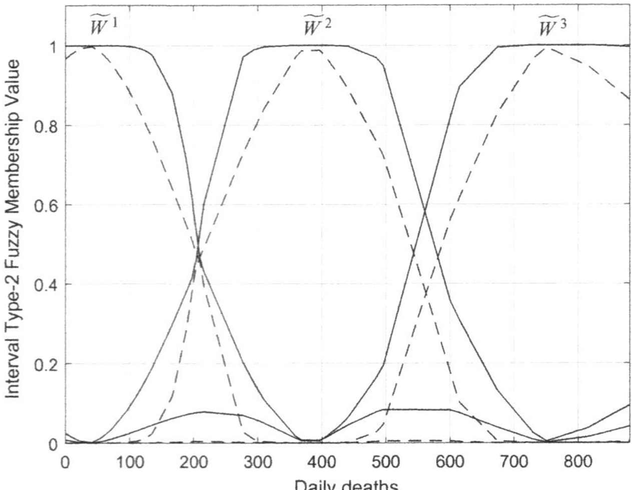

Fig. 5 The upper (solid line) and lower (dashed line) fuzzy membership functions estimated from the interval type-2 fuzzy clustering of daily death reports, in Brazil

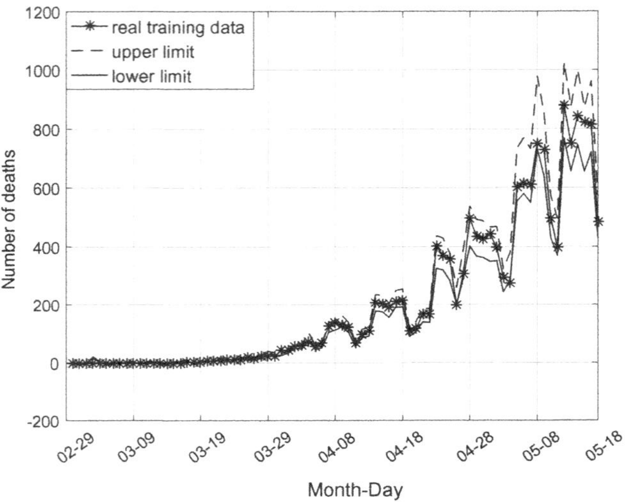

Fig. 6 The confidence region generated by interval type-2 fuzzy Kalman filter for tracking the experimental dataset of daily death reports, from 29 February 2020 to 18 May 2020, in Brazil

death reports, in Brazil, the following auxiliary information, and helpful for the Ministry of Health of Brazil, can be inferred:

- The proposed methodology can be helpful to the Ministry of Health of Brazil as auxiliary information in the diagnosis

regarding the flexibility of social activities, in Brazil. Fig. 7 depicts a time-based displacement of the interval projections as well as their amplitudes, as the daily death reports are processed by interval type-2 fuzzy Kalman filter. From the recursive updating on 13 October 2020, the forecasting interval projections indicate that the month of February 2021 is more adequate for reevaluating the requirements on the flexibility of social activities, in Brazil.

3.2 Comparative Analysis and Discussions

In this section, a more detailed discussion on the results shown in Sect. 3.1, according to comparative analysis of proposed methodology with the approaches in [69–73] as well as with the machine learning models LASSO, ARIMA and RNN, is presented.

The approach in [69] is based on Bayesian structural time series (BSTS) models for forecasting the COVID-19 dynamic propagation in Brazil, within the horizon of 30 days. The efficiency of interval type-2 fuzzy Kalman filter, compared to approach proposed in [69], according to RMSE (Root Mean Square Error), MAE (Mean Absolute Error), and RMSPE (Root Mean Square Percentage Error), is shown in Table 1. As it can be seen, although the Bayesian model in approach [69] be adaptive, it presents an inferior performance compared to interval type-2 fuzzy Kalman filter, once that it is based on Bayesian inference mechanism influenced by previously computed probability distributions, which contributes for increasing the forecasting errors [74].

The approach in [70] is based on Wavelet-Coupled Random Vector Functional Link (WCRVFL) network for forecasting the COVID-19 dynamic propagation in Brazil, within the horizon of 60 days, using a normalization procedure of dataset from the following formulation:

$$\check{z}_k = \frac{z_k - min\,(\mathbf{Z})}{max\,(\mathbf{Z}) - min\,(\mathbf{Z})}, \quad k = 1, 2, \ldots, N_b \qquad (57)$$

where $\mathbf{Z} = \left[z_1, z_2, \ldots, z_{N_b}\right]^T$ is the experimental dataset, $\check{z}_k$ is the normalized value of z_k, $min\,(\mathbf{Z})$ and $max\,(\mathbf{Z})$ are the maximum and minimum values of $\mathbf{Z}$, respectively. The efficiency of interval type-2 fuzzy Kalman filter, compared to approach in [70], according to RMSE (Root Mean Square Error), MAE (Mean Absolute Error) and coefficient of determination (R^2), is shown in Table 2. As it can be seen, once

Fig. 7 Performance of the interval type-2 fuzzy Kalman filter for adaptive tracking and real-time forecasting the COVID-19 dynamic propagation related to daily death reports, in Brazil: **a** updating based on training data from 29 February 2020 to 18 May 2020; **b** recursive updating on 24 June 2020; **c** recursive updating on 23 July 2020; **d** recursive updating on 28 August 2020; **e** recursive updating on 25 September 2020; **f** recursive updating on 13 October 2020

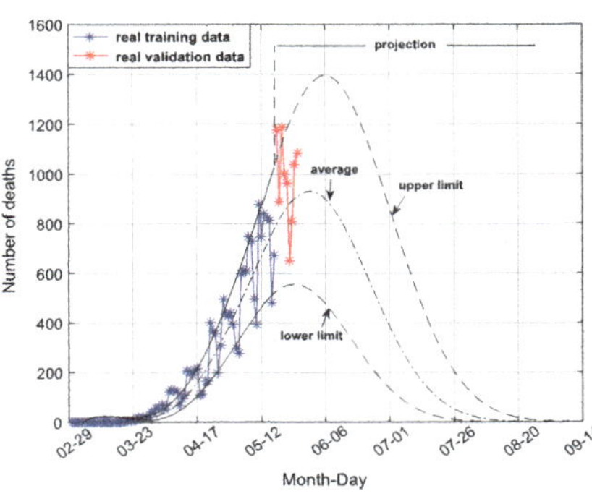

(a) The performance of interval type-2 fuzzy Kalman filter based on its initial estimation by training step for forecasting the daily deaths reports within the period ranging from 19 of May 2020 to 27 of May 2020, in Brazil.

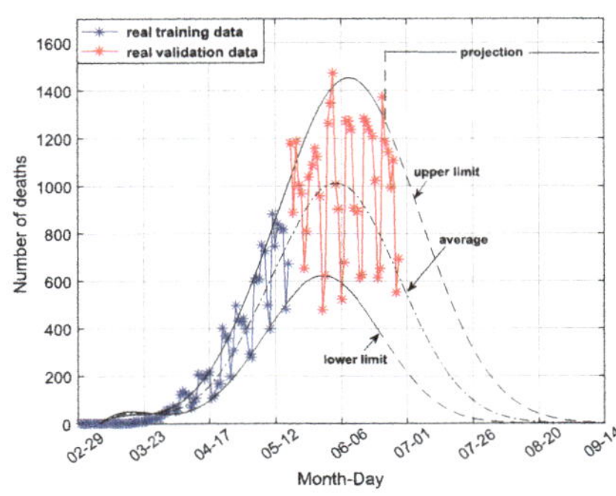

(b) The performance of interval type-2 fuzzy Kalman filter based on its recursive updating on 24 of June 2020 for forecasting the daily deaths reports within the period ranging from 25 of June 2020 to 30 of June 2020, in Brazil.

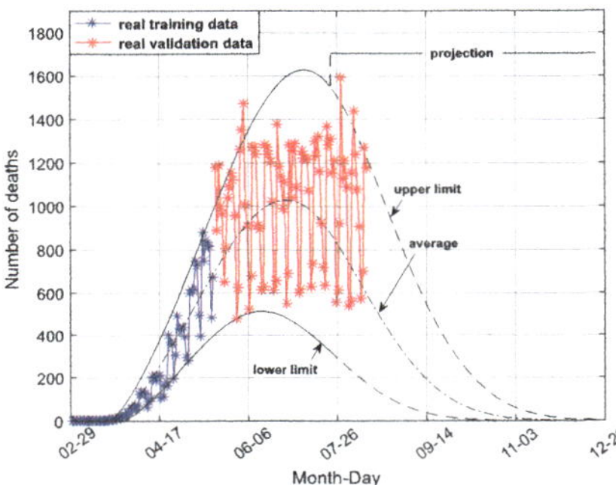

(c) The performance of interval type-2 fuzzy Kalman filter based on its recursive updating on 23 of July 2020 for forecasting the daily deaths reports within the period ranging from 24 of July 2020 to 14 of August 2020, in Brazil.

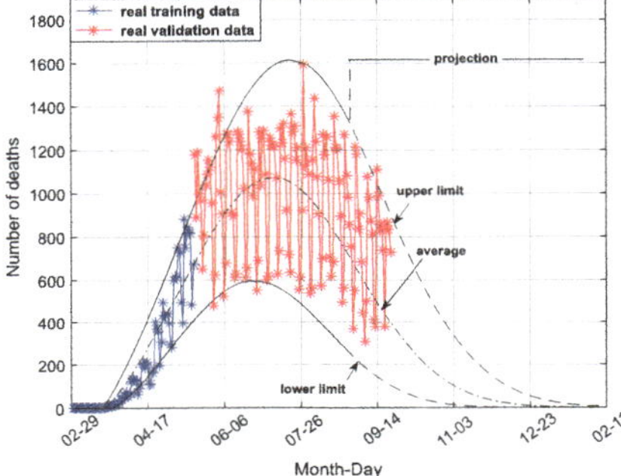

(d) The performance of interval type-2 fuzzy Kalman filter based on its recursive updating on 28 of August 2020 for forecasting the daily deaths reports within the period ranging from 29 of August 2020 to 25 of September 2020, in Brazil.

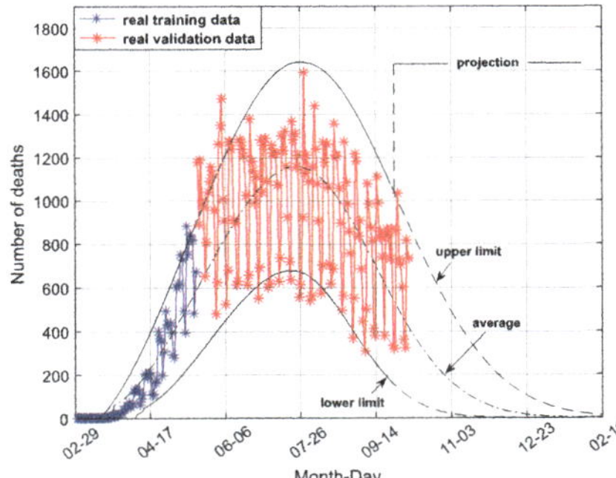

(e) The performance of interval type-2 fuzzy Kalman filter based on its recursive updating on 25 of September 2020 for forecasting the daily deaths reports within the period ranging from 26 of September 2020 to 13 of October 2020, in Brazil.

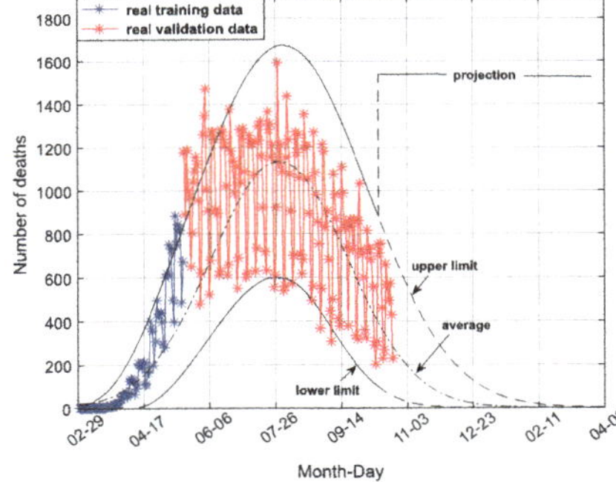

(f) The performance of interval type-2 fuzzy Kalman filter based on its recursive updating on 13 of October 2020 for forecasting the daily deaths reports within the period ranging from 14 of October 2020 to ahead, in Brazil.

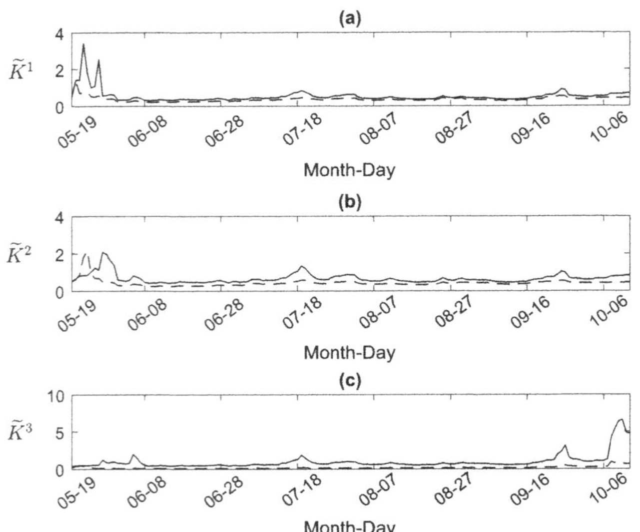

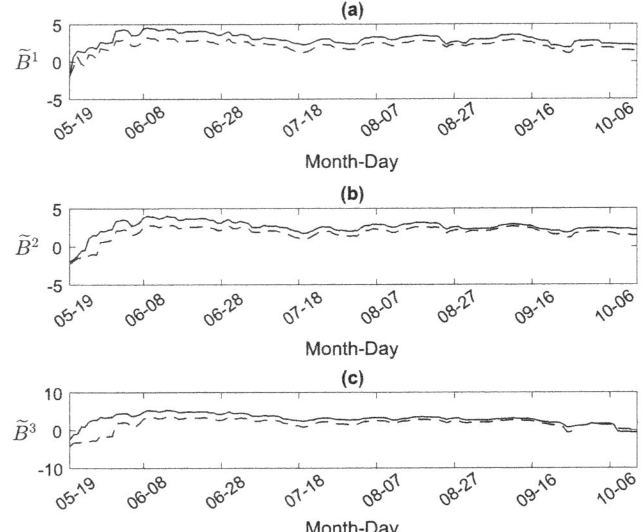

Fig. 8 Recursive estimation of interval type-2 fuzzy Kalman gains, in tracking and forecasting the COVID-19 dynamic propagation within period ranging from 19 May 2020 to 13 October 2020, in Brazil: **a** Rule 1, **b** Rule 2, **c** Rule 3

Fig. 10 Recursive estimation of interval type-2 fuzzy matrix $\widetilde{\mathbf{B}}^{i}$, in tracking and forecasting the COVID-19 dynamic propagation within period ranging from 19 May 2020 to 13 October 2020, in Brazil: **a** Rule 1, **b** Rule 2, **c** Rule 3

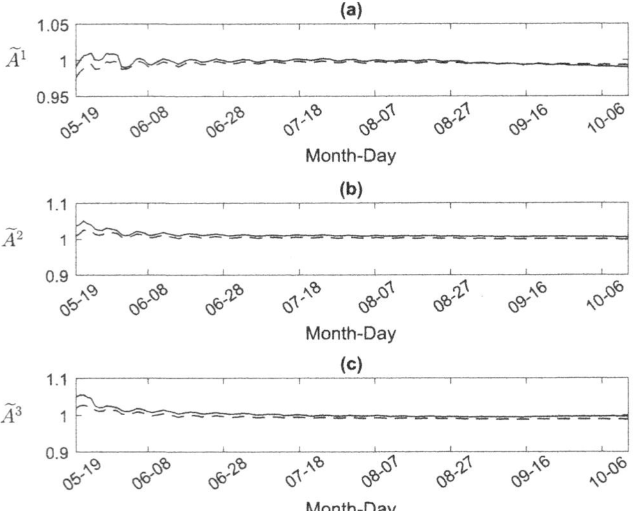

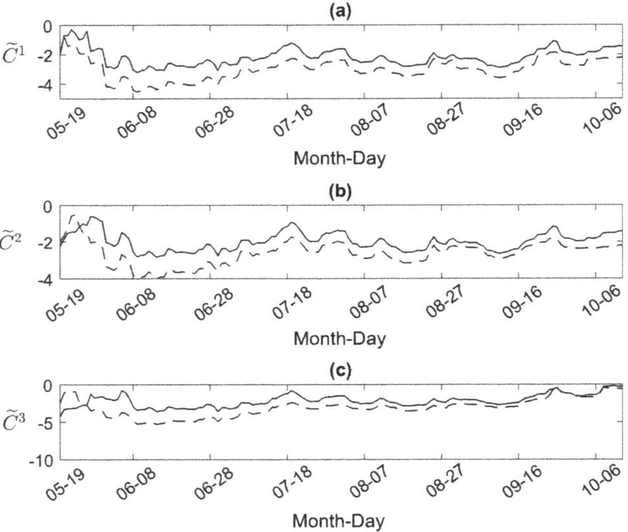

Fig. 9 Recursive estimation of interval type-2 fuzzy matrix $\widetilde{A}^{i}$, in tracking and forecasting the COVID-19 dynamic propagation within period ranging from 19 May 2020 to 13 October 2020, in Brazil: **a** Rule 1, **b** Rule 2, **c** Rule 3

Fig. 11 Recursive estimation of interval type-2 fuzzy matrix $\widetilde{C}^{i}$, in tracking and forecasting the COVID-19 dynamic propagation within period ranging from 19 May 2020 to 13 October 2020, in Brazil: **a** Rule 1, **b** Rule 2, **c** Rule 3

that the approach in [70] uses different types of wavelets to process non-stationarity of experimental dataset, it presents competitive results compared to interval type-2 fuzzy Kalman filter, but the performance is slightly inferior due to its computing limitation from determination of the optimal number of nodes in the hidden layer of the WCRVFL network, tuning the scaling of the uniform randomization range for wavelet estimator and accurate data availability.

The approach in [71] is based on the Autoregressive Integrated Moving Average (ARIMA) model for forecasting the

COVID-19 dynamic propagation in Brazil, within the horizon of 77 days. The efficiency of interval type-2 fuzzy Kalman filter, compared to approach in [71], according to MAD (Median Absolute Deviation) and MAPE (Mean Absolute Percentage Error), is shown in Table 3. The approach in [71] is fast in processing speed but presents performance more inferior than interval type-2 fuzzy Kalman filter due to consider only linear characteristics for modeling the COVID-19 dynamic propagation, which tends to increase forecasting errors in the

Table 1 Comparative analysis between the interval type-2 fuzzy Kalman filter and approach in [69] for forecasting the COVID-19 dynamic propagation in Brazil

Methodology	RMSE	MAE	RMSPE
Approach in [69]	3669.000	2533	0.0873
Interval type-2 *fuzzy* Kalman filter	531.472	97	0.0249

Table 2 Comparative analysis between the interval type-2 fuzzy Kalman filter and approach in [70] for forecasting the COVID-19 dynamic propagation in Brazil

Methodology	RMSE	MAE	R^2
Approach in [70]	0.006190	0.004880	0.999450
Interval type-2 *fuzzy* Kalman filter	0.003388	0.000701	0.999677

Table 3 Comparative analysis between the interval type-2 fuzzy Kalman filter and approach in [71] for forecasting the COVID-19 dynamic propagation in Brazil

Methodology	MAD	MAPE (%)
Approach in [71]	33614	3.701
Interval type-2 *fuzzy* Kalman filter	97	0.0025494

time-varying epidemiological data [75]. Differently from the approach in [71], the interval type-2 fuzzy Kalman filter considers a distributed and parallel compensation associated to each interval operating region defined on the experimental dataset for better approximating the time-varying fluctuation of COVID-19 dynamic propagation.

The approach in [72] is based on statistical modeling of daily new cases and daily new deaths caused by COVID-19 using the Weibull probability distribution, for forecasting the COVID-19 dynamic propagation in Brazil. The efficiency of interval type-2 fuzzy Kalman filter, compared to approach in [72], according to the coefficient of determination (R^2), is shown in Table 4. The approach in [72], although uses the Weibull distribution suitable for modeling real-life dataset, it presents slightly inferior results compared to interval type-2 fuzzy Kalman filter once it does not consider the variability in the dynamics of the experimental dataset to update the prop-

agation forecasts of COVID-19 [76]. On the other hand, the interval type-2 fuzzy Kalman filter presents greater efficiency due to its recursive parameterizing mechanism for adaptive tracking and real-time forecasting of the experimental dataset.

The approach in [73] is based on an age-structured SEIR (Susceptible–Exposed–Infectious–Recovered) model for forecasting the COVID-19 dynamic propagation in Brazil. According to approach in [73], the epidemic peak is on 05 June 2020 and the end of COVID-19 outbreak is on 23 July 2020. According to results obtained by interval type-2 fuzzy Kalman filter shown in Fig. 7b, in the same context and dataset used in approach [73], the epidemic peak is on 10 June 2020 and the end of COVID-19 outbreak is on 14 September 2020. The comparative analysis between the interval type-2 fuzzy Kalman filter and approach in [73] is shown in Table 5. The approach in [73], although considers the effect of the age of individuals in mortality rate

Table 4 Comparative analysis between the interval type-2 fuzzy Kalman filter and approach in [72] for forecasting the COVID-19 dynamic propagation in Brazil

Methodology	R^2	
	Daily new cases	Daily new deaths
Approach in [72]	0.87	0.989
Interval type-2 fuzzy Kalman filter	0.9809	0.9984

Table 5 Comparative analysis between the interval type-2 fuzzy Kalman filter and approach in [73] for forecasting the COVID-19 dynamic propagation in Brazil

Methodology	Epidemic peak	End of epidemic
Approach in [73]	05 June 2020	23 July 2020
Interval type-2 fuzzy Kalman filter	10 June 2020	14 September 2020

Table 6 Comparative analysis between the interval type-2 fuzzy Kalman filter and machine learning models LASSO, ARIMA and RNN for forecasting the COVID-19 dynamic propagation in Brazil

Model	RMSE	MAE	R^2
LASSO	191.5600	163.4643	0.7652
ARIMA	203.0832	140.9561	0.368
RNN	116.0065	94.9875	0.829
Interval type-2 *fuzzy* Kalman filter	10.3586	3.9000	0.9984

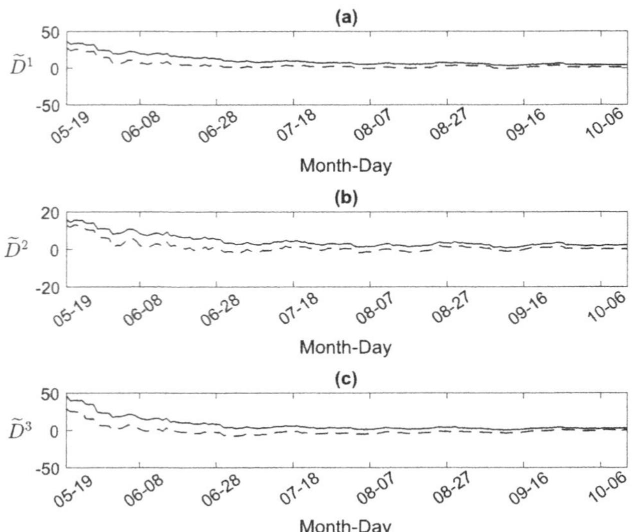

Fig. 12 Recursive estimation of interval type-2 fuzzy matrix $\widetilde{\mathbf{D}}^i$, in tracking and forecasting the COVID-19 dynamic propagation within period ranging from 19 May 2020 to 13 October 2020, in Brazil: **a** Rule 1, **b** Rule 2, **c** Rule 3

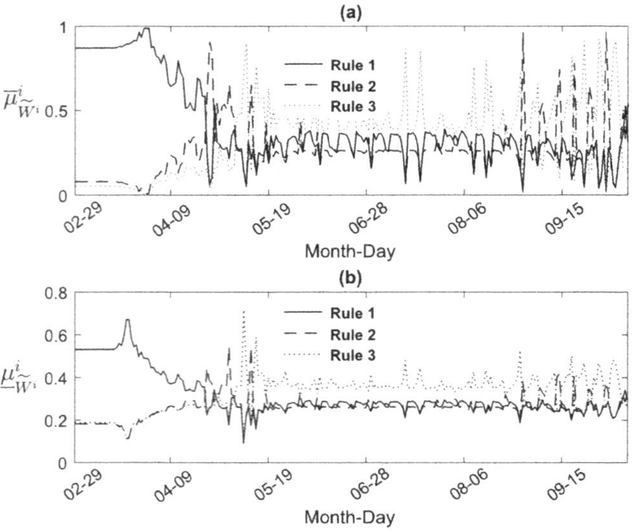

Fig. 13 Activation degrees of type-2 fuzzy Kalman inference system, in tracking and forecasting the COVID-19 dynamic propagation within a period ranging from 29 February 2020 to 13 October, in Brazil: **a** Upper fuzzy activation degrees, **b** Lower fuzzy activation degrees

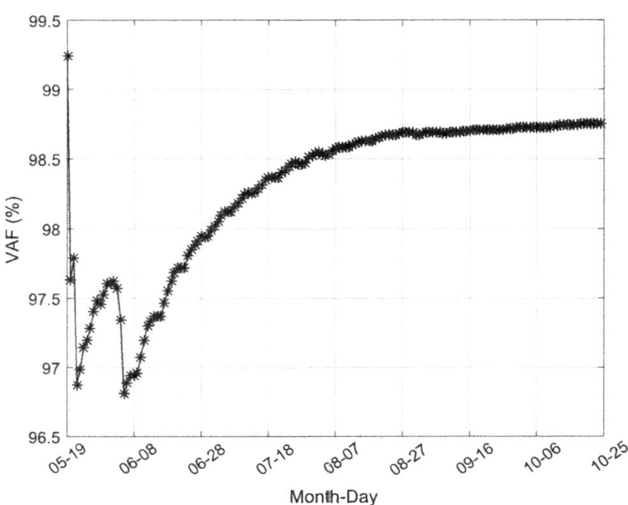

Fig. 14 Efficiency of interval type-2 fuzzy Kalman filter, in tracking and forecasting the COVID-19 dynamic propagation within a period ranging from 19 May to 25 October 2020

by COVID-19 for better suitability of the SEIR model, it presents low efficiency compared to the interval type-2 fuzzy Kalman filter once it does not considers the uncertainties in the experimental dataset and assumes a transmission rate of COVID-19 constant throughout the period of pandemic [77]. The interval type-2 fuzzy Kalman filter is more predictive to the real behavior of epidemiological dataset in Brazil than the approach in [73], due to its interval adaptive similarity measure to define interval operating fuzzy regions that best represent the dynamics and uncertainties of the dataset.

The comparative analysis between the interval type-2 fuzzy Kalman filter and the machine learning models LASSO, ARIMA, RNN, for forecasting the COVID-19 dynamic propagation in Brazil, within the horizon of 10 days, is shown in the Table 6. The machine learning model LASSO, although increases the model interpretability by eliminating irrelevant variables that are not associated to the COVID-19 dynamic propagation, it can allow to biased parametric estimations and, in consequence, an inferior performance compared to interval type-2 fuzzy Kalman filter [78]. The machine learning model ARIMA is fast in processing speed but it can lead to inaccurate estimations once it does not consider the non-stationarity correlated to the experimental dataset which causes its inferior performance compared to interval type-2 fuzzy Kalman filter [79]. The machine learning model RNN is capable to provide accurate estimations with the limitation of does not consider the uncertainties inherent to COVID-19 dynamic propagation that results in an inferior performance compared to interval type-2 fuzzy Kalman filter [79]. On the other hand, the uncertainties inherent to the experimental dataset are processed by the interval type-2 fuzzy Kalman filter through approximating the dynamic behavior in interval fuzzy operating regions defined on the dynamic fluctuations of the propagation of COVID-19, providing a reduction in tracking and forecasting errors.

A possible limitation of the interval type-2 fuzzy Kalman filter is the determination of some parameters (γ, β and q) for parametric estimation of its consequent proposition, which requires some intuition by experts and depends on the experimental dataset.

4   Conclusion

The results shown the applicability of machine learning approach based on interval type-2 fuzzy Kalman filter due to its recursive updating mechanism, for adaptive tracking and real-time forecasting COVID-19 dynamic propagation. For further works, the formulation and applicability of the proposed methodology in the context of evolving interval type-2 fuzzy systems is of particular interest.

Acknowledgements This work was developed in Computational Intelligence Applied to Technology Laboratory at the Federal Institute of Education, Science and Technology of Maranhão.The authors are grateful to Coordination for the Improvement of Higher Education Personnel (CAPES) for financial support and to the Graduate Program in Electrical Engineering at Federal University of Maranhão (PPGEE-UFMA) for their support in the development of this research.

References

[1] W. Mack and E. A. P. Habets, "Deep filtering: Signal extraction and reconstruction using complex time-frequency filters," *IEEE Signal Processing Letters*, vol. 27, pp. 61–65, 2020.

[2] R. Gomez-Garcia, L. Yang, J.-M. Munoz-Ferreras, and W. Feng, "Lossy signal-interference filters and applications," *IEEE Transactions on Microwave Theory and Techniques*, vol. 68, no. 2, pp. 516–529, feb 2020.

[3] W. Liu, Y. Liu, and R. Bucknall, "A robust localization method for unmanned surface vehicle (USV) navigation using fuzzy adaptive kalman filtering," *IEEE Access*, vol. 7, pp. 46 071–46 083, 2019.

[4] X. Zhu, T. Wang, Y. Bao, F. Hu, and S. Li, "Signal detection in generalized gaussian distribution noise with nakagami fading channel," *IEEE Access*, vol. 7, pp. 23 120–23 126, 2019.

[5] R. E. Kalman, "A new approach to linear filtering and prediction problems," *Journal of Basic Engineering*, vol. 82, no. 1, pp. 35–45, mar 1960.

[6] G. L. O. Serra, Ed., *Kalman Filters - Theory for Advanced Applications*. InTech, feb 2018.

[7] Z.-P. Wang and H.-N. Wu, "Robust guaranteed cost sampled-data fuzzy control for uncertain nonlinear time-delay systems," *IEEE Transactions on Systems, Man, and Cybernetics: Systems*, vol. 49, no. 5, pp. 964–975, may 2019.

[8] C. S. Chin and W. P. Lin, "Robust genetic algorithm and fuzzy inference mechanism embedded in a sliding-mode controller for an uncertain underwater robot," *IEEE/ASME Transactions on Mechatronics*, vol. 23, no. 2, pp. 655–666, apr 2018.

[9] H. J. Kim, J. B. Park, and Y. H. Joo, "Decentralized h_∞ sampled-data fuzzy filter for nonlinear interconnected oscillating systems with uncertain interconnections," *IEEE Transactions on Fuzzy Systems*, vol. 28, no. 3, pp. 487–498, mar 2020.

[10] J. Zhao and C.-M. Lin, "Wavelet-TSK-type fuzzy cerebellar model neural network for uncertain nonlinear systems," *IEEE Transactions on Fuzzy Systems*, vol. 27, no. 3, pp. 549–558, mar 2019.

[11] J. Khodaei-Mehr, S. Tangestanizadeh, R. Vatankhah, and M. Sharifi, "Optimal neuro-fuzzy control of hepatitis c virus integrated by genetic algorithm," *IET Systems Biology*, vol. 12, no. 4, pp. 154–161, aug 2018.

[12] T. D. Pham and K. Berger, "Automated detection of white matter changes in elderly people using fuzzy, geostatistical, and information combining models," *IEEE Transactions on Information Technology in Biomedicine*, vol. 15, no. 2, pp. 242–250, mar 2011.

[13] G. L. O. Serra, Ed., *Frontiers in Advanced Control Systems*. InTech, jul 2012.

[14] A. P. F. Evangelista and G. L. O. Serra, "Multivariable state-space recursive identification algorithm based on evolving type-2 neural-fuzzy inference system," *Journal of Control, Automation and Electrical Systems*, vol. 30, no. 6, pp. 921–942, oct 2019.

[15] J. M. Mendel, "Comparing the performance potentials of interval and general type-2 rule-based fuzzy systems in terms of sculpting the state space," *IEEE Transactions on Fuzzy Systems*, vol. 27, no. 1, pp. 58–71, jan 2019.

[16] Q. Liang and J. Mendel, "Interval type-2 fuzzy logic systems: theory and design," *IEEE Transactions on Fuzzy Systems*, vol. 8, no. 5, pp. 535–550, 2000.

[17] S. Ryu and B. C. Chun, "An interim review of the epidemiological characteristics of 2019 novel coronavirus," *Epidemiology and Health*, vol. 42, p. e2020006, feb 2020.

[18] S. Ryu and B. C. Chun, "Controlling the spread of covid-19 at ground crossings," World Health Organization, Tech. Rep., 2020. [Online]. Available: https://www.who.int/.

[19] S. Ryu and B. C. Chun, "Infection prevention and control for the safe management of a dead body in the context of covid-19: interim guidance," World Health Organization, Tech. Rep., 2020. [Online]. Available: https://www.who.int/.

[20] I. Chakraborty and P. Maity, "COVID-19 outbreak: Migration, effects on society, global environment and prevention," *Science of The Total Environment*, vol. 728, p. 138882, aug 2020.

[21] Y. Feng, Y. Ling, T. Bai, Y. Xie, J. Huang, J. Li, W. Xiong, D. Yang, R. Chen, F. Lu, Y. Lu, X. Liu, Y. Chen, X. Li, Y. Li, H. D. Summah, H. Lin, J. Yan, M. Zhou, H. Lu, and J. Qu, "COVID-19 with different severities: A multicenter study of clinical features," *American Journal of Respiratory and Critical Care Medicine*, vol. 201, no. 11, pp. 1380–1388, jun 2020.

[22] S. Fishbane and J. S. Hirsch, "Erythropoiesis-stimulating agent treatment in patients with COVID-19," *American Journal of Kidney Diseases*, may 2020.

[23] N. Sun, L. Wei, S. Shi, D. Jiao, R. Song, L. Ma, H. Wang, C. Wang, Z. Wang, Y. You, S. Liu, and H. Wang, "A qualitative study on the psychological experience of caregivers of COVID-19 patients,"

American Journal of Infection Control, vol. 48, no. 6, pp. 592–598, jun 2020.

[24] S. M. Brown, I. D. Peltan, B. Webb, N. Kumar, N. Starr, C. Grissom, W. R. Buckel, R. Srivastava, E. S. Harris, L. Leither, S. A. Johnson, R. Paine, and T. Greene, "Hydroxychloroquine vs. azithromycin for hospitalized patients with suspected or confirmed COVID-19 (HAHPS): Protocol for a pragmatic, open label, active comparator trial," *Annals of the American Thoracic Society*, may 2020.

[25] Y. Huang, S. Chen, Z. Yang, W. Guan, D. Liu, Z. Lin, Y. Zhang, Z. Xu, X. Liu, and Y. Li, "SARS-CoV-2 viral load in clinical samples from critically ill patients," *American Journal of Respiratory and Critical Care Medicine*, vol. 201, no. 11, pp. 1435–1438, jun 2020.

[26] H. Kang, L. Xia, F. Yan, Z. Wan, F. Shi, H. Yuan, H. Jiang, D. Wu, H. Sui, C. Zhang, and D. Shen, "Diagnosis of coronavirus disease 2019 (COVID-19) with structured latent multi-view representation learning," *IEEE Transactions on Medical Imaging*, pp. 1–1, 2020.

[27] F. Deeba, M. S. H. Haider, A. Ahmed, A. Tazeen, M. I. Faizan, N. Salam, T. Hussain, S. F. Alamery, and S. Parveen, "Global transmission and evolutionary dynamics of the chikungunya virus," *Epidemiology and Infection*, vol. 148, 2020.

[28] O. H. Price, S. G. Sullivan, C. Sutterby, J. Druce, and K. S. Carville, "Using routine testing data to understand circulation patterns of influenza a, respiratory syncytial virus and other respiratory viruses in victoria, australia," *Epidemiology and Infection*, vol. 147, 2019.

[29] M. R. Korcinska, K. D. Bjerre, L. D. Rasmussen, E. T. Jensen, T. K. Fischer, A. Barrasa, and S. Ethelberg, "Detection of norovirus infections in denmark, 2011–2018," *Epidemiology and Infection*, vol. 148, 2020.

[30] Y. Chen, K. Leng, Y. Lu, L. Wen, Y. Qi, W. Gao, H. Chen, L. Bai, X. An, B. Sun, P. Wang, and J. Dong, "Epidemiological features and time-series analysis of influenza incidence in urban and rural areas of shenyang, china, 2010–2018," *Epidemiology and Infection*, vol. 148, 2020.

[31] R. D. van Gaalen, J. van de Kassteele, S. J. M. Hahné, P. Bruijning-Verhagen, and J. Wallinga, "Determinants of rotavirus transmission," *Epidemiology*, vol. 28, no. 4, pp. 503–513, jul 2017.

[32] C. Sloan, R. Chandrasekhar, E. Mitchel, D. Ndi, L. Miller, A. Thomas, N. M. Bennett, S. Chai, M. Spencer, S. Eckel, N. Spina, M. Monroe, E. J. Anderson, R. Lynfield, K. Yousey-Hindes, M. Bargsten, S. Zansky, K. Lung, M. Schroeder, C. N. Cummings, S. Garg, W. Schaffner, and M. L. Lindegren, "Spatial and temporal clustering of patients hospitalized with laboratory-confirmed influenza in the united states," *Epidemics*, vol. 31, p. 100387, jun 2020.

[33] J. van de Kassteele, P. H. C. Eilers, and J. Wallinga, "Nowcasting the number of new symptomatic cases during infectious disease outbreaks using constrained p-spline smoothing," *Epidemiology*, vol. 30, no. 5, pp. 737–745, sep 2019.

[34] G. Chowell, R. Luo, K. Sun, K. Roosa, A. Tariq, and C. Viboud, "Real-time forecasting of epidemic trajectories using computational dynamic ensembles," *Epidemics*, vol. 30, p. 100379, mar 2020.

[35] D. S. Pires and G. L. O. Serra, "Methodology for evolving fuzzy kalman filter identification," *International Journal of Control, Automation and Systems*, vol. 17, no. 3, pp. 793–800, feb 2019.

[36] I. Eyoh, R. John, G. D. Maere, and E. Kayacan, "Hybrid learning for interval type-2 intuitionistic fuzzy logic systems as applied to identification and prediction problems," *IEEE Transactions on Fuzzy Systems*, vol. 26, no. 5, pp. 2672–2685, oct 2018.

[37] P. Gil, T. Oliveira, and L. Palma, "Adaptive neuro–fuzzy control for discrete-time nonaffine nonlinear systems," *IEEE Transactions on Fuzzy Systems*, vol. 27, no. 8, pp. 1602–1615, aug 2019.

[38] M. Bouhentala, M. Ghanai, and K. Chafaa, "Interval-valued membership function estimation for fuzzy modeling," *Fuzzy Sets and Systems*, vol. 361, pp. 101–113, apr 2019.

[39] C.-L. Hwang, H.-M. Wu, and J.-Y. Lai, "On-line obstacle detection, avoidance, and mapping of an outdoor quadrotor using EKF-based fuzzy tracking incremental control," *IEEE Access*, vol. 7, pp. 160 203–160 216, 2019.

[40] X. Wang, Z. Xu, X. Gou, and L. Trajkovic, "Tracking a maneuvering target by multiple sensors using extended kalman filter with nested probabilistic-numerical linguistic information," *IEEE Transactions on Fuzzy Systems*, vol. 28, no. 2, pp. 346–360, feb 2020.

[41] R. M. Asl, R. Palm, H. Wu, and H. Handroos, "Fuzzy-based parameter optimization of adaptive unscented kalman filter: Methodology and experimental validation," *IEEE Access*, vol. 8, pp. 54 887–54 904, 2020.

[42] F. Matía, V. Jiménez, B. P. Alvarado, and R. Haber, "The fuzzy kalman filter: Improving its implementation by reformulating uncertainty representation," *Fuzzy Sets and Systems*, nov 2019.

[43] S. Yang, B. Deng, J. Wang, C. Liu, H. Li, Q. Lin, C. Fietkiewicz, and K. A. Loparo, "Design of hidden-property-based variable universe fuzzy control for movement disorders and its efficient reconfigurable implementation," *IEEE Transactions on Fuzzy Systems*, vol. 27, no. 2, pp. 304–318, feb 2019.

[44] A. Rajaei, A. Vahidi-Moghaddam, A. Chizfahm, and M. Sharifi, "Control of malaria outbreak using a non-linear robust strategy with adaptive gains," *IET Control Theory & Applications*, vol. 13, no. 14, pp. 2308–2317, sep 2019.

[45] N. J. Watkins, C. Nowzari, and G. J. Pappas, "Robust economic model predictive control of continuous-time epidemic processes," *IEEE Transactions on Automatic Control*, vol. 65, no. 3, pp. 1116–1131, mar 2020.

[46] D. P. Martins, M. T. Barros, M. Pierobon, M. Kandhavelu, P. Lio, and S. Balasubramaniam, "Computational models for trapping ebola virus using engineered bacteria," *IEEE/ACM Transactions on Computational Biology and Bioinformatics*, vol. 15, no. 6, pp. 2017–2027, nov 2018.

[47] D. He, X. Wang, D. Gao, and J. Wang, "Modeling the 2016–2017 yemen cholera outbreak with the impact of limited medical resources," *Journal of Theoretical Biology*, vol. 451, pp. 80–85, aug 2018.

[48] R. X. Weng, H. L. Fu, C. L. Zhang, J. B. Ye, F. C. Hong, X. S. Chen, and Y. M. Cai, "Time series analysis and forecasting of chlamydia trachomatis incidence using surveillance data from 2008 to 2019 in shenzhen, china," *Epidemiology and Infection*, vol. 148, 2020.

[49] I. S. Koolhof, K. B. Gibney, S. Bettiol, M. Charleston, A. Wiethoelter, A.-L. Arnold, P. T. Campbell, P. J. Neville, P. Aung, T. Shiga, S. Carver, and S. M. Firestone, "The forecasting of dynamical ross river virus outbreaks: Victoria, australia," *Epidemics*, vol. 30, p. 100377, mar 2020.

[50] C. R. Hranac, J. C. Marshall, A. Monadjem, and D. T. Hayman, "Predicting ebola virus disease risk and the role of african bat birthing," *Epidemics*, vol. 29, p. 100366, dec 2019.

[51] T. Stocks, L. J. Martin, S. Kühlmann-Berenzon, and T. Britton, "Dynamic modeling of hepatitis c transmission among people who inject drugs," *Epidemics*, vol. 30, p. 100378, mar 2020.

[52] L. Zhong, L. Mu, J. Li, J. Wang, Z. Yin, and D. Liu, "Early prediction of the 2019 novel coronavirus outbreak in the mainland china based on simple mathematical model," *IEEE Access*, vol. 8, pp. 51 761–51 769, 2020.

[53] Q. Lin, S. Zhao, D. Gao, Y. Lou, S. Yang, S. S. Musa, M. H. Wang, Y. Cai, W. Wang, L. Yang, and D. He, "A conceptual model for the coronavirus disease 2019 (COVID-19) outbreak in wuhan, china with individual reaction and governmental action," *International Journal of Infectious Diseases*, vol. 93, pp. 211–216, apr 2020.

[54] M. H. Mohd and F. Sulayman, "Unravelling the myths of r0 in controlling the dynamics of COVID-19 outbreak: A modelling perspective," *Chaos, Solitons & Fractals*, vol. 138, p. 109943, sep 2020.

[55] X. Duan and X. Zhang, "ARIMA modelling and forecasting of irregularly patterned COVID-19 outbreaks using japanese and south korean data," *Data in Brief*, vol. 31, p. 105779, aug 2020.

[56] N. Chintalapudi, G. Battineni, and F. Amenta, "COVID-19 virus outbreak forecasting of registered and recovered cases after sixty day lockdown in italy: A data driven model approach," *Journal of Microbiology, Immunology and Infection*, vol. 53, no. 3, pp. 396–403, jun 2020.

[57] H. B. Fredj and F. Chrif, "Novel corona virus disease infection in tunisia: Mathematical model and the impact of the quarantine strategy," *Chaos, Solitons & Fractals*, p. 109969, jun 2020.

[58] S. Kim, Y. B. Seo, and E. Jung, "Prediction of COVID-19 transmission dynamics using a mathematical model considering behavior changes," *Epidemiology and Health*, p. e2020026, apr 2020.

[59] S. W. Park, D. M. Cornforth, J. Dushoff, and J. S. Weitz, "The time scale of asymptomatic transmission affects estimates of epidemic potential in the COVID-19 outbreak," *Epidemics*, vol. 31, p. 100392, jun 2020.

[60] K. Kanagarathinam and K. Sekar, "Estimation of reproduction number (ro) and early prediction of 2019 novel coronavirus disease (COVID-19) outbreak in india using statistical computing approach," *Epidemiology and Health*, p. e2020028, may 2020.

[61] F. Rustam, A. A. Reshi, A. Mehmood, S. Ullah, B. On, W. Aslam, and G. S. Choi, "COVID-19 future forecasting using supervised machine learning models," *IEEE Access*, pp. 1–1, 2020.

[62] Z. Zhao, X. Li, F. Liu, G. Zhu, C. Ma, and L. Wang, "Prediction of the COVID-19 spread in african countries and implications for prevention and control: A case study in south africa, egypt, algeria, nigeria, senegal and kenya," *Science of The Total Environment*, vol. 729, p. 138959, aug 2020.

[63] N. Piovella, "Analytical solution of SEIR model describing the free spread of the COVID-19 pandemic," *Chaos, Solitons & Fractals*, vol. 140, p. 110243, nov 2020.

[64] R. Takele, "Stochastic modelling for predicting COVID-19 prevalence in east africa countries," *Infectious Disease Modelling*, vol. 5, pp. 598–607, 2020.

[65] C. A. Varotsos and V. F. Krapivin, "A new model for the spread of COVID-19 and the improvement of safety," *Safety Science*, vol. 132, p. 104962, dec 2020.

[66] J. B. Elsner, "Analysis of time series structure: SSA and related techniques," *Journal of the American Statistical Association*, vol. 97, no. 460, pp. 1207–1208, dec 2002.

[67] R. Babuska, *Fuzzy Modeling for Control*. Springer, 1998.

[68] J. N. Juang, *Applied System Identification*. Prentice Hall, 1994.

[69] N. Feroze, "Forecasting the patterns of COVID-19 and causal impacts of lockdown in top five affected countries using bayesian structural time series models," *Chaos, Solitons & Fractals*, vol. 140, p. 110196, nov 2020.

[70] B. B. Hazarika and D. Gupta, "Modelling and forecasting of COVID-19 spread using wavelet-coupled random vector functional link networks," *Applied Soft Computing*, vol. 96, p. 106626, nov 2020.

[71] A. K. Sahai, N. Rath, V. Sood, and M. P. Singh, "ARIMA modelling & forecasting of COVID-19 in top five affected countries," *Diabetes & Metabolic Syndrome: Clinical Research & Reviews*, vol. 14, no. 5, pp. 1419–1427, sep 2020.

[72] V. H. Moreau, "Forecast predictions for the COVID-19 pandemic in brazil by statistical modeling using the weibull distribution for daily new cases and deaths," *Brazilian Journal of Microbiology*, vol. 51, no. 3, pp. 1109–1115, aug 2020.

[73] S. Djilali and B. Ghanbari, "Coronavirus pandemic: A predictive analysis of the peak outbreak epidemic in south africa, turkey, and brazil," *Chaos, Solitons & Fractals*, vol. 138, p. 109971, sep 2020.

[74] J. O. Berger, *Statistical Decision Theory and Bayesian Analysis*. Springer New York, 1993.

[75] G. Zhang, "Time series forecasting using a hybrid ARIMA and neural network model," *Neurocomputing*, vol. 50, pp. 159–175, jan 2003.

[76] C.-D. Lai, D. Murthy, and M. Xie, "Weibull distributions and their applications," in *Springer Handbook of Engineering Statistics*. Springer London, 2006.

[77] M. Martcheva, *An Introduction to Mathematical Epidemiology*. Springer US, 2015.

[78] R. H. Shumway and D. S. Stoffer, *Time Series Analysis and Its Applications*. Springer New York, 2000.

[79] C. M. Bishop, *Pattern Recognition and Machine Learning*. Springer, 2006.

Heart Failure Occurrence: Mining Significant Patterns and 10 Days Early Prediction

Jad Eid, Georges Badr, Amir Hajjam El Hassani,
and Emmanuel Andres

Abstract

Electronic health records containing patient's medical history, drug prescription, vital signs measurements, and many more parameters, are being frequently extracted and stored as unused raw data. On the other hand, machine learning and data mining techniques are becoming popular in the medical field, providing the ability to extract knowledge and valuable information from electronic health records along with accurately predicting future disease occurrence. This chapter presents a study on medical data containing vital signs recorded over the course of some years, for real patients suffering from heart failure. The first significant patterns that come along with heart failure occurrence are extracted and examined using data mining techniques that have already proven to be effective. In this study, FP-GROWTH and RULEGROWTH algorithms are employed to discover the most influencing patterns and series of vital signs recordings leading to a possible heart failure risk. Finally, as a first contribution, Long short-term memory (LSTM) recurrent neural network is used to predict a possible heart failure risk within a window of 10-days in the future, with 76% of correct predictions.

J. Eid · G. Badr (✉)
TICKET Lab, Antonine University, Hadat, Baabda, Lebanon
e-mail: georges.badr@ua.edu.lb

J. Eid
e-mail: eng.jad.eid@gmail.com

A. Hajjam El Hassani
Nanomedicine Lab, Université de Bourgogne Franche - Comté,
UTBM, Belfort, France
e-mail: amir.hajjam-el-hassani@utbm.fr

E. Andres
Université de Strasbourg, Centre Hospitalier Universitaire, Strasbourg,
France
e-mail: emmanuel.andres@chru-strasbourg.fr

1　Introduction

According to the world health care organization, 17.9 million people die yearly from cardiovascular diseases, making 30% of the total deaths around the globe. Cardiovascular diseases, more specifically heart failure causes a large number of deaths around the world. It occurs when the heart cannot pump enough blood to the parts of the body. Patients may develop several symptoms including dyspnea, fatigue, weight gaining because of fluid retention, and many more. Some Daily activities become more difficult, along with organs dysfunction such as kidney failure. Life- threatening complications may persist after being exposed to heart failure and patients with a heart failure condition have a short lifespan and are regularly hospitalized. In fact, researchers found that usually life expectancy of near half of patients diagnosed with heart failure is barely five years down to one year for advanced heart failure forms.

The process of diagnosing heart failure usually includes a review of the patient's medical history, symptoms, and risk factors along with a physical examination. Practitioners also may look for certain blood tests, heart electrical activity using electrocardiogram test, and monitoring heart response to an effort by performing the stress test. A classification of the heart failure risk is performed using two systems: the symptom-based New York Heart Association classification (NYHA), or the phase-based American College of Cardiology/American Heart Association guidelines (ACC/AHA). Each of these scoring models defines four heart failure classes. Determining a heart failure risk will lead to the most appropriate medical prescription.

Nowadays, large amounts of medical data are collected from patients. At the same time, machine learning artificial intelligence is merging in the medical field, proving some

© Springer Nature Switzerland AG 2021
J. Alja'am et al. (eds.), *Emerging Technologies in Biomedical Engineering and Sustainable TeleMedicine*,
Advances in Science, Technology & Innovation, https://doi.org/10.1007/978-3-030-14647-4_8

promising results. Applications vary from predicting, classifying, and mining significant knowledge from gathered electronic health records. The result of combining medical data with artificial intelligence and data mining techniques can be used to provide practitioners with meaningful insights to understand heart failure's most influencing risk factors. It also helps predict heart failure future occurrences, therefore, increasing patients' lifestyle by planning effective treatments, and preventing hospital readmission.

This chapter aims to reveal the most significant patterns and association rules standing behind heart failure risk classification. Data mining approaches are applied on electronic health records containing multiple vital signs gathered from real patients suffering from heart failure. Different patterns and association rules are further elaborated using the FP-GROWTH algorithm. Next, interdependencies between different clinical measurements of patients are extracted and presented using the RULE GROWTH algorithm. Finally, a time-series forecasting method based on long short-term memory recurrent neural networks is used to analyze sequences of historical medical records to predict the heart failure occurrence risk in a window of 10 days in the future. Risks will be classified as no risk, moderate, or high risk.

2 Literature Review

This section elaborates previous works done including heart disease occurrence predictions using machine learning techniques, then pattern and sequence extraction using data mining techniques. Finally, early predictions with time-series data and deep neural networks are presented.

2.1 Heart Diseases Classification

Many applications use decision trees to predict and classify patients suffering from heart disease, authors in [1] extracted significant patterns using CART classifier after preprocessing the data to remove uncertainty. Extracted patterns are used later for heart disease prediction. In [2], authors tested CART, Iterative Dichotomized 3 (ID3), and decision trees on the Cleveland Heart Disease Dataset (CHDD). The performance of each algorithm was tested based on precision true positive and true negative. Again CART has proved to have more accuracy.

To classify heart failure risk levels, authors in [3] gathered data from the Cleveland dataset and then enriched it with 3 new risk factor features that may cause higher heart failure risk with a total of 297 instances in the dataset. Using C4.5 decision trees, the model was built, achieved 86.53% accuracy classifying true risk levels.

In [4], researchers proposed the use of support vector machines SVM, to build a scoring model to help with heart failure diagnostic. This study aims to classify three HF classes: healthy group, heart failure prone group, and the heart failure group. First of all, medical records were collected from Zhejiang Hospital, missing values are handled using Bayesian principal component analysis which is reliable. Two SVM models were used along with a decision tree system for classification. Results show an accuracy of 87.5% for HF-prone group, 65% for HF group, and 78.79% for healthy groups (testing on 90 samples).

ECG[1] is the process of detecting heart electrical activity at rest. Physicians use these records in order to identify high risk factors of heart diseases.

In order to detect Congestive Heart Failure (CHF), several machine learning techniques in [5] were applied to ECG records that record heartbeat signals and might show some irregularities. Data were collected from several databases including both genders from different age trunks. The next step was feature extraction using Burg method for autoregressive parameter estimation. Several machine learning techniques are used to evaluate the CHT classification system, mainly Random forest outperformed the support vector machine, C4.5 decision tree, K-NN (K nearest neighbor), and neural networks, and reached 100% of accuracy classifying congestive heart failure, cases.

In [6], high and low-risk congestive heart failure patients are classified using heart rate variability measures and ECG records. Data is gathered from the BIDMC and Congestive Heart Failure RR Interval Database, some data preprocessing was done including sampling. The model was built using the CART algorithm and achieved 85.4% accuracy in grouping patient's risk.

Another experimentation was conducted in [7] on a dataset containing 13 attributes. The authors added two more attributes that are directly connected with heart diseases: obesity and smoking. They used three data classification techniques in order to build a heart disease prediction system. Data preprocessing including replacing missing values and splitting data to train and test was made. Neural networks provided more accurate classification results than Decision trees and Naïve Bayes techniques.

2.2 Frequent Itemset Mining

With the appearance of many data mining techniques, knowledge discovery and extracting significant information from the data is now possible. Nowadays these methods are used for identifying frequent item sets, especially when mining medical records.

Data mining algorithms are used for extracting frequent and significant itemsets and patterns, especially when mining

---

[1] Electrocardiogram.

medical records. Many surveys discussed sequential pattern mining, in [8]. This paper discussed the previous existing algorithms and the dataset types suitable for their application. After that, many temporal and time-dependent sequences like searching for events that occur simultaneously such as pattern-growth algorithm have been discussed, to end with incremental algorithms.

Another survey [9], also discussed recent sequential pattern mining and its applications. First, the sequential mining is discussed along with its various applications, while enumerating and explaining breadth-first and depth-first algorithms such as GSP, SPADE, SPAM, and many others. After that, the authors discussed the variations of the sequential pattern mining problems including closed sequential patterns, association rule mining, episode mining, and many others.

In [10], frequent itemsets are extracted to help with the early heart disease diagnostic. First specific symptoms are chosen and a minimum support value is set. After that frequent itemsets are generated and used in the heart disease risk evaluation, a dataset of 1000 patients suffering from heart problems was used and the results were encouraging.

Researchers in [11] applied the Apriori algorithm on a dataset of 1216 patients affected by diverse diseases. Association rules are mined from the dataset to detect disease frequency for these patients. Results could help doctors to make decisions and diagnose disease.

Knowledge extraction was also studied in [12] using Apriori, predictive-apriori, and tetrius algorithms. Different association rules leading to heart diseases for males and females are extracted. The approach was applied on the UCI Cleveland dataset [13], results identified many significant risk factors for both males and women.

Many diseases may be seen as an association of multiple symptoms, especially for coronary vascular disease (CVD). In [14] authors had a dataset of 1897 patients for each, 21 features are presented. The goal was to find strong associations among attributes. First, the dataset numerical attributes were transformed into intervals mapped into an object. After that categorical values are encoded to numerical ones. Valid association rules are generated and many attributes proved a strong association with CVD.

2.3   Time-Series Forecasting

Time-series data is a group of data points, captured over time. Let $x(t)$ be a variable that varies over time and $t = 0, 1, \ldots n$ indicates the total time passed. Therefore, the total sequences of $x(t)$ indicate the time series with a chronological order over time. The term univariate characterizes a time series that records the values of a single variable. Whereas multivariate specifies a time-series recording multiple variables over time.

Observations recorded on every time step t form a continuous time series, while recording observations over dis-continued chunks of time indicates discrete time series. In this project, univariate time series is used. Time-series analysis and forecasting serve nowadays in many domains, such as weather forecasts for the future, stock market predictions, and even health applications.

In [15] authors simulated a telehealth care scenario within an elderly environment. They created artificial scenarios such as daily diastolic blood pressure variations. ARIMA[2] model was applied, and near future diastolic pressure values were predicted with 91% accuracy.

Many prediction problems are solved using deep learning and recurrent neural networks like LSTM[3] networks. In [16], authors used LSTM to predict traffic flow in a real-time application scenario. The data used is a time-series data, collected every 30 s. Predictions were done for the upcoming data collected every 5 min. Compared to ARIMA, LSTM had a better performance.

2.4   LSTM Neural Networks

Many prediction problems are mapped with the Long Short term memory (LSTM) solution that has many applications, but none has mentioned predicting heart failure risk. Our solution is based on LSTM.

In [17], another real-time application for LSTM is proposed. The travel time from a start point to an end point was predicted. Since travel time is usually irregular, the authors decided to use LSTM rather than ARIMA which consists of a linear model. Data is provided by Highways England and it contains travel information of 66 highway links. The goal of this paper is to predict multiple-step ahead for each link. After training the model, multi-step ahead travel time predictions were performed. The 1-step ahead prediction shows a relatively small error. A 7.0% of median of the mean relative error was observed.

3   Methods

This work has mainly two objectives:

1. Significant patterns extraction via data mining techniques.
2. Early heart failure detection using LSTM neural networks.

The early heart failure model uses historical records that will be mapped as time-series data, about patients already diagnosed with heart failure. Before applying any method, data preprocessing and dataset enriching is required.

---

[2]AutoRegressive Moving Average.

[3]Long Short term memory.

3.1 Data Overview

Daily medical data observations for 31 real patients suffering from heart failure are gathered over few years making a total of 3568 records. For each observation, five basic vital signs presented in Table 1 are retrieved and stored as electronic health records in 31 CSV files, one for each patient containing the corresponding measurements.

3.2 Dataset Enriching

Data cleansing is performed to prevent data inconsistency and improve models and data mining accuracy the following steps are applied on every CSV file:

- Insure that the five basic parameters exist.
- Removing duplicated data points.
- Handling missing and null values.
- Checking that data has correct formats.

The next step is to enrich the dataset with 16 additional columns, including:

- Δ_i PAS/PAD/FC/O2/POIDS: Percentage difference for each vital sign on one, three, and seven days, therefore, adding 15 new columns.
- Risk class: Heart failure classes in Table 2 are determined based on a sheet provided by a medical expert, indicating for each parameter variation a possible heart failure class.

To detect heart failure class, we wrote a JAVA code, that reads the CSV files, calculates the day difference parameters. Next, we will find the heart failure class based on a sheet provided by a medical expert, that indicated for each parameter variation a possible heart failure class.

4 Mining Significant Patterns

The first method aims to identify frequent patterns and association rules occurring along with corresponding itemsets. The extracted patterns will be used later to reveal the most influencing patterns leading to determine the heart failure risk class. Before proceeding to implementation, additional data transformation and preprocessing is required.

Following are the algorithms used:

- FP-GROWTH for mining frequent itemsets and association rules.
- RULEGROWTH algorithm to mine sequential patterns taking into consideration an ordering factor.

4.1 Data Discretization

First of all, we have collected all of our 31 CSV files and made a new dataset containing records of all patients making a total of 3568 rows of observations. This new file will be used to mine the frequent patterns.

After observing our data, we can see that each column contains a large number of different values. For example, the 7 days difference of systolic blood pressure noted as Δ_7PAS, contains 1268 unique values, and the 7 days heart rate difference column Δ_7FC, contains 916 unique values. Therefore, in order to increase the frequency of each item/value to appear, we proposed a data transformation.

To increase the chance of mining significant itemsets, a data transformation is performed as mentioned in [14]. The transformation consists of assigning each numerical data point to a specific categorical range. These categorical ranges are defined based on a medical sheet provided by the medical expert. Figure 1 represents a chunk of the original dataset, while Fig. 2 illustrates the chunk after transformation.

4.2 Algorithms

Let X$\Rightarrow$Y be a rule with a support indicating the count of X (antecedent) and Y (consequent) in the same transaction. The confidence, indicating how often this rule is found true, is calculated as support$(X \cup Y)$/support(Y).

We should note that X$\Rightarrow$Y, is not always true even if the confidence is high, it depends on X and Y. The reason is that the standard algorithm does not take into consideration the items ordered. This problem will be solved in the second implemented algorithm. The consequent item that we are targeting is the heart failure class, and the antecedent items might be any parameter that is leading to the heart failure occurrence.

D1Poids	D1PAS	D1PAD
0	0	0
0	3.45	10.61
0.6	1.79	5.08

Fig. 1 Original dataset

D1PoidsN	D1PasN	D1PadN
0.0 <= D1Poids < 2	0.0 <= D1PAS < 10	0.0 <= D1PAD < 10
0.0 <= D1Poids < 2	0.0 <= D1PAS < 10	10 <= D1PAD < 20.0
0.0 <= D1Poids < 2	0.0 <= D1PAS < 10	0.0 <= D1PAD < 10

Fig. 2 Transformed dataset

Table 1 Vital signs captured

Sign	Measure unit
PAS: systolic blood pressure	mmHg
PAD: diastolic blood pressure	mmHg
FC: heart rate	Beats per minute
O2: blood oxygen saturation	Percentage %
POIDS: weight	Kilogram

Table 2 Heart failure classes

Classes	Risk
Blue	Low
Orange	Possible
Red	High

FP-Growth

Frequent-pattern tree noted as FP-growth [18], is an efficient way to mine frequent patterns with specified minimum pattern support and confidence in a transaction dataset.

Comparing to a traditional algorithm for mining frequent itemsets like the Apriori algorithm which requires n+1 dataset scans where n is the length of the longest pattern. FP-growth reduces dataset scan numbers to two, therefore, achieving high efficiency and fast low memory usage, because of a special structure called FP-Tree.

Input

The algorithm accepts as an input a transaction database, in our case each record in the dataset is considered as a transaction. We should take into consideration that a transaction should not contain the same item twice. For implementing this algorithm, we use the SPMF graphical interface tool [19], which allows us to test the algorithm, along with tuning the min support and min confidence parameters.

Output

After running, the algorithm will mine the frequent itemsets, along with all the possible association rules, that will be directly visualized as the output. Finally, we will save the outputted rules in a text file along with the support and confidence values. The expected output contains all the possible rules including those leading to heart failure, which will be discussed later.

Rule Growth

RuleGrowth as described in [20], is a sequential pattern mining algorithm designed to detect common sequential rules between different transactions. Using the pattern-growth approach.

Let's assume that we have a sequence dataset noted as $DS = \{S_1, S_2, ..., S_n\}$, and each sequence S contains multiple unordered itemsets such as $S = \{X_1, X_2, ..., X_n\}$. If X$\Rightarrow$Y, such as items of X and Y will probably not be appearing in the same itemset of any sequence Sn, we can conclude that items of Y will appear in an itemset regardless of the order, after the appearance of the items of X in any order. A specific confidence level is taken into consideration. We calculate the confidence of the rule X$\Rightarrow$Y, by counting how many sequences contains all the items of X followed by all the items of Y. Therefore, regardless of the support count of the rule, if the confidence is 100%, then we are sure that this association is always true in the dataset.

In the example presented in Fig. 3, we can extract to following rule:

- $(1) (4) \Rightarrow (3)$

That means, when item 1 and 4 occurs in any order in any itemset, they are followed by 3 with a confidence of 100%, and a support of 75% because this rule is present in 3 out of 6 rows.

Input

The SPMF toolkit provides a full implementation of the Rule-Growth algorithm with the ability to tune rules with minimal support and confidence, plus visualizing the outputted rules. As already mentioned, the Rule Growth algorithm deals with a sequence dataset, therefore, we should adapt our dataset

ID	Sequences
S1	(1), (1 2 3), (1 3), (4), (3 6)
S2	(1 4), (3), (2 3), (1 5)
S3	(5 6), (1 2), (4 6), (3), (2)
S4	(5), (7), (1 6), (3), (2), (3)

Fig. 3 Sample sequence dataset

into an acceptable format. The input is a text file, containing a series of itemsets containing positive integers, separated by a space. A -1 value indicates the end of an itemset, and -2 value indicated the end of a single sequence. Using python, we have mapped the categorical values in the transformed dataset, into numerical values, but we have ensured to group certain parameters in the same itemsets:

- Difference for one day is grouped in the first itemset.
- Difference for three days is grouped in the second itemset.
- Difference for one day is grouped in the third itemset.
- Heart failure class is placed in the final itemset.

The main objective behind this grouping strategy is to let the algorithm find any possible $X \Rightarrow Y$ rule where Y is the heart failure class and X can contain any item The second objective is to probably find other $X \Rightarrow Y$ rules between the items different than the heart failure class items, which might help in the early heart failure occurrence.

Output

The results will be our mined sequential rules as $X \Rightarrow Y$, along with the support and confidence levels. The expected output will confirm the results of the FP-growth algorithm and will reveal new patterns and interdependencies between different parameters.

5 Early Heart Failure Prediction

The second objective of this project is to find a method for predicting the heart failure class for 10-days ahead. This will help doctors to provide a suitable precaution process for the patients.

5.1 Conception and Modeling

First of all, we must ask this question: under which category we should classify our prediction problem? Taking into consideration that the heart failure class is deduced from the values of specific parameters, then our model must predict these parameters before we can classify the heart failure class based on the output predictions. We can say that we are fac-

ing a situation where we must apply regression to predict the first five vital signs 10 days in the future, and then calculate other parameters and deduce the heart failure class. We are trying to predict the future, so the problem can be classified as forecasting the near future. More specifically 10-days ahead.

As we said before, the datasets contain daily observations for multiple parameters, along with the date of observations (DD/MM/YY). Therefore, we can index each data point or observation in a time order, making a series of historical observations separated by an equal timestamp (1 day in our data). Now we can reference our data as a time series over a specific time depending on each patient.

Based on the previous observations, the problem of early heart failure class prediction is modeled as Time-series forecasting. This refers to predict future vital signs values for 10 days ahead, based on the historical previous observations. This might be valid because some patterns of how the observation values are variating may appear in the historical data, thus based on the past behavior we will predict the future behavior.

5.2 Data Statistics

We have calculated the correlation matrix using python which indicates the linear relationship between any two parameters and if these variables tend to increase or decrease in a parallel way. Positive coefficients between variable X and Y indicates that when X increases, Y also increase, while negative correlations indicated that if X increase, Y will decrease and so on. The maximum value of correlation between two values is 1 meaning a perfect relation and values equal to 0 indicates no correlation. We must mention that -1 indicates a perfect negative relation. Table 3 resumes the coefficient interpretation process.

After examining the correlation matrix applied to all patients' records, we found that the data linearity cannot be taken into consideration while adopting a forecast method.

Another observation of the data was to plot the set of data points for each column in the datasets, representing a specific feature. For example, while checking the weight variations of a patient over time in Fig. 4, we found sudden fluctuations in the values from 68 KG to 64 KG for the next day.

Table 3 Vital signs captured

Coefficient	Interpretation
1	Full positive correlation
$0.4 \Rightarrow 0.7$	Moderate positive correlation
0	No correlation
$-0.4 \Rightarrow -0.7$	Moderate negative correlation
-1	Full negative correlation

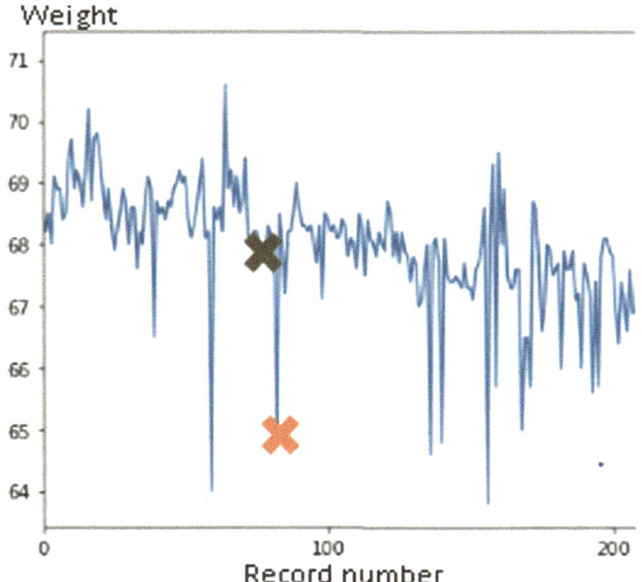

Fig. 4 Suddent weight variations for patient number 1

Input

We will use the univariate model to make predictions for the next time step. As mentioned in the state of art, the univariate data records observations for a single feature only. We will input a series of sequential values referring to 30 days of data history that we call a window of previous information, along with the 10 days in the future value that the model should learn to predict.

Steps to prepare the training data are enumerated as following:

1. Load the dataset.
2. Select the desired feature that could be one of the five vital signs.
3. Assign the date column as the index.
4. Split the training and testing data (80% for training and 20% for testing).
5. Create a series of windows contacting 30 observations and specify the time step to predict (10 days in our case).

5.4   Neural Network Architecture

After preparing the data, we built a multiplayer neural network that contains a single LSTM layer and three other dense layers, making a total of four layers stacked as the following:

1. Input dense layer containing 10 nodes.
2. LSTM layer containing 8 memory cells activated with the Relu function.
3. Dense layer containing 10 nodes activated with the Relu function.
4. Dense layer for output contacting a single node.

Using hidden layers gives the ability for the network to perform in a nonlinear behavior. Setting the Relu activation function will help the network to learn from the nonlinear data, and extract some significant knowledge and build interdependencies between provided input parameters. The output of the LSTM network is a 10-step prediction of the future.

These fluctuations should be taken into consideration, and therefore, could not be considered as data noise. Patients suffering from heart failure are prone to these fluctuations. In this case, the patient might have fluid retention because of a heart failure, and the next day this retention gets reduced. This explains the sudden drop in weight.

5.3   LSTM Model

Based on the previous results and observations, we used the Long Short-Term memory, which derives from the recurrent neural networks that can handle time-series data. Data points might have an interdependency and forms a special pattern, therefore, it can learn complex and nonlinear relations. Recurrent neural networks use an internal memory to integrate some kind of bias from the previous input, such as input at time $t - 1$ affects the decisions taken by the network at time t. LSTM's, are more efficient than normal recurrent neural networks, because of the ability to remember data behavior for longer time periods. This memory feature provides the capability to accept a longer sequence of inputs. This method is adopted for this part and using python and TensorFlow [21] open source library, we will build our multilayer neural networks. A total of five LSTM models are needed, one for each vital sign (Weight, Systolic arterial pressure, Diastolic arterial pressure, Heart rate, O2 blood saturation) to predict a 10 days value in the future.

6   Results and Discussion

In this section, the experimentation process of the proposed methods and algorithms is presented, then results are explained and discussed. We will start by explaining some observations about data correlation, after that, we discuss association rule and sequential pattern algorithms for extracting significant knowledge about heart failure causes. Finally, time-series forecasting predictions for future heart failure is presented.

Table 4 Correlation value observations

Red class	Orange class
Δ_1POIDS: moderated $\Rightarrow$ +0.34	Δ_1PAD: low $\Rightarrow$ +0.2 correlation
Δ_3POIDS: moderated to strong $\Rightarrow$ +0.66	Δ_1FC: low $\Rightarrow$ +0.1
Δ_7POIDS: moderated $\Rightarrow$ +0.36	Δ_3PAS: low $\Rightarrow$ +0.17
Δ_7FC: moderated negative $\Rightarrow$ -0.5	Δ_3PAD: low $\Rightarrow$ +0.21
Δ_1PAS: low $\Rightarrow$ +0.2	Δ_7POIDS: low $\Rightarrow$ +0.15
Δ_1PAD: low $\Rightarrow$ +0.18	Δ_7O2: Strong $\Rightarrow$ -0.83

6.1 Data Correlation

Table 4 presents the relation between heart failure classes and some variables. These results can be used to pick some parameters to perform the itemset and association rule mining, rather than mining all the dataset parameters. Also, by only looking at these values, we can notice the most influencing parameters to decide which class the patient is suffering from.

6.2 Association Rule Mining

We proposed the FP-Growth algorithm to mine frequent itemsets and association rules. The experimentation process can be resumed by these steps:

1. Concatenate all the CSV file into one file containing all medical records.
2. Transform the dataset to ranged values form (as discussed earlier).
3. Tune the min support and min confidence parameters.
4. Observation and analysis.

We have divided our dataset into two new separate files, the first one containing all the records with red heart failure class with a total of 901 records. The second one containing all the records with orange heart failure class with a total of 1729 records.

6.3 Results

1. Minimum support was set to 0.05 or 5%.
2. Minimum confidence is set to 100%.
3. Maximum consequent length is set to one.
4. Maximum antecedent length set to three.

The support parameter was set to 5% because we want to know the most influencing parameter in the classification of heart failure (red or orange), therefore, we should extract rules with the less and the highest correlation between a parameter and the class determined.

We set the consequent length to 1 in order to simplify the observation task, because we are only interested in finding rules X $\Rightarrow$ Y, where Y is the heart failure class. To simplify the observation step we set the consequent to three.

Orange Class

After executing the algorithm, we got a total of 265,155 association rules, after filtering the output to only get the patterns with consequent as the orange class, we reduced the count to 14,870 rule. The first step is to observe the mined rules, to calculate the frequency of each item with the associated class. In Table 5 we can observe each rule mined along with the frequency of occurrence in the dataset. For simplification, we define PA as total blood pressure, which is PAS and PAD combined. All the rules have a confidence of 1.

As we can see, after observing the results, we had verified 6 out of 8 conditions presented by the medical sheet, the unverified conditions are:

- Δ_TPAS > 10%, Δ_TPAD > 10% a and Δ_TFC > 20%.
- 10% < Δ_TO2 < -5%.

This may be explained by the low correlation between these conditions and the orange class. Furthermore, if we examine Table 4, we can explain the second unverified condition because O2 concentration percentage difference over days and orange class have a negative correlation coefficient. That means that when this class will not appear when Δ_TO2 tends to increase.

From the above Table 5, we can conclude that the orange class condition is mostly influenced by the heart rate parameter (FC) and heart rate difference (DFC), appearing in 40.65 and 42.3% of the causes of orange class occurrence.

New Association Rules

After observations, new rules appeared and can be referred as additional causes, or associated with orange class appearance.

Table 5 Observation results orange class

Condition $\Rightarrow$ Orange	Count		Percentage of total orange classes (%)
PA $> 13/8$ (mmHg)	126		7.2
FC > 70(bpm),$(70 < FC < 80)$	703		40.6
Δ_TPA $> 10\%$, FC > 70	52		3
Δ_7POIDS > 2 (kg)	74		4.2
Δ_TPA$>10\%$	$10 <= \Delta_1$ PA $<= 20$	117	23.3
	$10 <= \Delta_3$ PA $<= 20$	136	
	$10 <= \Delta_7$ PA $<= 20$	150	
	Total	403	
Δ_TFC $> 20\%$	$20 < \Delta_1$ FC $<= 30$	120	23.3
	$30 < \Delta_1$ FC $<= 50$	84	
	$20 < \Delta_3$ FC $<= 30$	154	
	$30 < \Delta_3$ FC $<= 50$	115	
	$20 < \Delta_7$ FC $<= 30$	151	
	$30 < \Delta_7$ FC $<= 50$	109	
	Total	733	

- $0 < \Delta_1$Poids<0.5 kg, PA$>13/8$ mmHg $\Rightarrow$ Orange. Support:85, confidence:1

The above rule means that a variance of patients' weight is occurring in 5% of the total cases in the orange class.

- $80\% < \Delta_1$FC$<90\% \Rightarrow$ Orange. Support:294, confidence:1

In 17% of the cases, a heartbeat rate between 80 and 90 is accompanying the orange class appearance.

Red Class

The same process will be applied to verify the medical conditions in the sheet, that would provoke the red heart failure class appearance. After running the algorithm, a total of 31152 association rules appeared, and after filtering the output to get the red class as a consequent, we got 3507 mined patterns that should be examined to verify the conditions preceding red heart failure class occurrence. The following Table 6 resumes the observations. Note that all the rules have a confidence equal to 1.

These observations have specified the most influencing parameters of a red heart failure class. Furthermore, we can correlate with the high correlation coefficient (0.66) of D3POIDS Table 4, and what we found, because Δ_3POIDS>2kg appears in 38.8% of the red class causes. Three unverified conditions remained:

- Δ_7Poids > 2 kg, Δ_TPA $> 10\% \Rightarrow$ Red.
- $-5\% < \Delta_T$O2 $< -10\%$, $\Delta_7$7Poids > 2kg $\Rightarrow$ Red.

The above rules did not appear in the observations, this can be explained by the low rate in which these parameters appears and causes a red class.

New Association Rules

While examining the patterns, new rules and associations appeared that can be resumed as the following:

- $20\% < \Delta_3$PA $< 40\%$, $0 < \Delta_1$O2 $< 10\% \rightarrow$ Red. Support:49, confidence:1.

This rule is true in 5.4% of the total cases where the red class appears.

- $2\% < \Delta_3$POIDS $< 4\%$, $10\% <= \Delta_3$PA $< 20\% \rightarrow$ Red. Support:24, confidence:1.

This rule means that the patient must have fluid retention because of the large weight difference for three days which is highly associated with red class appearance. In 2.6% of the cases, this rule will be associated with a red heart failure class.

6.4   Sequential Pattern Mining

The RuleGrowth algorithm will mine the frequent sequential patterns, and find the sequential rules $X \Rightarrow Y$ in which all the items of X appeared before the items of Y. We must recreate the same steps to run the algorithm, as we did in the previous part, while only formatting our dataset to the acceptable format.

Result

First of all after running the algorithm with two input files, the first one for the red class and the second containing all records with the orange class. Results were the same as Tables 5 and 6 with the same support and frequency values, which confirms the medical sheets of heart failure conditions.

Table 6 Observation results red class

Condition $\Rightarrow$ Red	Count			Percentage of total Red classes (%)
PA $>$ 14/9 (mmHg)	128			14.2
Δ_TPA $>$ 20%	63			7
FC$<$50 (bpm)	145			16
FC$>$=100 (bpm)	145			12.4
Δ_7POIDS $>$ 2 (kg), Δ_TFC $>$ 20%	19			2.1
$-10\% < \Delta_3$O2 $< -5\%$, Δ_TFC $>$ 20%	22			2.4
Δ_3POIDS $>$ 2 (kg)	323			38.8
Δ_1O2 $> -10\%$	34			3.7
Δ_1O2 $> -10\%$	34			3.7
Δ_3O2 $> -10\%$	37			4.1
Δ_7O2 $> -10\%$	43			4.7
O2 $<$ 90%	80 $<=$ **O2** $<$ 86	31		8.4
	86 $<=$ **O2** $<$ 90	45		
	Total	76		

What if we want to determine the heart failure class of a patient, but we are missing some influencing parameters in the classification process of the heart failure class. Can we predict the value of the missing parameters based on the values of the existing ones? To answer this question, we had executed this algorithm using several input file versions of red class (901 records) and orange class (1729 records). Rearranging the parameter ordering in the file to get the desired output is required. Table 7 contains a part of the founded patterns.

These results might be used to predict some missing parameters. Confirmation or denial of these rules will take place in the future works after testing.

6.5 Time-Series Forecasting

The second objective of the project is to build a model capable of predicting a possible future heart failure class for a patient. As mentioned before, LSTM recurrent neural network was implemented to achieve this task. For each vital sign including patients weight, systolic and diastolic blood pressure, heart beat rate, and oxygen saturation in blood, a unique model was built to predict future values for 10 days ahead. All the implementation process is done using Python and Tensorflow for building models.

Experimentation Process

The experimentation process can be resumed by the following steps:

- Load data.
- Split data 80% for training and 20% for validation.
- Index data by date and create a univariate series containing values of the desired parameter to predict.

- set up the input to a series of batches, each one contacting 30 days of history $(t - 30)$, followed by the value at $t + 10$ days.
- Build the neural network and shape data to the acceptable format by the model, then train and save the model with the lowest validation loss.
- Load the model and test it.

After getting the predicted values, we create a new CSV file containing them. The next step is to calculate the day difference for each one of them for 1, 3 and 7 days. Finally, a new CSV file is created containing predicted vital signs along with day differences column. Using this file and Python, the heart failure class is calculated based on the previously mentioned medical sheet.

6.6 Results

For testing, we used 3 patients, and after predicting the five vital signs for each one, we calculated the 1, 3, 7 days difference parameters the determined the class. Results in Table 8 resumes the results. For each patient we have tested the model on the last 10 days of observations, as shown in the previous Table 7. The average model accuracy for all predictions is 76%, which is considered a good result taking into consideration the small amount of data we got (173 records for patient 1, 144 for patient 2, 309 for patient 3). And the type of data we are handling.

Our model clearly proved the ability to extract significant patterns from the 30-days window provided to make the 10-days ahead predictions. These are primary results and the model will be susceptible for more testing in future on the

Table 7 Sequential patterns between parameters

Parameter	Pattern	Support	Confidence (%)
Δ_T POIDS (Kg)	Δ_1 POIDS $> 2 \Rightarrow \Delta_3$ POIDS > 2	75	42
	Δ_1 POIDS $> 2, 10 <=$ PAS $<= 13 \Rightarrow \Delta_3$ POIDS > 2	47	50
	$10 <= \Delta_3$ PAS $< 20 \Rightarrow 2 < \Delta_7$ POIDS < 4	70	32
PAS (mmHg)	$0 < \Delta_3$ PAD < 5, PAD $> 9 \Rightarrow$ PAS > 14	48	96
	FC < 60 bpm $\Rightarrow$ PAS > 14	74	51
	$0 < \Delta_3$ O2 $< 10, 8 <=$ PAD $< 9 \Rightarrow$ PAS > 14	96	41
PAD (mmHg)	PAS > 14, FC $< 70 \Rightarrow$ PAD > 9	50	51
	80 bpm $<$ FC < 90 bpm $\Rightarrow 6 <=$ PAD < 8	118	85
Δ_T PAS (%)	$20 <= \Delta_3$PAD$<40 \Rightarrow 10\% <= \Delta_7PAS<20$	50	35
Δ_T PAD (%)	$10 <= \Delta_1$PAD$<20 \Rightarrow 10 <= \Delta_3PAD<20$	69	33

Table 8 10 days class prediction results

Patient 1		Patient 2		Patient 3	
Actual class	Predicted	Actual class	Predicted	Actual class	Predicted
Orange	Blue	Orange	Orange	Orange	Orange
Orange	Orange	Red	Red	Red	Red
Orange	Blue	Red	Red	Red	Red
Orange	Orange	Red	Red	Red	Red
Orange	Orange	Red	Orange	Red	Red
Orange	Orange	Red	Red	Red	Red
Orange	Orange	Red	Orange	Red	Red
Orange	Orange	Orange	Orange	Red	Red
Orange	Orange	Red	Red	Orange	Red
Orange	Orange	Red	Orange	Orange	Red
Accuracy	80%		70%		80%

remaining patients to confirm the prediction's accuracy. These results are the first of its kind in heart failure early prediction, and by this work, we provide a baseline study for future works.

7 Conclusion

In this work, we have used several data mining techniques to extract knowledge from the datasets. Data preprocessing and data transformation is applied first. Then using data mining techniques, the most influencing medical conditions leading to heart failure are extracted. Additional rules are defined and explained. The second algorithm had found some interesting interdependency between data parameters. These rules will help in understanding the heart failure occurrence. In the second part, we have built a special type of recurrent neural network model using LSTM to predict the occurrence of heart failure within a 10 days window. We used only the five basic vital signs provided by the dataset of real patients. Results show good accuracy of 76% when testing on 3 patients.

In future, we should consider improving the LSTM model by performing some parameter tuning and modifying the internal architecture of the multilayer neural network. For the sequential pattern mining, the result could be more refined by retransforming the dataset and finding a new range of values. Adding and acquiring new data with more recorded observations would be a huge plus, and will definitively improve the results.

By finishing this project, we hope to provide a baseline model to researchers in the field to build on and achieve more advancements in the Heart failure domain.

References

[1] Suganya, S.: A proficient heart disease prediction method using fuzzy-cart algorithm. (2016)

[2] Chaurasia, V., Pal, S.: Early prediction of heart diseases using data mining techniques. Caribbean Journal of Science and Technology **1** (2013) 208–217

[3] Aljaaf, A.J., Al-Jumeily, D., Hussain, A.J., Dawson, T., Fergus, P., Al-Jumaily, M.: Predicting the likelihood of heart failure with a multi level risk assessment using decision tree. In: 2015 Third International Conference on Technological Advances in Electrical, Electronics and Computer Engineering (TAEECE), IEEE (2015) 101–106

[4] Yang, G., Ren, Y., Pan, Q., Ning, G., Gong, S., Cai, G., Zhang, Z., Li, L., Yan, J.: A heart failure diagnosis model based on support vector machine. In: 2010 3rd International Conference on Biomedical Engineering and Informatics. Volume 3., IEEE (2010) 1105–1108

[5] Masetic, Z., Subasi, A.: Congestive heart failure detection using random forest classifier. Computer methods and programs in biomedicine **130** (2016) 54–64

[6] Melillo, P., De Luca, N., Bracale, M., Pecchia, L.: Classification tree for risk assessment in patients suffering from congestive heart failure via long-term heart rate variability. IEEE journal of biomedical and health informatics **17**(3) (2013) 727–733

[7] Dangare, C.S., Apte, S.S.: Improved study of heart disease prediction system using data mining classification techniques. International Journal of Computer Applications **47**(10) (2012) 44–48

[8] Mooney, C.H., Roddick, J.F.: Sequential pattern mining–approaches and algorithms. ACM Computing Surveys (CSUR) **45**(2) (2013) 1–39

[9] Fournier-Viger, P., Lin, J.C.W., Kiran, R.U., Koh, Y.S., Thomas, R.: A survey of sequential pattern mining. Data Science and Pattern Recognition **1**(1) (2017) 54–77

[10] Ilayaraja, M., Meyyappan, T.: Efficient data mining method to predict the risk of heart diseases through frequent itemsets. Procedia Computer Science **70** (2015) 586–592

[11] Ilayaraja, M., Meyyappan, T.: Mining medical data to identify frequent diseases using apriori algorithm. In: 2013 International Conference on Pattern Recognition, Informatics and Mobile Engineering, IEEE (2013) 194–199

[12] Nahar, J., Imam, T., Tickle, K.S., Chen, Y.P.P.: Association rule mining to detect factors which contribute to heart disease in males and females. Expert Systems with Applications **40**(4) (2013) 1086–1093

[13] UCI Heart Disease Data Set. https://archive.ics.uci.edu/ml/datasets/Heart+Disease

[14] Srinivas, K., Rao, G.R., Govardhan, A.: Analysis of attribute association in heart disease using data mining techniques. International Journal of Engineering Research and Applications (IJERA) **2** (2012)

[15] Billis, A., Bamidis, P.D.: Employing time-series forecasting to historical medical data: an application towards early prognosis within elderly health monitoring environments. In: AI-AM/NetMed@ECAI, Citeseer (2014) 31–35

[16] Fu, R., Zhang, Z., Li, L.: Using lstm and gru neural network methods for traffic flow prediction. In: 2016 31st Youth Academic Annual Conference of Chinese Association of Automation (YAC), IEEE (2016) 324–328

[17] Duan, Y., Yisheng, L., Wang, F.Y.: Travel time prediction with lstm neural network. In: 2016 IEEE 19th international conference on intelligent transportation systems (ITSC), IEEE (2016) 1053–1058

[18] Han, J., Pei, J., Yin, Y., Mao, R.: Mining frequent patterns without candidate generation: A frequent-pattern tree approach. Data mining and knowledge discovery **8**(1) (2004) 53–87

[19] SPMF tool. https://www.philippe-fournier-viger.com/spmf/index.php?link=download.php

[20] Fournier-Viger, P., Nkambou, R., Tseng, V.S.M.: Rulegrowth: mining sequential rules common to several sequences by pattern-growth. In: Proceedings of the 2011 ACM symposium on applied computing. (2011) 956–961

[21] tensorFlow. https://www.tensorflow.org/api_docs/python/tf/keras/layers/LSTM

The Efficiency of the Reverse Engineering to Fabricate a New Respirator Technology Compatible with the COVID-19 Pandemic

Mohamed Zied Chaari, Rashid Al-Rahimi, Abdulaziz Aljaberi, Mohamed Abdelfatah, and Christopher Loreno

Abstract

This research will present reverse engineering's utility to provide assistance systems and rehabilitation technology in the medical field [34]. According to the fast and widespread COVID-19 contagion globally, the demand for ventilators and PPE materials is very high after the factories look-down. There are limitations in the chain of supply and delivery of critical medical equipment thought worldwide. In this urgent drum, reverse engineering is the right solution at a low price and a short time to provide safety equipment to healthcare professionals, hospitals, and pharmaceuticals. Reverse manufacturer necessitates a series of phases to collect precise information on a product's dimensions. 3D printing, 3D scanning, and PCB fast prototyping it is the best solution and low cost with a short time of prototyping for most existing technologies. We are looking forward to making a new design of the Powered Air Purifier with Hood (PAPR) Ventilator, which features a lightweight, long-lasting battery and three airflow rates that change according to the doctor's need. Therefore, this work aimed to explore the possibility of reverse engineering, such as the speed of obtaining the biomedical and healthcare device's prototype in a critical time. We are working on upgrading the existing PAPR from regular use to COVID-19 use with high performance. We will add the germicidal ultraviolet light between the HE filter and hood to ensure the airbreathing purifier from any virus. A UV drum for sanitizing different respirator parts after used and charging it battery wirelessly inside the drums simultaneously. We are also adding IoT technology in the respirator for physical distancing and healthcare staff tracking and recording.

M. Zied Chaari (✉) · R. Al-Rahimi · A. Aljaberi · M. Abdelfatah · C. Loreno
Qatar Scientific Club, Doha, Qatar
e-mail: chaari_zied@ieee.org

1 Introduction

The impact of Coronavirus has influenced every corner of life. COVID-19 outbreak has caused hundreds of millions of lives around the world. In this situation, all the global shut down, and only the healthcare industry is battling against the virus. To control the COVID-19 from propagating, many states, including the USA, European Union, UK, and others, are currently in some level of lockdown, with the closure of companies, gyms, airports, universities, and schools. Reverse engineering obtains three-dimensional data in a computerized form of the original healthcare device with a high accuracy 3D scanner or a redesign CAD file. The reverse engineering method is named as such because it involves working backward through the actual design process. It has clear benefits of practical use and additive technologies and vacuum casting in silicone, FDM plastic, or titanium molds. 3D printing, also known as rapid manufacturing technology, creates an object package with high precision and low cost [46]. 3D printers can produce more complicated geometry than traditional manufacturing techniques (Lather and CNC three-axis machines) at a low price and short period [30]. Since the Coronavirus outbreak, 3D printing currently involves manufacturing individual surgical templates, fabrication of individual swabs, air-purifying respirator, and face shied for COVID-19 [48]. The medical instrument's intricate geometric form complicates measuring the control size and determination of the exact geometry. Swabs used in the pandemic test are subject to frequent changes in design appearance. Scientific groups are thinking about how they could print critical medical supplies as part of the organization's response to the COVID-19 pandemic [18]. There are limitations in the chain of supply and delivery of critical medical equipment thought worldwide. Scientific teams from Europe, the US, Middle East, and Fab Lab Foundation and open-source platforms work together and share many 3D models of healthcare devices like face shields, masks, and swabs in the open-source platform. In this research, we will present the utility of reverse engineering to decrease the impact of the COVID-19 and help countries respond to this pandemic [39,43]. We are not interested in replicating the original devices to make money, but we have looking to help health professionals [6,25].

2   Common Uses for Reverse Engineering

Reverse engineering can be used for educational purposes and much further, improving product documentation, corporate espionage and competitor intelligence, replacing legacy parts, part improvement, forensics, and problem-solving, as presented below [3,32,35,41].

– Education to improve future production:
  Engineers can learn a variety of data by reverse engineering devices, products, parts, and more. The more items they reverse engineering, the more skills and methods they learn to create something new. Reverse engineering encourages engineers to keep redesigning and repurposing products until they cannot improve on them anymore.
– Improving product documentation:
  Machinery documentation can be deficient, missing, or hard to understand. Reverse engineering makes it feasible to determine how a product was made and how it works to create new documentation.
– Corporate espionage and competitor intelligence:
  Reverse engineering powers innovation, as noticed in the case research. Companies can discover how a competitor's product works and then improve to create their own, better product. This helps the companies gain a competitive edge and inspires engineers to make the best possible product to serve a specific purpose.
– Replacing legacy parts:
  Machinery and devices are expensive purchases. To get the most return on investment for those purchases, the company needs to keep them up and run for as long as possible. When elements malfunction or break, the company needs to be able to replace them. Sometimes, this is not possible because the plant may be out of business or stopped producing for some reason. Reverse engineering provide companies the power to replicate and reproduce those parts by senior staff, so they can keep their machinery running longer.
– Part improvement:
  The same methods that are used for forensics and problem-solving can use to improve parts. Engineers can take pieces that are no longer useful and reverse engineer them to discover any defects. The element can be redesigned to fix those flaws or remodeled to operate another objective.

– Forensics and problem-solving:
  Reverse engineering can detect product defects or help engineers understand why machinery or equipment is malfunctioning. Long ago, scientists would have to take a device apart and put it back together manually to understand how it works and learn flaws. With technology evolutions, engineers can now trace over existing parts and assemblies and input them into a CAD file. This gives them a big image view to pinpoint problem areas and develop solutions to fix them.

The reverse engineering method helps scientists determine how a part was fabricated to recreate it. In many cases, the only way to achieve an original device design is through reverse engineering. Regularly, there will be no way to contact the actual companies or their long discontinued production because of the lockdown [44]. Often, engineers will improve the design with new developments and innovations. Fabrication of swabs necessitated using reverse engineering to create a 3D model, as shown in Fig. 1. Many laboratories and university labs share the 3D model swabs in the open-source platform, and many users printed it with SLS technology, as shown in Fig. 2.

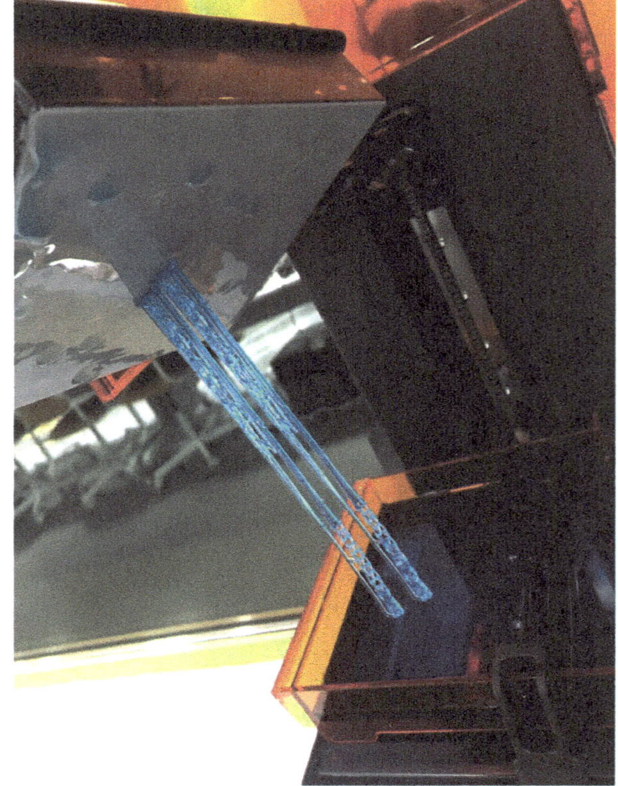

Fig. 1 3D model swab

Fig. 2 Swab 3D printed with SLS technology

3   Powered Air-Purifying Respirator

The medical staff needs PAPR that can safeguard both themselves and their infected peoples [23]. In COVID-19, we decide to re-engineer a device and make a significant effort to obtain technical data. Because of the global crisis and the absence of medical products. COVID-19 proved the efficiency of reverse engineering in medical device. Reverse engineering is a logical approach for evaluating the design of existing healthcare devices to tackle the virus. We are creating a new strategy focused on the work we are doing to assess and potentially reverse engineer replacement PAPR. We study different parts of the powered air-purifying respirator, as shown in Fig. 3. This solution would be a fast way to fill the gaps in the air-purifying respirator supply chain. In our cases, we can use the original device as an initial step to repurposing a new device that can use it in this pandemic. To remake PAPR should be following the process below:

– Observe and evaluate the mechanisms that make the respirator work.
– Analyze and study the inner components of the respirator (Electrical and Mechanical).

– Develop the part or product geometry in a CAD model from the original devices.
– Redesign the electronic PCB board and any mechanical parts similar to the original device according to the new application.

The powered air-purifying respirator consists of two parts; Mechanical parts:

– High durability belt,
– Filters and breathing tube,
– Hood (Head cover).

Electronics parts:

• PCB motherboard a air flow rate controller,
• The intelligent air flow regulator,
• Blower unit a two air flow rate 6CFM and 8CFM,
• Battery pack (11.1 V/4.8AH).

Therefore, the task is to gain a working knowledge of the initial device by disassembling the product into parts, as shown in Figs. 4a, 4b, and 4c respectively. In this research, we will

Fig. 3 Different parts of the powered air-purifying respirator

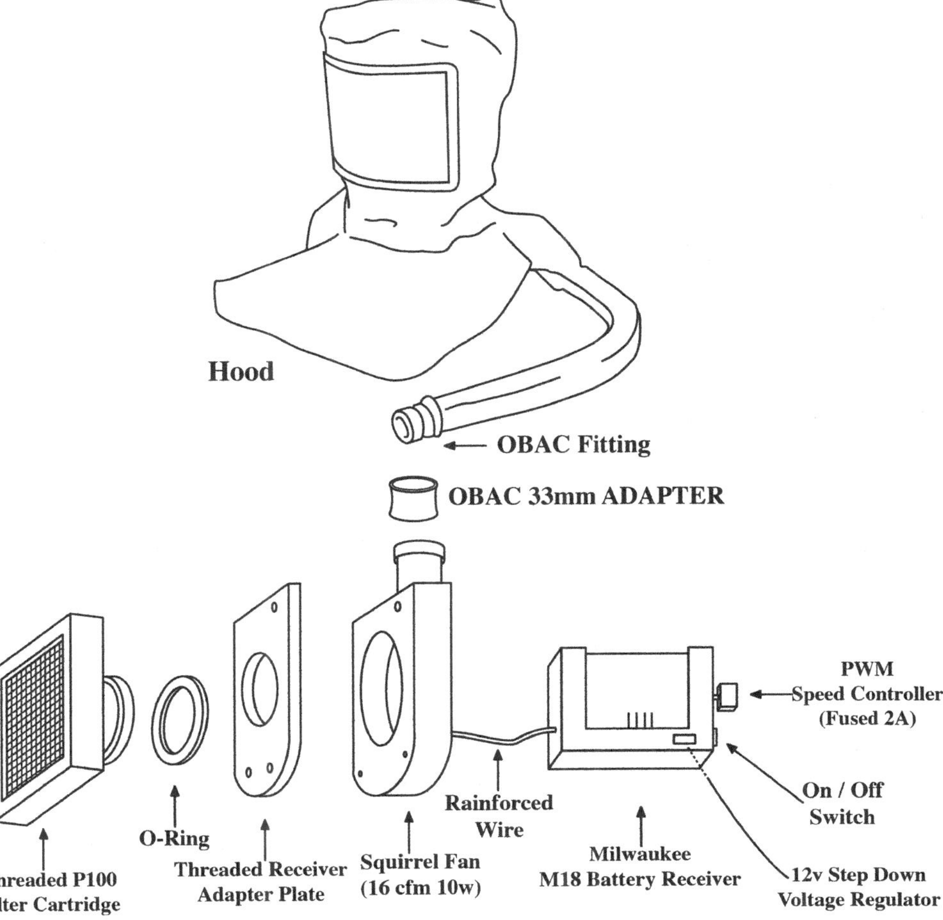

Fig. 4 Disassemble the original PAPR piece-by-piece

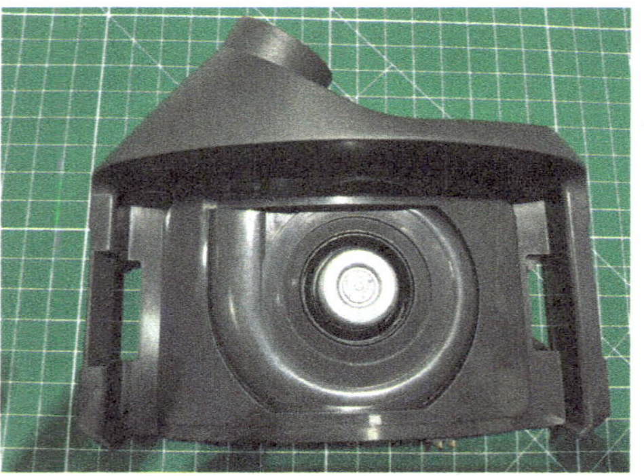

(a) A front view of the blower unit

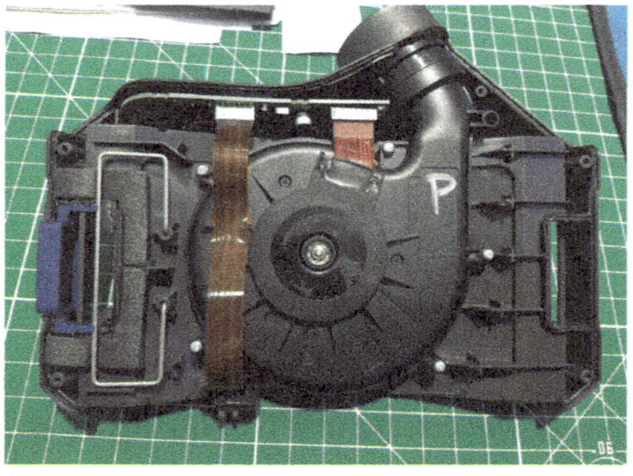

(b) A back view of the blower unit

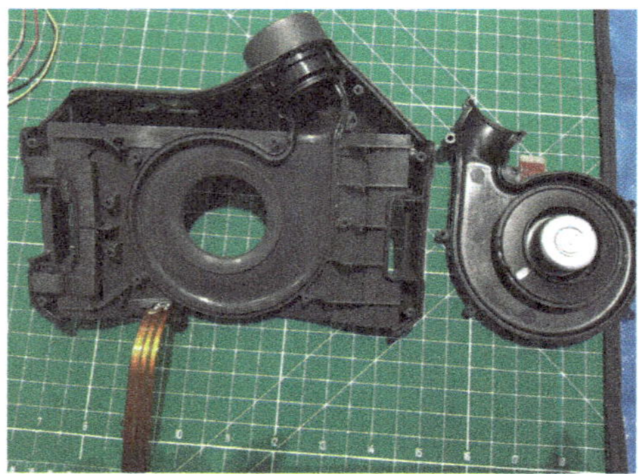

(c) Disassemble the air blower unit

fabricate all these parts and fix them inside the 3D package. When we started the new PAPR manufacturing phase, we discovered slight limitations in the current device that could not be compatible with this pandemic. There are minor limitations in this current product that it cannot protect healthcare staff a high efficiency from this pandemic. The TR300 protects against vapors or gasses and not intrinsically for the COVID-19 virus.

4 Repurposing a New PAPR Compatible with COVID-19

The TR-300 belt-mounted assemblies consist of a blower unit, HE filter, lithium battery, waist belt, and hood. In this part, we study and analyze all steps to make a new PAPR as per the characteristics of COVID-19. The process starts from the DC blower, PCB board, assembly programming, 3D model, and sewing of the head cover (Full hood) [40]. This phase needs to understand very well the mechanical parts included the CAD and the electronic PCB board of the original device. In the first next subsection, we study the mechanical aspects of the PAPR. Second, we analyze the electronic part of the device.

4.1 Mechanical Components of the Air-Purifying Respirator

In the following subsection, we study and examine the different mechanical parts of the PAPR. Engineers use solid-works to redesign the CAD drawings.

Air Flow Measurement and Analysis

PAPR purifying provides a constant air flow rate of 205 LPM to health professionals, as shown in Fig. 5a. The blower and intelligent air flow regulator unit is the central part of this device. This section presents an analysis of the output of air flow, the model used for analyzing the influence of the air flow inside the hood. We have measured the air flow from the original device to know the air flow rate. The soft air distribution on the head hood air flow sensor concerning the air flow rate and relative humidity of air is computed for system stability. The moisture in the air will decrease the upstream and downstream resistance temperature and increase the temperature difference between the two resistances and the motor's power consumption. In this phase, we approximately calculated the reverse engineering air blower's air flow. After determined the technical specification of the original blower's capacity, we are looking for a similar air blower that can use in our new reverse engineering device [45,50], as shown in Fig. 5b.

Fig. 5 Measure and determine the air flow rate

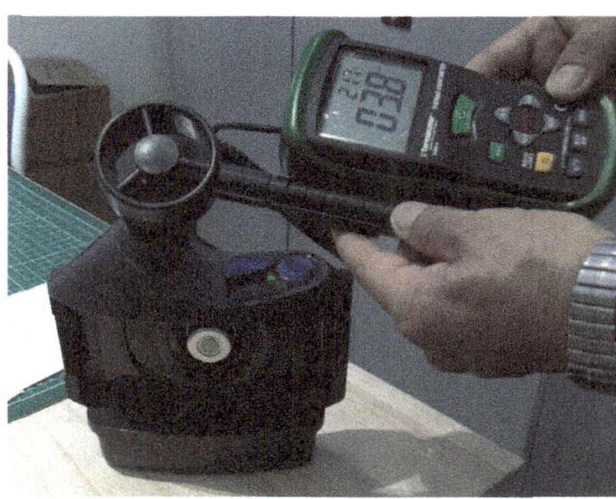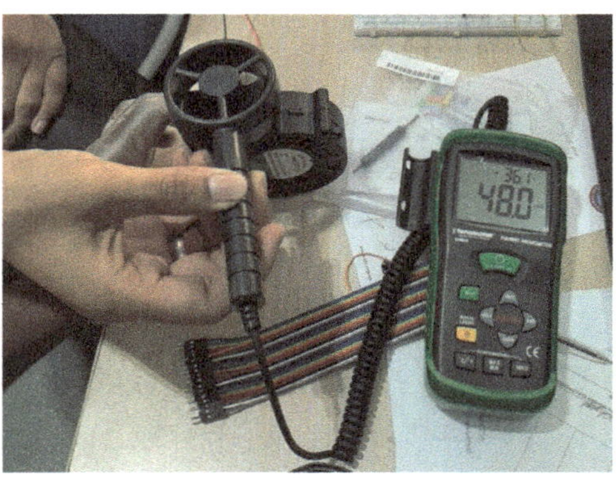

(a) Provide a constant air flow rate of 205 LPM (7.3 CFM)

(b) Provide a constant air flow rate of 237 LPM

Table 1 A list of similar blowers can provide air flow rate comfort to healthcare staff

Digi-key part number	Voltage (V)	Air flow rate (CFM)
1688-1908-ND	12	8
PF97331BX-B00U-A99	12	13
381-3126-ND	12	17

Table 1 shown three different DC blowers similar to the original device and can provide enough air flow and comfortable situations for doctors to work with the COVID-19 cases with high efficiency.

HE Particulate Filter

The COVID-19 can be move via particles in the air [12, 33, 49]. The existing HE Filter (TR-3712N) of powered air-purifying respirator plays several vital roles. The filter is placed in several positions in the PAPR circuit to filtration air-breathing from the bacteria and COVID-19 viruses and protecting healthcare patients [13, 47]. However, the HE Filters can block at least 99.97% of airborne particles according to NIOSH-approved filtering facepiece respirator classifications, as shown in Fig. 6. HE filters must remove at least 99.97% of all particles that are 1.55 μm–0.2 μm [14, 16, 36]. Coronavirus is reported to be 60–140 nm (0.06 μm–0.14 μm) in size. Although the CDC has advised using HEPA filters in powered air-purifying respirators for effective purifiers of SARS-CoV-2,8 at present, the CDC has not offered any suggestions for utilizing portable HEPA filtration for decontamination of SARS-CoV-2 in clinical areas [15]. This percentage of 99.97% to blocking viruses is not enough in our application and design. It does not respect our work scope to protect healthcare professionals working in the first defense line. According to many research and WHO reports, HE filters are not enough to prevent the COVID-19 virus from crept into the air ventilation system [51]. So reverse engineering only is not the right solution in this case. Many health experts ask to add in additional requests to have an ultraviolet light or another decontaminating agent to destroy viruses and microbes that deposit the filter itself. So we are thinking about many solutions to upgrade this device. One of these solutions is adding UV light 222 nm in the air circulation system to ensure the air-breathing from outside pure and avuncular from viruses and bacteria. The Care222 UV light includes a power supply, full housing, and a DC power source connection. They were designed to be mounted on the air circulation system between to hood and the blower. The UV circuit has three activation settings. These are simple on/off switch duty control, continuous output, or activation through the built-in human sensor,

Fig. 6 The HE filter is not capable of blocking 100% Coronavirus

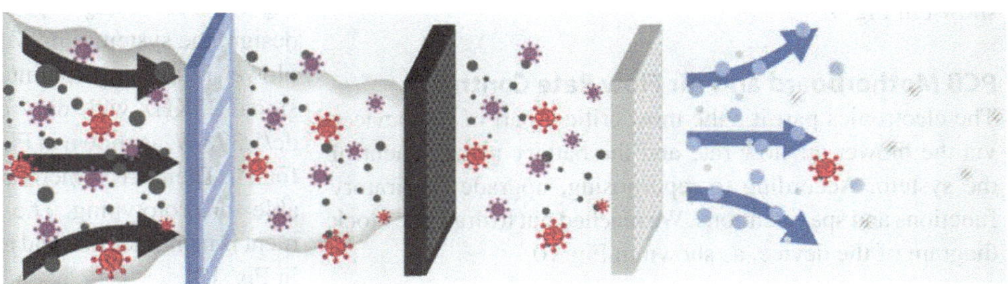

Fig. 7 Implement of UV light inside the respirator

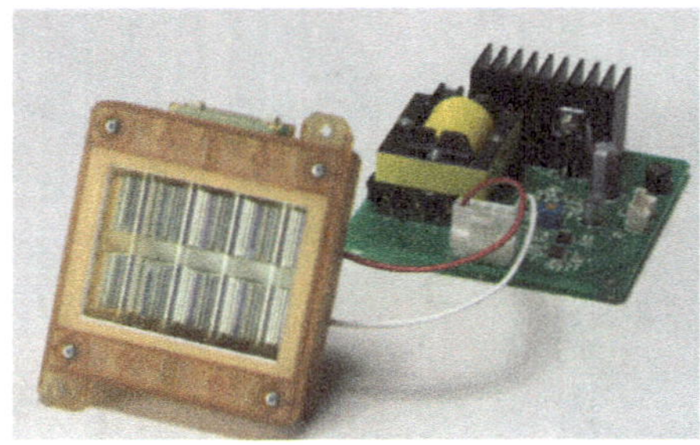
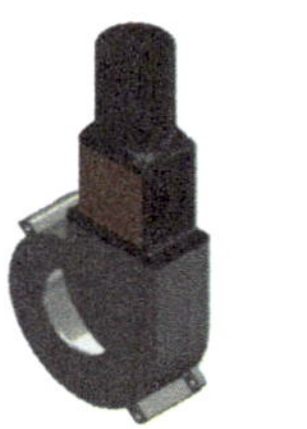
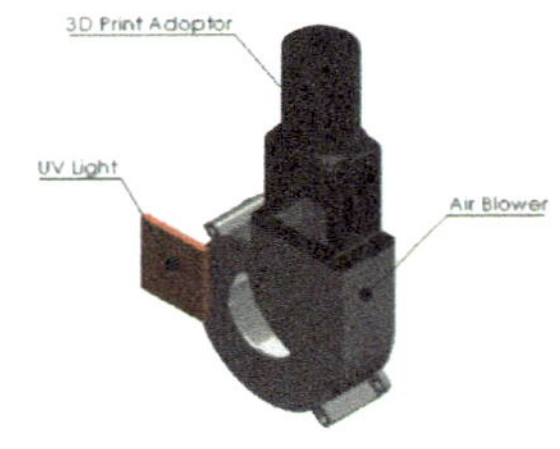

(a) UV light (Care222)

(b) Fixing the UV light in the air circulation system.

as shown in Fig. 7a. The specifications of the UV light it's below:

– Light Source: Mercury-free krypton chloride (KrCl) excimer lamp,
– Emitted wavelength: 203 nm ∼ 220 nm,
– Peak wavelength: 222 nm Far UV-C,
– Output: 5.4 mW/cm^2.

We place the UV-C in the breathing tube because it has harmful effects on the human body. We are making a design to ensure not UV leak and reflection during use [7,9]. This idea guaranty the air-breathing by doctors pure and 100% without a virus, as shown in Fig. 7b. With UV light 222nm, we upgrade, and we are making high efficient PAPR device that can use in COVID-19 [8].

Hood (Head cover)

The simplest way is to make a complete system for a hospital, healthcare, and pharmacy application. We used waterproof Non-Woven material with anti-fog precise view acrylic thickness 0.3 mm to fabricate the hood with low weight within 90 gm, as shown in Fig. 8b. Everyone's face and head are different, so how is one eyewear model fit everybody. With the 3D design of the headbands, we've carefully avoided sensitive areas of the head while designing self-adapting twin pads for the browband, as shown in Fig. 8.

4.2 Electronics Part

In this section, we study and make a PCB required to an upgrade PAPR compatible with COVID-19 specification, as shown in Fig. 9.

PCB Motherboard and Air Flow Rate Control

The electronics part it's the most critical part of the devices via the blower air flow rate and the battery management of the system. According to repurposing, upgrade respiratory functions and specifications. We reached out to draw the block diagram of the device, as shown in Fig. 10.

We have to control the air rate to get proper air flow for head cover air circulation. We are using PF97331BX-B00U-A99 fan blower as centrifugal DC Blower, 12VDC, 54.7CFM, 42 W, 63.2dBA, 6800RPM. We use Arduino nano with a TB6612FNG DC-motor driver to control blower speed with a PWM control signal of 25KHz with a pk voltage of 5vdc and a programmable duty cycle to control blower speed according to mode switch in three different air flow rate (Low, Medium, and High). For accurate PWM 25KHz frequency, we used the Arduino built-in timer to generate the PWM signal, as shown in Fig. 10b. The TB6612FNG is an H-Bridge driver. I will study the specifics of how it works, but the result is that it can turn a connected DC blower in either direction and variable speed. Breadboard timer frequency is defined by the selected Prescaler, where

$$\frac{16\,\text{MHz}}{Prescaler \times (TOP + 1)} = 25\,\text{KHz} \tag{1}$$

$$Prescaler \times (TOP + 1) = \frac{16\,\text{MHz}}{25\,\text{KHz}} = 640 \tag{2}$$

If we select a prescaler of 8, we get that

$$TOP + 1 = \frac{640}{8} = 80 \tag{3}$$

According to Eqs. 1 and 2, TOP = 80 to summarize, using Arduino running at 16 MHz, and use an 8-bit timer 2 to generate a 25 kHz PWM with a Prescaler of 8 (TCCR2B = 0x09) and a TOP of 79 (OCR2A = 79). Then we change the duty cycle during timer running using OCR2B register. The output PWM signal with 25 kHz and 30% duty cycle, as shown in Fig. 11a. According to practical measurements of our reverse design, the system runs with a battery of 12vdc 1.8Ah. If the blower is working continuously in high-rates level 3 (PWM signal 25KHz with duty cycle 30%), it will draw 0.448 A dc/5.378 W, as shown in Fig. 11b. The battery at least will stay for 4 h. There are numerous PCB fabrication techniques available for prototyping. The standard PCB prototyping equipment is manufactured and tested for its performance, as shown in Fig. 12.

Fig. 8 Manufacture of the hood (Head cover)

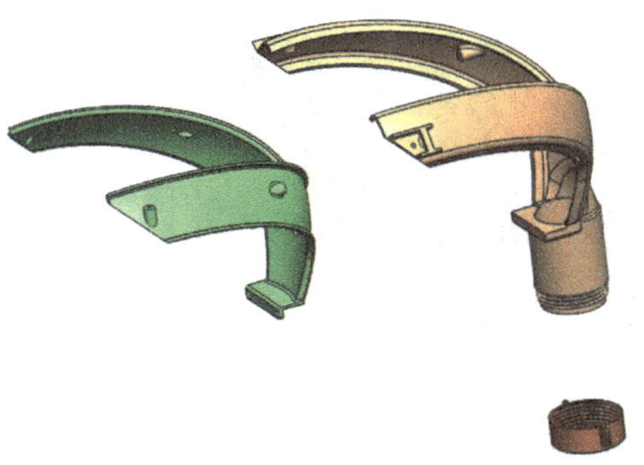

(a) 3D Printed hood support

(b) Sewing hood (Headcover)

Fig. 9 The block diagram of the upgrade respirator

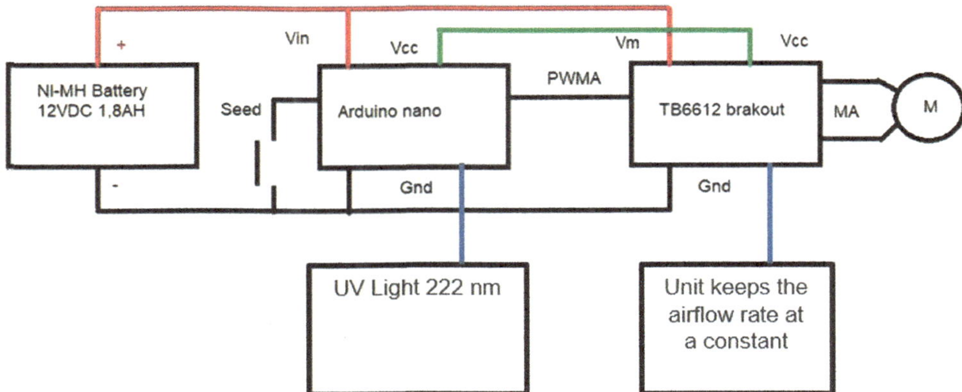

Fig. 10 Electronics circuit of the air-purifying respirator

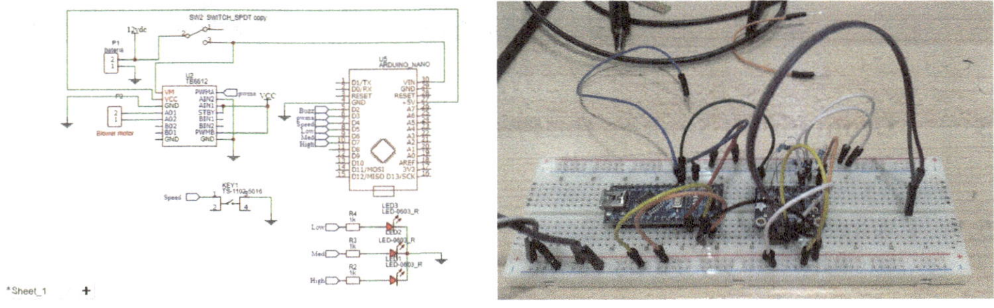

(a) Intelligent air flow regulator

(b) Building a reverse circuit on breadboard

Intelligent Air Flow Regulator

So powered air-purifying respirator operation will be like Power on wait mode select, after mode switch, pressed it will start blowing air with a low rate (6 CFM). 2nd press will select a medium rate (8 CFM), 3rd the press will choose the high rate (10 CFM). One more press will stop the blower unit and turn it back to standby mode. We have shown the upgrade air-purifying respirator with UV light for air sanitizing and air flow control unit, as shown in Fig. 10a. Users can choose the air source according to the temperature and the situation.

Fig. 11 Electronics circuit of the air-purifying respirator

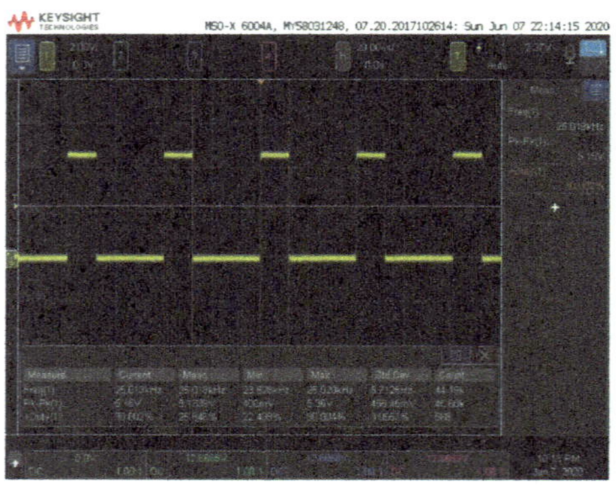

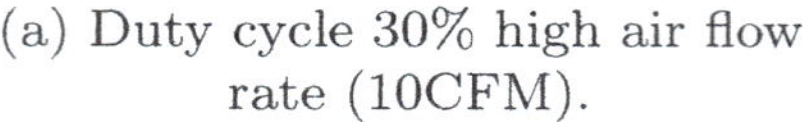

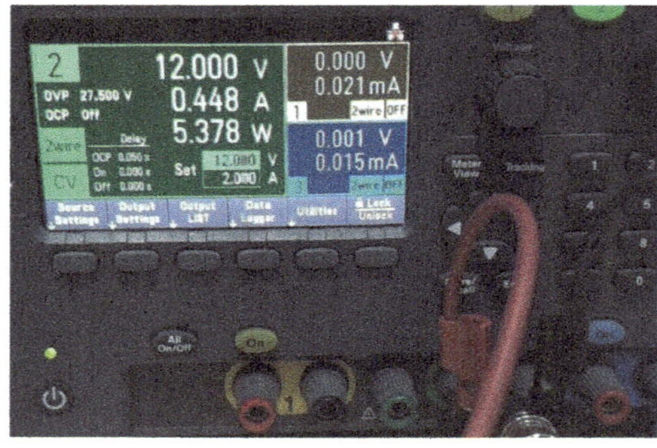

(a) Duty cycle 30% high air flow rate (10CFM).

(b) System practical electrical measurement.

Fig. 12 The PCB board of the upgrade PAPR

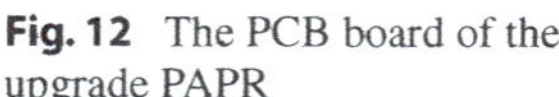

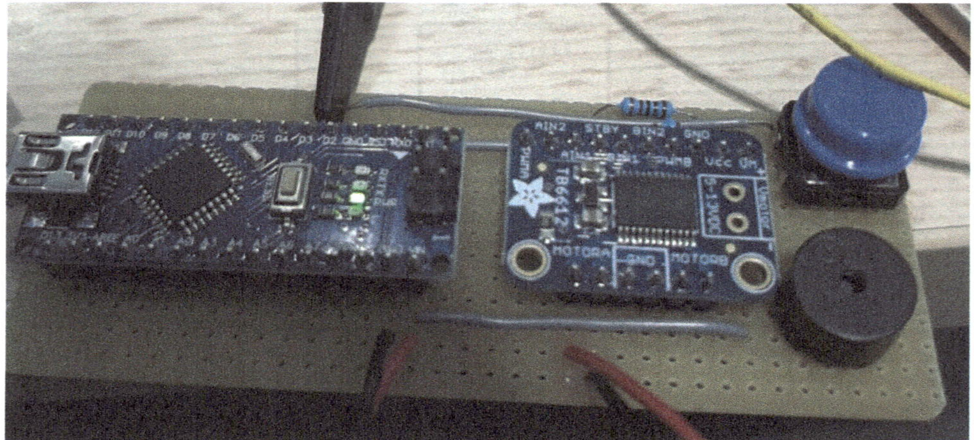

5 Drum for UV Sanitize the PAPR and Charge Wirelessly It

5.1 Wireless Charging the Battery for Air-Purifying Respirator

We ensure wireless power charging reduces the contact directly with the air-purifying respirator, and we minimize the spread of COVID-19. In this device, wireless power transmission relies on electromagnetic resonance, as shown in Fig. 14b [21,24]. Wireless power charging (WPT) range is just a few centimeters, which represents a significant obstacle towards its practical implementation, as shown in Fig. 13a. The analytical model of a WPT scheme can be developed through coupled-mode theory (CMT). Magnetic resonant coupling uses the same principles as inductive coupling, but it uses resonance to increase the scale at which the energy transfer can efficiently occur. A higher-quality factor indicates a lower rate of energy loss relative to the energy of the generator. The quality factor is an important parameter that describes a square generator resonator's character and characterizes a resonator bandwidth relative to its center frequency (50KHZ). Initially, we make two coils (Rx, Tx), each of which I wrapped 25 turns of insulated copper wire around a 25mm diameter. Each coil has an internal resistance R and inductance L, two coils tuned at the same frequency. A capacitor is put in parallel with each coil. The oscillator circuit produces a square-wave signal. A complete high-efficiency transmit amplifier unit designed to be implemented in on-coil transmit. The load coil Tx, tuned at the same resonant frequency, receives the power through the source coil Rx's magnetic field.

5.2 Transmission Circuit

We manufactured both an emitter coil (Rx) and a square oscillator generator. The frequency signal is the device that will create electromagnetic radiation that will permit the transmitter through the source coil to exchange energy [1,29,31], as shown in Fig. 13b.

Fig. 13 Block diagram of wireless air-purifying respirators charger

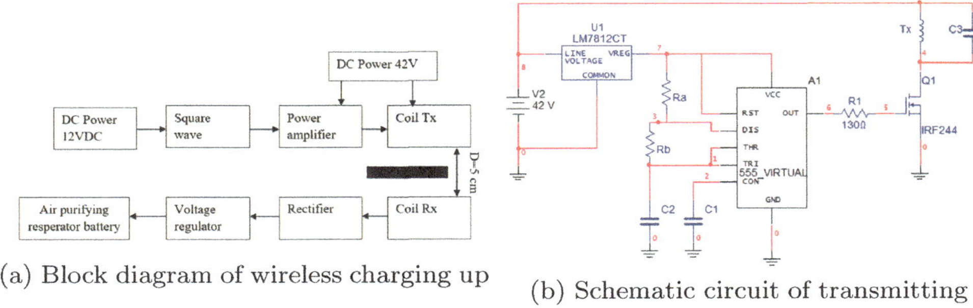

(a) Block diagram of wireless charging up

(b) Schematic circuit of transmitting section

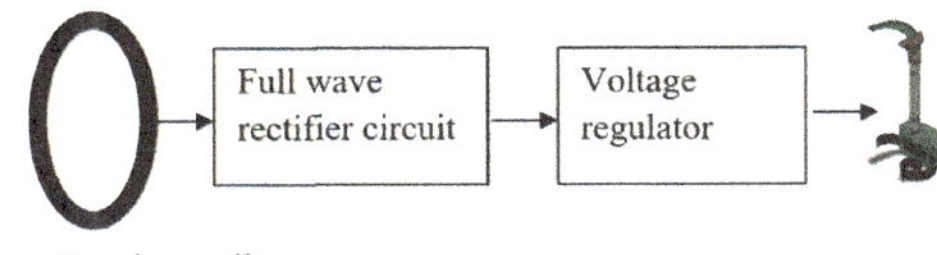

(c) Block diagram of the rectifier circuit

Frequency Oscillator

Many shapes can be used for configuring a square wave signal. After search and simulation, we choose and purchase the timer NE555. The schematic for the NE555 square wave generator, as shown in Fig. 13b. This device will be composed of components such as a battery, resistors, and capacitors. The output was insufficient to transfer power range 5cm, for that we will think to add power stage in our emitter circuit [10, 11].

Switched Mode Power Amplifier Circuit

In order for a PAPR to be functional, it needs to receive sufficient power. The energy received from the square wave generator is not sufficient to charge up the battery wirelessly. We want to try several solutions in this research to increase the efficiency of power transmission inside the drum. We can use a power amplifier to increase the output voltage, and electromagnetic radiation [22]. However, we need to find a balance between the need for high power and preventing the circuit temperature from going above safe levels. We are using an IRFZ44N power MOSFET to drive a source coil [2,5]. We prove from the datasheet that the IRFZ44N transistor has an ampere rating of 49A; however, it heats up very quickly. I have attached the schematic here. IRFZ44N is driven from a square wave signal with a frequency of around 55 kHz and duty cycles 50%. This device supply a voltage of 12 V DC to operate the transmitter coil through the power amplifier. We added a voltage regulator to reduce to voltage to 12 V DC to run the oscillator. When the voltage in the power stage increases, the range of wirelessly power transmission increases, the receiver circuit connected with the respirator consists of the load coil with attached capacitor and rectifier stage to receive power.

5.3   Receiver Circuit Section

The receiver circuit connected with the battery charger; it consists of the receiver coil (Rx) with an attached capacitor and full bridge rectifier circuit to harvest power, as shown in Fig. 13c. A rectifier is an electrical stage that converts alternating current (AC) to direct current (DC). The process is known as rectification.

Power was successfully transferred and rectified at significant distances in this prototype. At the end of the work, we could conceive a system for transmitting energy wirelessly from the emitter coil to the receiving ring that was enough to charge the PAPR battery. We designed discrete components such as the square oscillator, switch power amplifier, and a rectifier bridge for the system. We were able to develop the receiver also. The object to be powered has a wireless power source. In its drum, the respirator automatically wirelessly charge without having to be plugged in. Future work includes connecting the square oscillator with the power amplifier using the current amplifier chip to provide enough current. Also, the size of the transmitting and receiving coils and study can increase the electromagnetic radiation zone that the respirator can recharge at any position inside the drum. The drum should non-ferrous material to reduce the eddy-current forces.

5.4   Discussion and Results

Electromagnetic radiation charging technology is a non-radioactive energy transmission mode, relying instead on the near magnetic field. The energy received from the square wave oscillator is not sufficient to LED lit up wirelessly with

Fig. 14 UV sanitizer and wireless charging drum

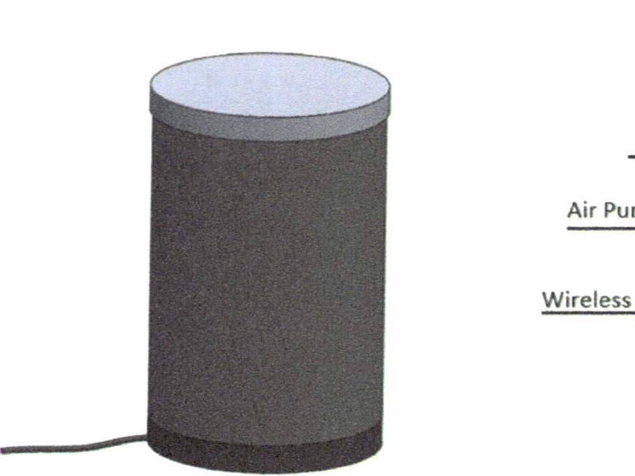

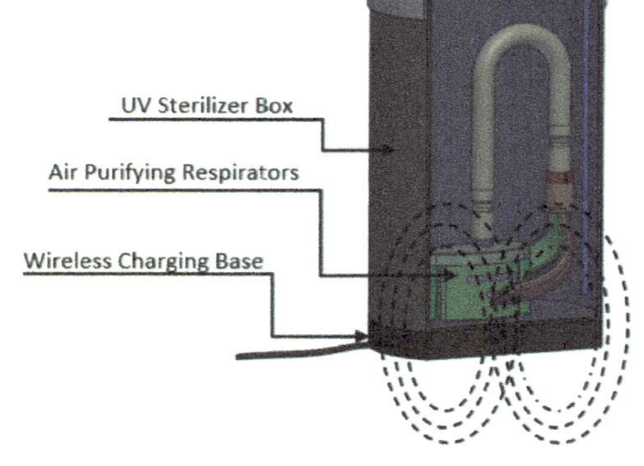

(a) UV sanitizer drum to kills viruses

(b) Cut-view of the UV sanitizer and wireless charging drum

more range distance. Efficiency was identifying from the source power measurements. We have successfully transported power wirelessly from the experiments at a distance of 50 mm. The receiver and the transmitter accomplish the inductive coupling. We approved that the PAPR was work with high efficiency. More work and studies are needed to increase the electromagnetic radiation zone that the battery can charge at any drum position.

5.5 Sanitizing Drum for the Upgrade Air-Purifying Respirator

After doctors wear the PAPR inside the infected COVID-19 area, the virus may be sticking to the device. So we are thinking about keeping the device disinfected. To clean up the respirator and kill the covid-19 virus with a high-efficiency solution. According to studies, these short wavelengths of light measuring between 200 and 300 nm are strongly absorbed by microorganisms' nucleic acid. Moreover, just like how stronger UV rays damage skin cells that result in sunburns, UV-C light equally hurts and kills microorganisms on a cellular level destroying the nucleic acids and interrupting the germs' DNA. Scientists have been using UV light to destroy viruses and bacteria. These days, anyone, not just award-winning scientists, can use light to prevent germs. After any contact with patients affected by COVID-19, the doctors and healthcare staff should remove the ventilator and put it inside the drum. And then turning up the UV and wireless battery charging working simultaneously, as shown in Fig. 14a. UV mobile drum can be used to clean up two or more respirators with all accessories at a time. The system uses ultraviolet light 222 nm, a short-wavelength light capable of converting the virus into harmless carbon compounds and water. Traditional UV-C tubers are also in short supply because of the COVID-19 pandemic. The prototype system uses a more readily available LED tuber capable of achieving the needed frequency for disinfectant, as shown in Fig. 14a. This technique can help the medical staff inside laboratories remove the respirator and immediately put it inside the drum. Through this system, we guarantee two options; Firstly, sterilize all parts of the ventilator, and secondly, wirelessly charge the PAPR battery as shown in Fig. 14.

6 Real-Time Monitoring of Indoor Healthcare Tracking Using the Internet of Things-Based E-BEACON

So, diffusion of the COVID-19 virus can occur by direct contact with an infected person or indirect contact with surfaces in the immediate atmosphere or with items used on the infected people. In this device, we are adding IoT technology in the respirator for physical distancing and healthcare staff tracking. A new device implanted inside the air-purifying respirator could register the details of other PAPR that come into its small area. The specification of the PAPR real-time localization system (RTLS) is below:

- Wireless indoor pallet tracking system,
- Accurate location of moving and stationary healthcare staff,
- Accuracy of 50 cm × 50 cm meters for locating indoor objects,
- Asset monitoring system,
- No electrical or wiring or networking cables need to be laid,
- Physical distancing,
- Strengthening of security surrounding the clinical area.

Real-time localization system (RTLS) to locate doctors and healthcare staff inside the hospital area, as shown in Fig. 15.

This section aims to develop new indoor doctors tracking to improve positioning accuracy [27,42]. There are some

Fig. 15 The architecture of the Bluetooth healthcare staff tracking system

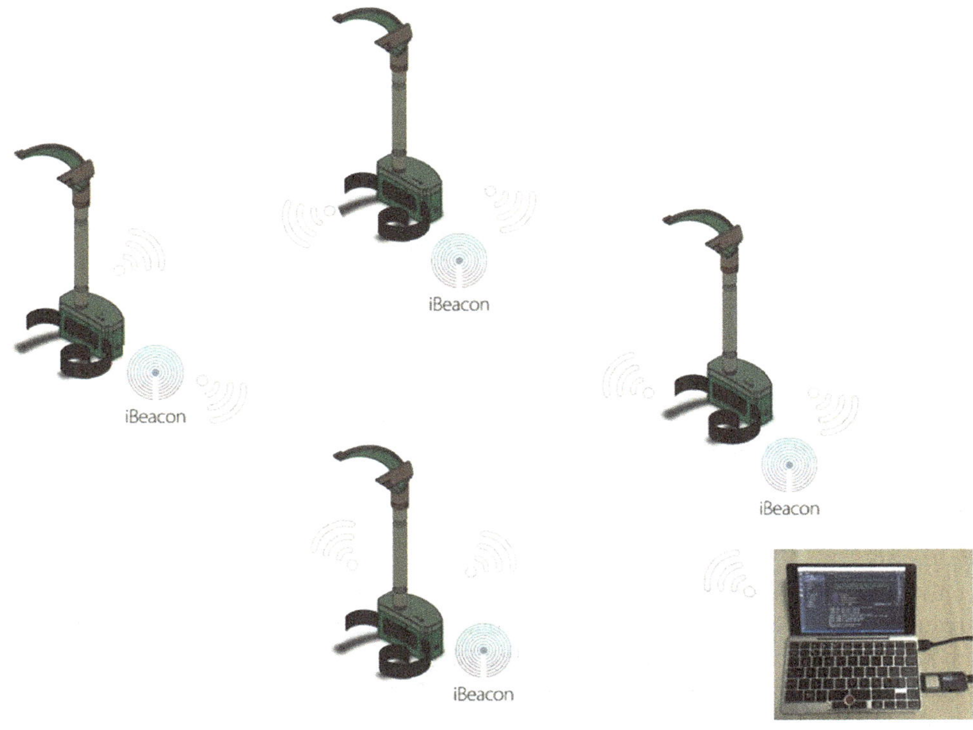

Fig. 16 Block diagram of the tracking system

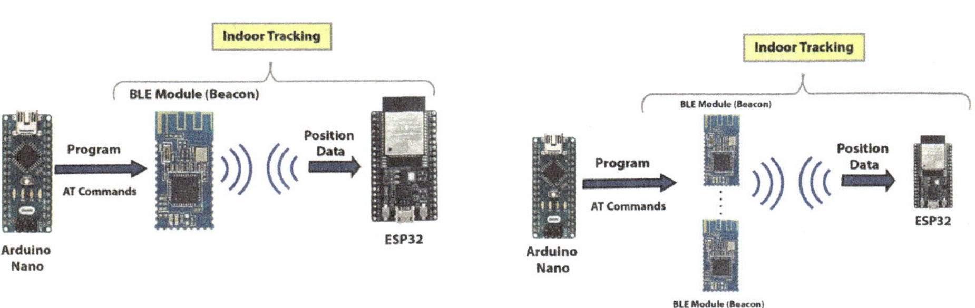

(a) Tracking system directly with one beacon.

(b) Tracking system with multi-beacon.

introduced indoor tracking systems. However, the rapid technology improvement opens for us new ways, which might be more effective. Unfortunately, there are no methods for indoor tracking that is being approved. Nevertheless, this thesis came to improve and prove that an indoor doctor's tracking system is essential. Moreover, offering a new solution to assist doctors. The purpose of this research is to design a system that uses Bluetooth for laboratory tracks. This prototype proposes and evaluates the possibility of using a new approach to allocate doctors. Nearly, it will be done by providing the doctors with the most accurate latitude and longitude, as shown in Fig. 16b. The importance of tracking the doctors in the hospital is to increase the matter of doctor's safety. The low strength Bluetooth uses low radio frequency, which has a lower health hazard to the surrounding individuals.

The prototype is to design a doctor's tracking system for indoor settings (hospitals, laboratories, and Quarantine.) based on Bluetooth technology. The system will identify the current position of a PAPR with a Bluetooth module attached to it. Multiple Bluetooth low Energy modules will broadcast the position data that will serve as beacons placed across the hospital. Whenever the PAPR passes by a beacon, the Bluetooth module on the ventilator receives the place data and passes it to the Arduino NANO to evaluate. Kalman filter will use to the received data for more precise results [19,37]. With extensive and complete hospital and laboratory, the alternative indoor tracking becomes expansive. Significantly, this project offers a better solution, including lower prices and high efficiency. Bluetooth low energy (BLE) is inexpensive to install and programming. BLE provided 40 channels. On the other hand, the Wi-Fi tracking system as an alternative includes

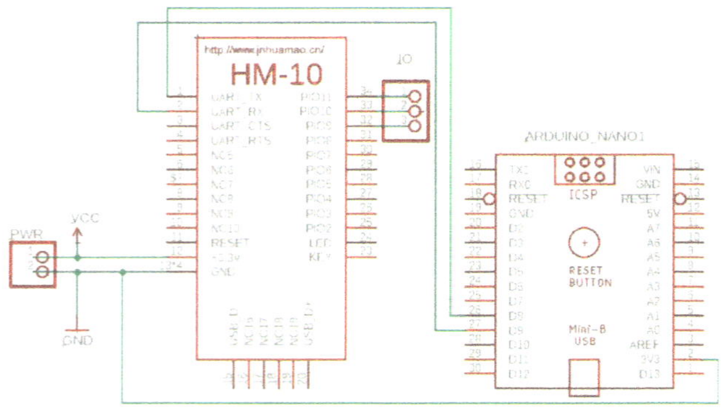

(a) iBeacon schematic diagram (Setup HM-10 BLE module as iBeacon).

(b) ESP32 tracking system.

Fig. 17 Electronics circuit of the real-time location system

only three channels, which have a terrible effect gap that reduces tracking quality. Use Bluetooth modules as beacons to advertise the location of the nearby PAPR. Bluetooth acts as an aided localization system where it uses the electronics to allocate the doctors. The BLE communication technology will broadcast a radio frequency in a low range. The passing doctors will receive these signals. The Low range radio frequency of 40 channel signals will result in maximum location precision. The iBeacons will propagation its location, and it will do its job to evaluate the location by the distance gap. The Kalman filter will use in this phase to ensure the estimation value is being calculated. Use a relatively cheap technology to develop a tracking PAPR. It compares alternative technology based on their precision, energy consumption, and compatibility with the local area. The alternative technique will be compared based on previous features. Bluetooth-based PAPR tracking could be the best smart low cost. It is cheap to implemented and maintain. It operates along with the same band as 802.11b/g/n Wi-Fi, the 2.4 GHz ISM; although, there is no significant RF interference because of the low broadcast energy. There are three main channels for Bluetooth to propagate, of which (39, 38, and 37). These channels have been selected not to interfere with the Wi-Fi channels (11, 6, and 1). This technique deployed numerous sensor nodes at fixed spots inside laboratories. The target person will fix in the PAPR device; it transmits a unique code every 20s via an infrared sensor. A location manager for correction views the nodes of the sensor. This centralized manager technique calculates the active badge's real position and provides location information to the users [4,28]. The system's primary function is to determine the current position using multiple BLE-enabled modules located along with the lab and act as beacons that broadcast the position information to be received and interpreted by the microcontroller. The HM-10 module can use the advertisement principle, which allows the mod-

ule, as a BLE device, to broadcast data to adjoining devices periodically. The HM-10 module will be programmed using AT commands that will send through using UART pins on the Arduino Nano (TX and RX), as shown in Fig. 17a.

Every beacon consists of a BLE module and battery holder with a 3V battery to power the module.

To find the beacon location data, the ESP32 microcontroller on the tracking system must receive the advertisement communication from the beacon, identify the beacon's name, and read the latitude and longitude values embedded in the advertisement, as shown in Fig. 17b. The ESP32 components establish an international hub to follow Bluetooth low energy devices using ESP32 node.

TX Power value advertised by the module is a hexadecimal value that represents the RSSI (Received Signal Strength Indication). This value is required to determine the proximity of the beacon to the tracking device. Therefore, the system will identify the nearest beacon whenever there is more than one beacon available, as shown in Fig. 16b. AT commands are simple commands used to communicate with specific devices. For this prototype, the commands will communicate with the Bluetooth modules to configure them as beacons and assign the UUID to each HM-10. Such configuration is done by connecting RX and TX pins of the beacon to pins 9 and 8 of the Arduino Nano to create UART communication. The ESP32 will scan for nearby beacons and receive the location data from the nearest beacon.

The Bluetooth ability of ESP32 will allow the device to scan the area for nearby beacons [26].

When the tracking device discovers multiple beacons available nearby, it has to decide which beacon to receive the position data. This is succeeded by comparing the RSSI value of each detected HM-10 beacon. The RSSI value is negative and indicates the strength level of the received signal. The additional the beacon is from the tracking system, the higher the RSSI absolute value. So, when the tracking system discovers multiple beacons nearby, it will accept location data from the beacon with the lowest RSSI value.

The system received the advertised data from the beacon and converted the hexadecimal data into decimal values that can be interpreted as position data. Bluetooth Low Energy components, serve as beacons, placed along the laboratory will have information about their location, and they will continuously advertise this information to the passing healthcare staff wear the air ventilator system. When the healthcare staff, which is attached to a Bluetooth module, passes by a beacon on the lab or Quarantine area, it will receive the position data and send it directly to the microcontroller. Gateway is placed around PAPR users. A battery powers the gateways. They connect via Wi-Fi. The gateways detect beacons implemented already in the upgraded PAPR device and send this information (PAPR Name, PAPR Serial number) to the computer for recording and diagnostic. The RTLS circuit received the advertised data from the beacon that be interpreted as location data. Moreover, the system can receive the location data from the absolute nearest beacon tested to ensure accuracy.

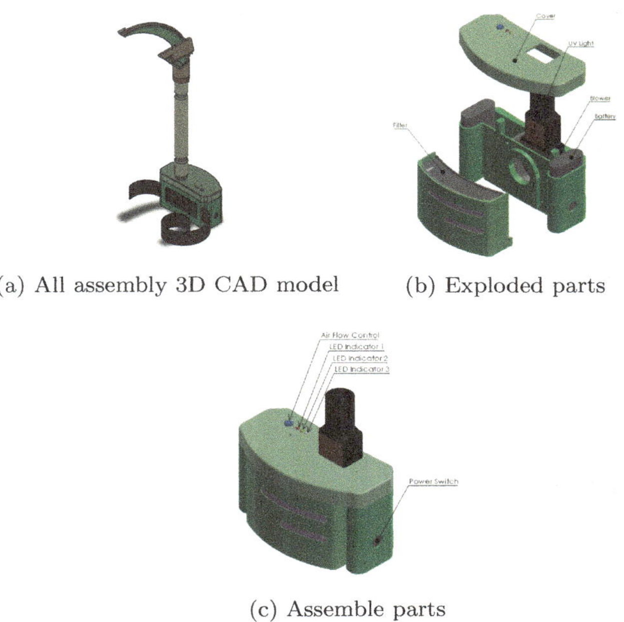

(a) All assembly 3D CAD model   (b) Exploded parts

(c) Assemble parts

Fig. 19 All assembly

7   Power Air-Purifying Respirators Prototyping and Testing Phase

After understanding very well the different components of the PAPR, we start the fabrication and prototyping process. The power air-purifying respirator consists of two significant parts; the blower unit (always install the HE filter into the blower unit) and the Hood (Head cover). We determine the airflow rate, and we are making the PCB circuit, as shown in Fig. 18. The package and the 3D design of the device should

respect the medical fabrication standard, as shown in Fig. 19. After 3D printing using FDM technology will fix these components (PCB, Blower, battery, and HE filter) inside the 3D package for testing and validation, as shown in Figs. 19a, 19b, and 19c, respectively. In this prototype, we are sure that we can see easily around us, available head and a lightweight of the upgrade PAPR to breathe fresh air, and we guaranty 100% without a virus. Table 2 shows the air flow rate measurement for the first device and the upgraded PAPR. Our device is better and more safe than the original one; our helmet is a little higher, and our head cover is less than the original equipment, as shown in Table 3. Evenly distributes clean air throughout the entire breathing zone of the hood. The intelligent regulator unit is designed to keep the air flow at a constant preset level. The stage of testing and wearing the device, as shown in Fig. 20.

Power was successfully transferred and rectified at significant distances in this drum (distance = 5 cm). At the end of the work, we could conceive a system for transmitting energy wirelessly from the transmitting coil (Tx) to the receiving coil (Rx) enough to charge the PAPR battery. We designed discrete components such as the square oscillator, switch power amplifier, and a rectifier bridge for the system. We were able to design the receiver also. The object to be powered has a wireless power source. Future work includes connecting the square oscillator with a power amplifier using the current amplifier chip to provide enough current. Air-purifying respirator not matching with COVID-19, as shown in Fig. 21a. Upgrade

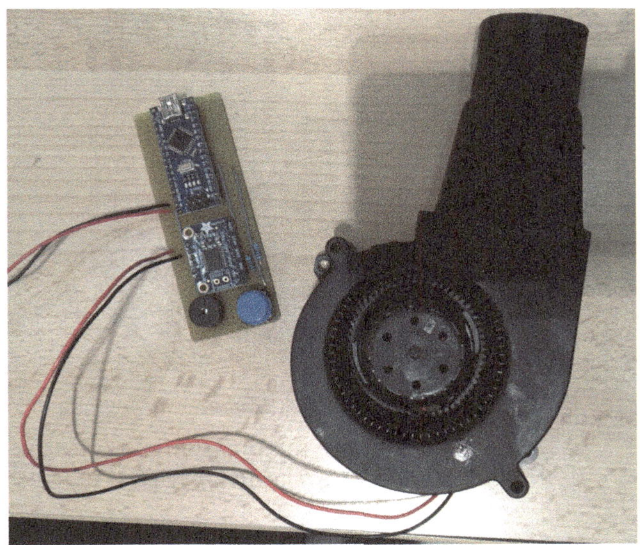

Fig. 18 The blower connected to intelligent air flow regulator

Table 2 Intelligent air flow regulator measurement

Air flow rate	Original device	Repurposing upgrade device (CFM)
Level 1	6 CFM	6
Level 2	8 CFM	8
Level 3	N/A	10

Table 3 Device weight

Parts	Original device (gm)	Repurposing upgrade device (gm)
Respirator casing	1200	1200
Helmet	200	270
Head cover	100	90

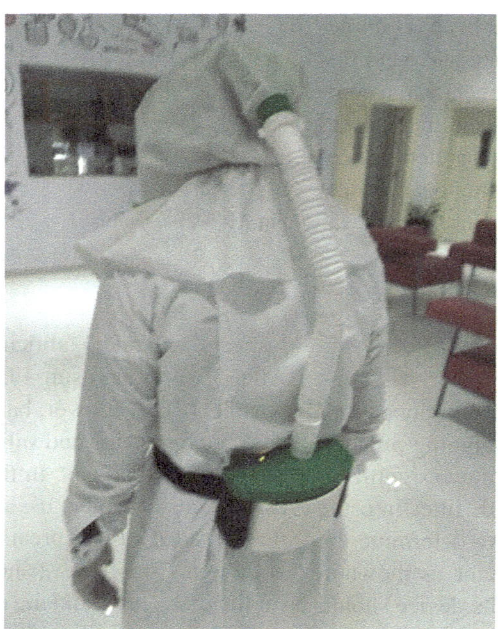
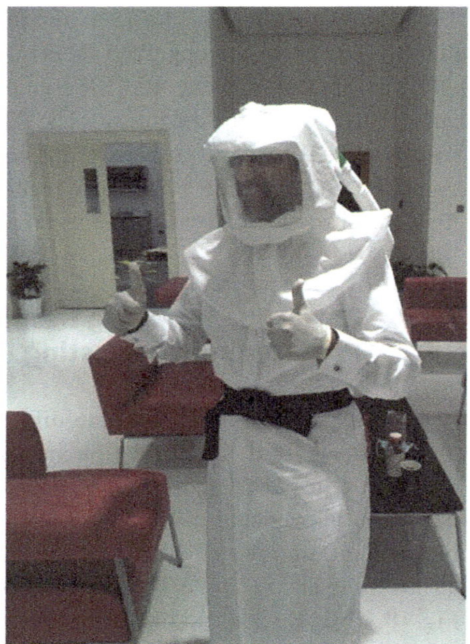

Fig. 20 One of our team wear and test the air-purifying respirator with hood

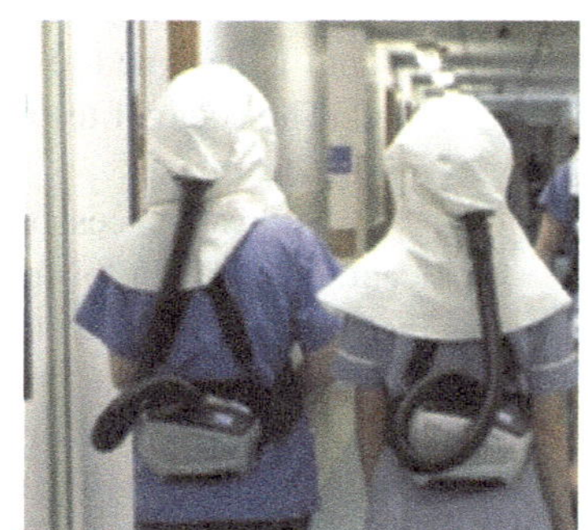

(a) Air purifying respirator not matching with COVID-19

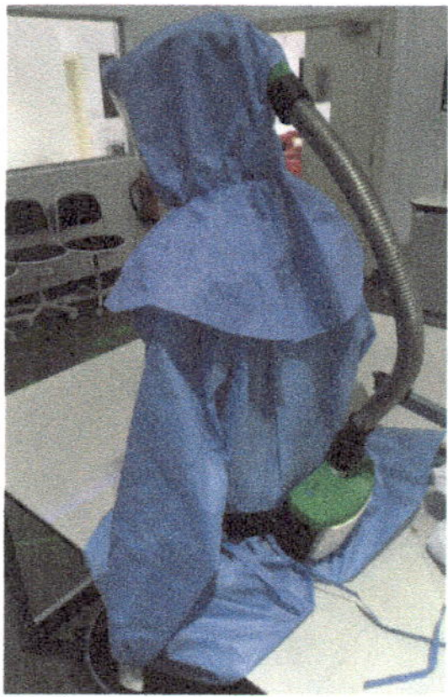

(b) Upgrade air-purifying respirator with UV air sanitizing (COVID-19 compatible)

Fig. 21 The anti-fog hood shield with air-purifying respirator

Table 4 Comparison between the original device and the upgrade prototype

Function	The original device	The repurpose device (Prototype)
Air flow rate	198–205 LPM	198–225 LPM
Battery charger	Charger battery with cable	Inductive charging solution
Tracking system	Without	Existing tracking solution to reduce the contact between healthcare staff
UV light	Without	With in

air-purifying respirator with UV air sanitizing (COVID-19 match), as shown in Fig. 21b.

8   Conclusion

In this research, we approved that with reverse engineering, we are repurposing a new local respirator with more air flow lightweight and anti-fog hood shield using available resources in Fab Lab in a short time and low cost. In this research, we made and tested the new respirator, the essential tool of the first defense line, an additional UV light to improve the quantity of air. We proved that reverse engineering in a medical device is the right solution in the COVID-19 crisis. In future, we will make respirators with less weight, longer battery lifetime, more air flow at a low price, and increase filter efficiency with a long lifetime using bipolar ionization technique. We add UV light between the HE filter and helmet to ensure the air-breathing one hundred germicides and UV drums for sanitizing different respirator parts after use and wireless charging simultaneously. We have also added IoT technology in the respirator for physical distancing and healthcare staff tracking and recording. We are not interested in replicating the original devices to make money, but we have looking to help health professionals.

Table 4 shows the comparison between the original air-purifying respirator and the repurposing upgrade device.

Acknowledgements This work was made possible by NPRP11S-0113-180276 from the Qatar National Research Fund (a member of the Qatar Foundation). The findings achieved herein are solely the responsibility of the author. The authors would like to acknowledge the support of the Qatar Scientific Club for creating an environment that encourages academic research and providing the hardware components.

References

[1] Abdolkhani A (2017) Single-switch soft-switched power flow controller for wireless power transfer applications. In: 2017 IEEE Wireless Power Transfer Conference (WPTC), IEEE, 10.1109/wpt.2017.7953804

[2] Alinikula P, Choi K, Long S (1999) Design of class e power amplifier with nonlinear parasitic output capacitance. IEEE Transactions on Circuits and Systems II: Analog and Digital Signal Processing 46(2):114–119, 10.1109/82.752911

[3] Alnuaimi MS, Ziout A (2018) The use of reverse engineering in a comparison between engineered and solid hardwood 10.13140/RG.2.2.29488.81925

[4] Bahl P, Padmanabhan V (????) RADAR: an in-building RF-based user location and tracking system. In: Proceedings IEEE INFOCOM 2000. Conference on Computer Communications. Nineteenth Annual Joint Conference of the IEEE Computer and Communications Societies (Cat. No.00CH37064), IEEE, 10.1109/infcom.2000.832252

[5] Belmili H, Cheikh SMA, Haddadi M, Larbes C (2010) Design and development of a data acquisition system for photovoltaic modules characterization. Renewable Energy 35(7):1484–1492, 10.1016/j.renene.2010.01.007

[6] Brosseau LM (2020) Are powered air purifying respirators a solution for protecting healthcare workers from emerging aerosol-transmissible diseases? Annals of Work Exposures and Health 64(4):339–341, 10.1093/annweh/wxaa024

[7] Buonanno M, Ponnaiya B, Welch D, Stanislauskas M, Randers-Pehrson G, Smilenov L, Lowy FD, Owens DM, Brenner DJ (2017) Germicidal efficacy and mammalian skin safety of 222-nm UV light. Radiation Research 187(4):493–501, 10.1667/rr0010cc.1

[8] Buonanno M, Welch D, Shuryak I, Brenner DJ (2020) Far-UVC light (222nm) efficiently and safely inactivates airborne human coronaviruses. Scientific Reports 10(1), 10.1038/s41598-020-67211-2

[9] Cadet J (2020) Harmless effects of sterilizing 222-nm far-UV radiation on mouse skin and eye tissues. Photochemistry and Photobiology 96(4):949–950, 10.1111/php.13294

[10] Chaari MZ, Rahimi R (2017) Light led directly lit up by the wireless power transfer technology. In: 2017 International Conference on Radar, Antenna, Microwave, Electronics, and Telecommunications (ICRAMET), IEEE, pp 137–141

[11] Chaari MZ, Lahiani M, Ghariani H (2017) Energy harvesting from electromagnetic radiation emissions by compact flouresent lamp. In: 2017 Ninth International Conference on Advanced Computational Intelligence (ICACI), IEEE, pp 272–275

[12] Chen H, Guo J, Wang C, Luo F, Yu X, Zhang W, Li J, Zhao D, Xu D, Gong Q, Liao J, Yang H, Hou W, Zhang Y (2020) Clinical characteristics and intrauterine vertical transmission potential of COVID-19 infection in nine pregnant women: a retrospective review of medical records. The Lancet 395(10226):809–815, 10.1016/s0140-6736(20)30360-3

[13] Choi B, Choudhary MC, Regan J, Sparks JA, Padera RF, Qiu X, Solomon IH, Kuo HH, Boucau J, Bowman K, Adhikari UD, Winkler ML, Mueller AA, Hsu TYT, Desjardins M, Baden LR, Chan BT, Walker BD, Lichterfeld M, Brigl M, Kwon DS, Kanjilal S, Richardson ET, Jonsson AH, Alter G, Barczak AK, Hanage WP, Yu XG, Gaiha GD, Seaman MS, Cernadas M, Li JZ (2020) Persistence and evolution of SARS-CoV-2 in an immunocompromised host. New England Journal of Medicine 10.1056/nejmc2031364

[14] Christopherson D, Yao W, Lu M, Vijayakumar R, Sedaghat R, Surgery N, et al. (????) High-efficiency particulate air (hepa) filters in the era of covid-19: function and efficacy. otolaryngol neck surg [internet]. 2020

[15] Christopherson DA, Yao WC, Lu M, Vijayakumar R, Sedaghat AR (2020) High-efficiency particulate air filters in the era of covid-19: Function and efficacy. Otolaryngology–Head and Neck Surgery p 0194599820941838

[16] for Disease Control C, Prevention, et al. (2020) Considerations for optimizing the supply of powered air-purifying respirators (paprs): for healthcare practitioners (hcp). Published April 19

[17] Elston DM (2020) Occupational skin disease among health care workers during the coronavirus (COVID-19) epidemic. Journal of the American Academy of Dermatology 82(5):1085–1086, 10.1016/j.jaad.2020.03.012

[18] Emanuel EJ, Persad G, Upshur R, Thome B, Parker M, Glickman A, Zhang C, Boyle C, Smith M, Phillips JP (2020) Fair allocation of scarce medical resources in the time of covid-19. New England Journal of Medicine 382(21):2049–2055, 10.1056/nejmsb2005114

[19] Faragher R (2012) Understanding the basis of the kalman filter via a simple and intuitive derivation [lecture notes]. IEEE Signal Processing Magazine 29(5):128–132, 10.1109/msp.2012.2203621

[20] Filho ECC, Castro R, Fernandes FF, Pereira G, Perazzo H (2020) Gastrointestinal endoscopy during the COVID-19 pandemic: an updated review of guidelines and statements from international and national societies. Gastrointestinal Endoscopy 92(2):440–445.e6, 10.1016/j.gie.2020.03.3854

[21] Haldar S, Mondal S, Mondal A, Banerjee R (2020) Battery management system using state of charge estimation: An IOT based approach. In: 2020 National Conference on Emerging Trends on Sustainable Technology and Engineering Applications (NCETSTEA), IEEE, 10.1109/ncetstea48365.2020.9119945

[22] He F, Xie Q, Zhuang Z, Wang Z (2019) The design of a high-efficiency mode-switching power amplifier with a parallel combining transformer for LTE application. In: 2019 IEEE International Conference on Integrated Circuits, Technologies and Applications (ICTA), IEEE, 10.1109/icta48799.2019.9012888

[23] Holland M, Zaloga DJ, Friderici CS (2020) COVID-19 personal protective equipment (PPE) for the emergency physician. Visual Journal of Emergency Medicine 19:100740, 10.1016/j.visj.2020.100740

[24] Huang M, Lu Y, Martins RP (2019) A reconfigurable bidirectional wireless power transceiver for battery-to-battery wireless charging. IEEE Transactions on Power Electronics 34(8):7745–7753, 10.1109/tpel.2018.2881285

[25] Kempfle JS, Panda A, Hottin M, Vinik K, Kozin ED, Ito CJ, Remenschneider AK (2020) Effect of powered air-purifying respirators on speech recognition among health care workers. Otolaryngology–Head and Neck Surgery p 019459982094568, 10.1177/0194599820945685

[26] Khalid A, Memon I (????) Bluetooth-based traffic tracking system using esp32 microcontroller. In: Advances in Machine Learning and Computational Intelligence, Springer, pp 737–746

[27] Kodali RK, Jain V, Bose S, Boppana L (2016) IoT based smart security and home automation system. In: 2016 International Conference on Computing, Communication and Automation (ICCCA), IEEE, 10.1109/ccaa.2016.7813916

[28] Lu M, Chen W, Shen X, Lam HC, Liu J (2007) Positioning and tracking construction vehicles in highly dense urban areas and building construction sites. Automation in Construction 16(5):647–656, 10.1016/j.autcon.2006.11.001

[29] Luo B, Long T, Guo L, Mai R, He Z (2019) Analysis and design of hybrid inductive and capacitive wireless power transfer system. In: 2019 IEEE Applied Power Electronics Conference and Exposition (APEC), IEEE, 10.1109/apec.2019.8722140

[30] Miles LF, Chuen J, Edwards L, Hohmann JD, Williams R, Peyton P, Grayden DB (2020) The design and manufacture of 3d-printed adjuncts for powered air-purifying respirators. Anaesthesia Reports 8(2):84–86, 10.1002/anr3.12055

[31] Minnaert B, Stevens N (2018) Maximizing the power transfer for a mixed inductive and capacitive wireless power transfer system. In: 2018 IEEE Wireless Power Transfer Conference (WPTC), IEEE, 10.1109/wpt.2018.8639265

[32] Monroy ME, Arciniegas JL, Rodríguez JC (2017) Caracterización de los contextos de uso de la ingeniería inversa. Información tecnológica 28(4):75–84, 10.4067/s0718-07642017000400010

[33] Murthy S, Gomersall CD, Fowler RA (2020) Care for critically ill patients with COVID-19. JAMA 323(15):1499, 10.1001/jama.2020.3633

[34] Organization WH, health organization W, et al. (2020) Coronavirus disease (covid-2019) situation reports

[35] Palka D (2020) Use of reverse engineering and additive printing in the reconstruction of gears. Multidisciplinary Aspects of Production Engineering 3(1):274–284, 10.2478/mape-2020-0024

[36] Perry JL, Agui J, Vijayakimar R (2016) Submicron and nanoparticulate matter removal by hepa-rated media filters and packed beds of granular materials

[37] Pop MD, Proştean O, David TM, Proştean G (2020) Hybrid solution combining kalman filtering with takagi–sugeno fuzzy inference system for online car-following model calibration. Sensors 20(19):5539

[38] Ramanathan K, Antognini D, Combes A, Paden M, Zakhary B, Ogino M, MacLaren G, Brodie D, Shekar K (2020) Planning and provision of ECMO services for severe ARDS during the COVID-19 pandemic and other outbreaks of emerging infectious diseases. The Lancet Respiratory Medicine 8(5):518–526, 10.1016/s2213-2600(20)30121-1

[39] Ranney ML, Griffeth V, Jha AK (2020) Critical supply shortages — the need for ventilators and personal protective equipment during the covid-19 pandemic. New England Journal of Medicine 382(18):e41, 10.1056/nejmp2006141

[40] Shaikh JG, Daimiwal NM (2017) Respiratory parameter measurement and analysis using differential pressure sensor. In: 2017 International Conference on Communication and Signal Processing (ICCSP), IEEE, 10.1109/iccsp.2017.8286485

[41] Sikorska-Czupryna S, Mazurkow A (2020) The use of reverse engineering to create FEM model of spiroid gears. Advances in Manufacturing Science and Technology 44(3):71–73, 10.2478/amst-2019-0013

[42] Singh H, Pallagani V, Khandelwal V, Venkanna U (2018) IoT based smart home automation system using sensor node. In: 2018 4th International Conference on Recent Advances in Information Technology (RAIT), IEEE, 10.1109/rait.2018.8389037

[43] Sohail A, Nutini A (2020) Forecasting the timeframe of 2019-nCoV and human cells interaction with reverse engineering. Progress in Biophysics and Molecular Biology 155:29–35, 10.1016/j.pbiomolbio.2020.04.002

[44] Sun X, Wandelt S, Zhang A (2020) How did COVID-19 impact air transportation? a first peek through the lens of complex networks. Journal of Air Transport Management 89:101928, 10.1016/j.jairtraman.2020.101928

[45] Tien TN, Thai NH (2019) A NOVEL DESIGN OF THE ROOTS BLOWER. Vietnam Journal of Science and Technology 57(2):249, 10.15625/2525-2518/57/2/13094

[46] Tino R, Moore R, Antoline S, Ravi P, Wake N, Ionita CN, Morris JM, Decker SJ, Sheikh A, Rybicki FJ, Chepelev LL (2020) COVID-19 and the role of 3d printing in medicine. 3D Printing in Medicine 6(1), 10.1186/s41205-020-00064-7

[47] Ullah S, Ullah A, Lee J, Jeong Y, Hashmi M, Zhu C, Joo KI, Cha HJ, Kim IS (2020) Reusability comparison of melt-blown vs nanofiber

face mask filters for use in the coronavirus pandemic. ACS Applied Nano Materials 3(7):7231–7241, 10.1021/acsanm.0c01562

[48] Wang CJ, Ng CY, Brook RH (2020a) Response to COVID-19 in taiwan. JAMA 323(14):1341, 10.1001/jama.2020.3151

[49] Wang D, Hu B, Hu C, Zhu F, Liu X, Zhang J, Wang B, Xiang H, Cheng Z, Xiong Y, Zhao Y, Li Y, Wang X, Peng Z (2020b) Clinical characteristics of 138 hospitalized patients with 2019 novel coronavirus–infected pneumonia in wuhan, china. JAMA 323(11):1061, 10.1001/jama.2020.1585

[50] Xu C, Guo X, Jiang H, Liu S, Cao W (2015) Analysis of measurement reliability of hot-film air flow sensor influenced by air contaminant. In: 2015 IEEE 65th Electronic Components and Technology Conference (ECTC), IEEE, 10.1109/ectc.2015.7159920

[51] Yu L, Peel G, Cheema F, Lawrence W, Bukreyeva N, Jinks C, Peel J, Peterson J, Paessler S, Hourani M, Ren Z (2020) Catching and killing of airborne SARS-CoV-2 to control spread of COVID-19 by a heated air disinfection system. Materials Today Physics 15:100249, 10.1016/j.mtphys.2020.100249

Exploiting Egocentric Cues for Action Recognition for Ambient Assisted Living Applications

Adrián Núñez-Marcos, Gorka Azkune, and Ignacio Arganda-Carreras

Abstract

Being the elder population in constant growth, governments have to cope with higher expenses for elder care from year to year. Helping the elderly to extend their independent lifestyle is of pivotal importance to minimise those costs. That is the goal of the Ambient Assisted Living research field. Through the use of Information and Communication Technologies, it is possible to provide solutions to help the elderly live independently for as long as possible or to predict mental health issues that could seriously harm their independence. The key enablers for these solutions are the egocentric cameras and the egocentric action recognition techniques for the analysis of egocentric videos. This chapter proposes various of those techniques focused on the exploitation of intrinsic egocentric cues.

1 Introduction

With the growth of the elder population, governments have to cope with higher expenses due to elder care, medicines, treatments, and so on. These are becoming more worrying with the expectation of the elder population duplicating by 2050,[1] making the issue unmanageable for the authorities. That is why, foreseeing that situation, governments are investing in research projects that will help elder people extend their independence for as long as possible, having to cope with problems related to ageing such as mental health issues. For example, some projects aim to mitigate serious illnesses such as Mild Cognitive Impairment (MCI) [2,47] or frailty [21] of elderly citizens using unobtrusive Information and Communication Technologies (ICT). That is, sensor or camera technologies are used to monitor people's activities and behaviour and correlate their evolution with MCI and frailty. This is useful to predict the possibility of those diseases or to plan interventions to minimise the consequences. Besides, these kinds of approaches are contained in the Ambient Assisted Living (AAL) field, which promotes the healthy and active ageing of people using the ICT, allowing elder people to avoid being dependent on someone else in their daily tasks.

In particular, automatic Human Action Recognition (HAR) is one of the main enablers of AAL approaches. The methods contained within that field are divided into two categories: the sensor-based HAR [11,63] and the vision-based HAR [7,68]. In the first one, multiple sensors are located in the environment and are activated when the user performs concrete movements and actions. Approaches

A. Núñez-Marcos (✉)
Deustotech Institute, University of Deusto, Avenida de las Universidades, No. 24, 48007 Bilbao, Spain
e-mail: adrian.nunez@deusto.es

G. Azkune · I. Arganda-Carreras
Department of Computer Science and Artificial Intelligence, University of the Basque Country, P. Manuel Lardizabal 1, 20018 San Sebastian, Spain
e-mail: gorka.azcune@ehu.eus

I. Arganda-Carreras
e-mail: ignacio.arganda@ehu.eus

G. Azkune
IXA NLP Group, Faculty of Computer Science, University of the Basque Country, P. Manuel Lardizabal 1, 20018 San Sebastian, Spain

I. Arganda-Carreras
Ikerbasque, Basque Foundation for Science, Maria Diaz de Haro 3, 48013 Bilbao, Spain

Donostia International Physics Center (DIPC), Manuel Lardizabal 4, 20018 San Sebastian, Spain

---

[1] https://www.nih.gov/news-events/news-releases/worlds-older-population-grows-dramatically.

© Springer Nature Switzerland AG 2021
J. Alja'am et al. (eds.), *Emerging Technologies in Biomedical Engineering and Sustainable TeleMedicine*, Advances in Science, Technology & Innovation, https://doi.org/10.1007/978-3-030-14647-4_10

using this technology suffer from the poor scalability of the sensors. The other approach, the vision-based one, uses cameras to record the activities, specially third-person vision cameras, such as the surveillance ones. However, some problems arise from them: the occlusions created due to the environment, the difficulty to keep all the body parts visible, and the limited field of view of third-person cameras [44]. To solve these, the first-person or egocentric vision can be very relevant to recognise self-performed activities [44]. In this type of vision, cameras are attached to the user's body or clothes, recording activities from their point of view.

The state-of-the-art approaches for the vision-based Egocentric Action Recognition (EAR) are currently based on Deep Learning (DL) techniques. These have demonstrated to be very effective for video-related tasks [3]. Thanks to the way DL models learn, they do not need hand-engineered features and can automatically learn these and classify instances altogether in an end-to-end fashion. Moreover, they are able to output a probabilistic view of the possible predictions for a given video, being the final prediction the one with the highest probability. In general, the EAR using DL is a very suitable tool for the AAL and the monitorisation of activities of daily living of elderly people. Therefore, in this chapter, we propose various EAR solutions to recognise daily actions such as "opening the fridge" or "cutting a cucumber" using DL methods and exploiting the intrinsic features that the egocentric vision offers. Furthermore, due to the importance of recognising the active object of the scene, we propose to extend the experiments to include the active object recognition task.

The remainder of the chapter is organised as follows. Section 2 reviews the related literature, and Sect. 3 presents the experimental setup in which the datasets and the object detector are described. For the experiments, Sect. 4 shows the first set of them using the SpatialNet baseline, Sect. 5 includes experiments using object features, and Sect. 6 covers the set of experiments that exploit hand location for attention. Finally, Sect. 7 summarises the conclusions.

2 Related Works

The EAR field has steadily grown since the introduction of the first wearable camera [38], having nowadays more mainstream cameras such as Google Glass or GoPro. During its two decades of history, several milestones have been achieved, increasing the eagerness of researchers to further explore this area of knowledge. Solutions from third-person vision have been used for first-person problems, but solutions tailored to egocentric characteristics have been the ones that have obtained state-of-the-art results.

In fact, an analysis of the literature reveals that there are various special cues or characteristics intrinsic to egocentric videos. These can be used to steer the learning of models towards the recognition of actions or active objects, i.e., those that are being manipulated and, thus, are relevant for actions. For example, [29] stated and used (i) the hand pose and its movement, (ii) the head motion, and (iii) the gaze direction as egocentric cues in their work. In addition, they also stressed the importance of objects in the egocentric setting.

In fact, the literature is highly dominated by works that focus on objects and, specially, on active objects. These are deemed as relevant for an action and, thus, their recognition is crucial. Fathi et al. [14] stressed that the egocentric setting is specially suitable for the analysis of actions that involve objects due to them being visible most of the time (occlusion is minimised), having consistent viewing directions with respect to the camera, and the focus that egocentric cameras have on objects, being usually centred and/or close to them.

How to recognise active objects is still a challenge, specially due to the background clutter (many objects may appear in a scene). To diminish the effect of the latter, [14, 16] proposed to detect a Region of Interest (RoI) before actually localising objects. There are other authors that aimed at detecting active objects in an unsupervised way (without assigning a label). Sun et al. [54] exploited the fact that the eyes always look directly at the objects being manipulated [22, 28] to track the position of hands and active objects. Kang et al. [24] generated a pool of segmentations, in which each object was individually searched (enforcing constraints such as geometric consistency). Mishra et al. [41] created a probabilistic boundary map of the scene and retrieved the contour that included the fixation point. Damen et al. [12] used a gaze tracker to detect relevant objects and analysed the interactions with them. In fact, all of these approaches could be integrated in an action recognition system that aims to use active objects' information.

The importance of objects is such that many proposals focused around the presence or absence of objects. These were called Bag-of-objects approaches. Works such as those of [39, 46] made use of bags of active and passive objects to infer actions. The objects were first detected by means of an object detector and, then, classified into active and passive. Another possibility is the one explored by [55], in which a set of observable objects and another one of manipulable objects were created. McCandless et al. [40] extended the bag-of-objects to the spatio-temporal binning, capturing space-time relations. To create spatio-temporal partitions that were the most discriminative they used a boosting approach. Then, they created object-centric partitions (regions of videos where active objects are supposed to appear), generating a histogram of active objects. For the classification phase, features from each of the best spatio-temporal proposals were computed and used to train the classifier.

Another extension of the usual bag-of-objects approach is the introduction of object fluents: the possible variations or states across time of objects or groups of objects [17, 33, 42].

For instance, a mug can take the *empty* and *full* fluents or states. Fathi and Rehg [13] used sequences of visual patches of objects (representing the change across time) instead of a static bag-of-objects. Liu et al. [33] proposed representing actions as concurrent and sequential objects fluents. Beam search was used to recognise the fluents per frame. In the work of [1], a Convolutional Neural Network (CNN) extracted visual features from a pool of frames from K segments (uniformly sampled across videos). Then, two branches arose from a point-wise convolution: one for nouns and another one for states or fluents. A global average pooling was used to get feature vectors from the branches. For the noun branch, a point-wise convolution led to a single feature vector. For the state branch, the same convolution left two channels, representing the change from the pre-state to the post-state. A Fully-Connected (FC) layer was used for the action classification. Kapidis et al. [26] explored the use of the object detections from YOLO [48] to recognise indoor actions. They observed that the object presence is highly correlated with the action. Therefore, errors in the detections could be potentially harmful. To alleviate this, they used detections from various frames. This is done using a bag-of-objects approach per frame (for the physical place) and a Long-Short-Term Memory (LSTM) network to infer the location. Another LSTM predicted actions using the location and shape of the bounding boxes (BBs) of the detected objects and the bag-of-objects.

Novel approaches to represent bag-of-objects are also appearing, such as that of [43]. In their preliminary work on object-based action recognition, they detected objects using a pre-trained CNN. No other model was trained for the detection of actions. Specifically, to estimate the latter, they exploited web data to compute the semantic similarity between the detected object names and the names action classes.

Another key feature of egocentric videos is the presence, pose, and shape of hands. Moreover, their interaction with objects (movement pattern) is of the utmost importance. Behera et al. [6] presented their bag of relations that included, not only the objects, but also the body part that interacted with them and the object-object relations. Later, [5] proposed a Histogram of Oriented Pairwise Relations, including the distances, orientations, and alignments between visual-words. Cartas et al. [9], in order to capture hands and manipulated objects, employed the R*CNN of [20] for primary regions (hands) and secondary regions (objects). An LSTM was in charge of the temporal evolution. Tekin et al. [56] presented a model that could estimate 3D hand and object poses given a single RGB image. Features were extracted using a Fully Convolutional Network (FCN), in which each cell predicted 3D hand poses and objects BBs. The cells were linked with vectors that contained the target values (for hand and object pose, object and action classes, and the confidence values). There also exists research that does not include interactions, only information about hands. For example, [4] masked out regions without hands to infer actions, using a CNN as the feature extractor. They showed that there is a high correlation between hands and actions in their experiments. Focusing more on the interaction between objects, [37] proposed to model the relation between arbitrary subgroups of objects using attention mechanisms.

Compared with the literature, our proposed solutions for EAR exploit some of the aforementioned egocentric cues: objects and hands.

3 Experimental Setup

This section introduces the fundamental aspects for the following experiments. First, the action recognition datasets, the GTEA dataset family, in Sect. 3.1 and the object detection model, the Faster R-CNN, for later sections, in Sect. 3.2.

3.1 GTEA Action Recognition Datasets

The Georgia Tech Egocentric Activity (GTEA) datasets are a family of egocentric datasets developed by the Georgia Institute of Technology, having four versions when this work was developed: the GTEA dataset [15,29], the GTEA Gaze dataset [16], the GTEA Gaze+ dataset [16,29], and the newest version at that moment, the Extended GTEA (EGTEA) Gaze+ dataset [30]. The last two were employed for the experiments carried out in the next sections. Therefore, this section aims at providing a presentation to these datasets and any necessary detail concerning them.

These datasets were collected at the Georgia Tech's Aware-Home, a living lab within the Aware Home Research Initiative (AHRI). The latter is an interdisciplinary research facility since 1998, mainly used for health and well-being related research. The AwareHome is a 5040 square foot facility that provides a realistic home scenario. Specifically, these datasets were recorded within the kitchen of this living lab and they consist in several videos, in which some subjects were recorded preparing meals following pre-defined recipes.

The GTEA Gaze+ dataset has 6 persons preparing seven different meals: an american breakfast, a pizza, a snack, a greek salad, a pasta salad, a turkey sandwich, and a cheese burger. It is important to note that the preparation of each meal is considered an activity while all the steps or sub-objectives required to prepare it are the actions: "taking a vegetable", "turning on the heat", and so on. Concerning the recording, they employed SMI eye-tracking glasses to record HD videos with 24 FPS and used the ELAN software for the annotations.

Each video contains several action annotations. These are composed of start and end frames, as well as verb and object annotations. The combination of a verb and an object can express an action when combined. A verb is simply a name to tag the type of motion of the action (e.g., "cut", "take",

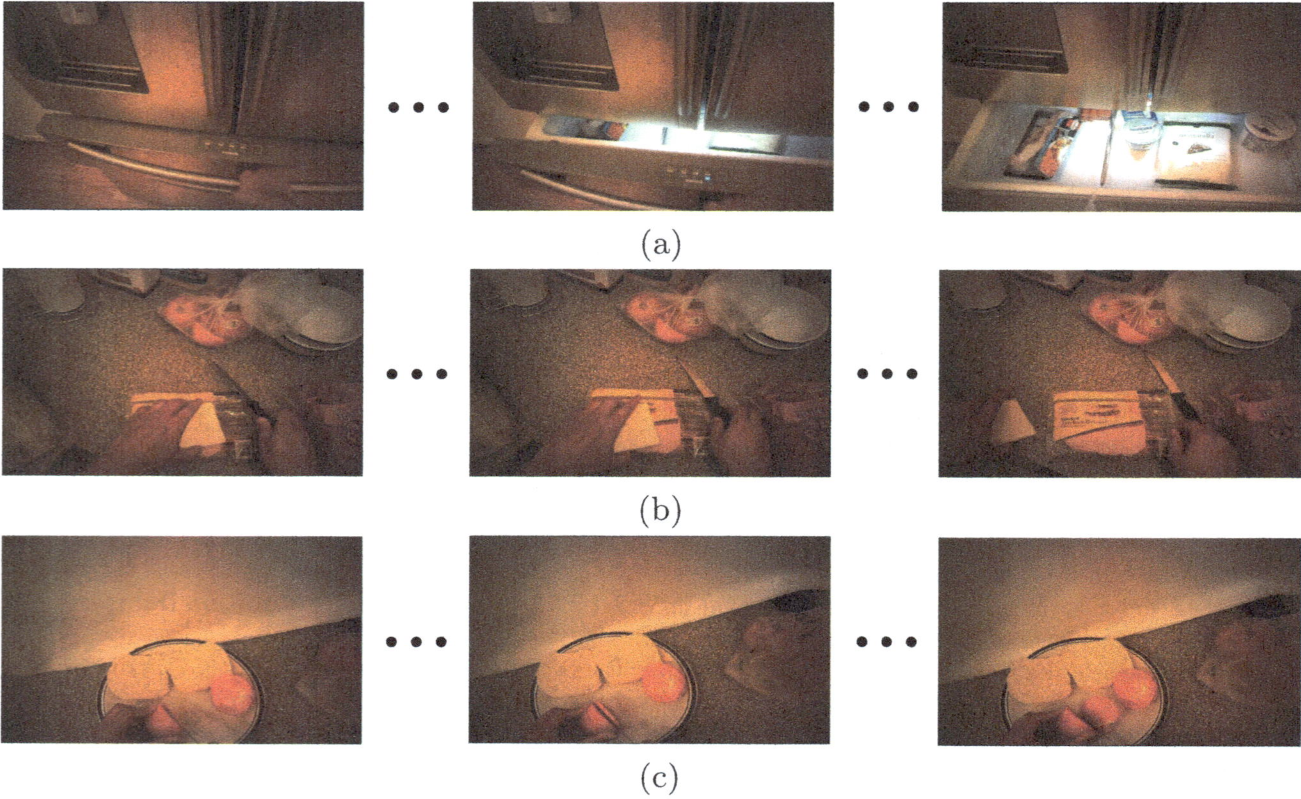

Fig. 1 GTEA Gaze+ action examples sampled from the dataset: **a** "open freezer" action, **b** "put knife" action, and **c** "cut tomato" action

"put", and so forth). The object, or more specifically, the active object, is the element that is interacted with, being the motion the type of interaction that is given with the object. In fact, in these datasets, there are not actions without objects (such as "walk" or "jump"), so it is assumed that there will always be a verb and an object. In addition, verbs and objects are presented in a stemmed way rather than in a legible or natural way. For instance, the label comes in the form "take knife" and not "take that big knife". Concerning the visual part, the clips used to learn actions are trimmed from their respective videos using the given beginning and ending annotations. A few samples of these trimmed videos from the GTEA Gaze+ dataset can be seen in Fig. 1.

The evaluation strategy defined for the GTEA Gaze+ dataset by its authors is the leave-one-subject-out validation. Taking into account that 6 subjects (Ahmad, Alireza, Carlos, Rahul, Shaghayegh, and Yin) are performing the actions and activities, each subject's clips (in which the subject performs actions) compose a fold. However, as specified by the authors, Shaghayegh's and Yin's videos (two of the subjects performing activities) are always part of the training set and, thus, are not used for evaluation. The reason for this is that they do not perform every activity and action in the dataset. Taking all this into account, four iterations or train/test splits are used within this leave-one-subject-out cross-validation.

Table 1 summarises the distribution and amount of data per fold. Without loss of generality, when mentioning Ahmad's fold we are referring to his data; in contrast, Ahmad's split is the one in which Ahmad's data is used for evaluation and the remaining subjects' data for training. This distinction is important, as we may be referring to both terms throughout the chapter. In the table, it can be seen that Shaghayegh's and Yin's folds have less actions than the rest, as mentioned earlier in the evaluation, and that their number of sequences (action instances) is quite low compared to the rest, although Alireza has remarkably fewer number of samples despite having all the 44 actions. Concerning the average of sequences, it can be seen that both Shaghayegh's and Yin's folds have less instances of each action. In contrast, Ahmad's and Rahul's folds are significantly larger than the rest and it is possible that, whenever their folds are used for testing and not for training, the performance drops due to the lower number of training samples.

The EGTEA Gaze+ dataset is an updated version of the GTEA family that was launched in 2017. This new dataset subsumes GTEA Gaze+, i.e., its data is contained within EGTEA Gaze+. It comes with HD videos (1280×960), audios, gaze tracking data, frame-level action annotations, and pixel-level hand masks at sampled frames, having 15, 176 hand masks from 13, 847 frames. In total, it has 28 hours of

Table 1 GTEA Gaze+ distribution per fold (subject). A subject's fold contains all their data, i.e., all the videos in which the subject was recorded performing actions

	Subjects					
	Ahmad	Alireza	Carlos	Rahul	Shaghayegh	Yin
Actions	44	44	44	44	35	40
Sequences	504	298	475	361	146	240
Seq./class	11.45 (±11.88)	6.77 (±8.25)	10.79 (±10.85)	8.20 (±11.18)	4.17 (±4.02)	6.00 (±5.52)

Table 2 EGTEA Gaze+ distribution per split

Split	Training videos	Test videos
Split 1	8299	2022
Split 2	8299	2022
Split 3	8300	2021

video with 32 subjects and 10, 325 instances of fine-grained actions. As with the GTEA Gaze+, EGTEA Gaze+ comes with several action annotations per video in the form of start frame, end frame, verb, object, and action label. Moreover, rather than having separate subject data for the cross-validation strategy, this dataset has three official train and test splits. In each split, the test set follows a distribution similar to that of the training set. The number of clips per split is summarised in Table 2. Furthermore, a few samples of the dataset can be seen in Fig. 2.

For the evaluation of both datasets, and for both active object and action classification, the accuracy and the macro-F1 metrics are used. The accuracy, as seen in Eq. 1, takes into account the TPs, TNs, FPs, and FNs. These values are determined by the evaluation protocol established for an algorithm and, hence, they will be defined in each section. In general terms, each sample's ground truth and its prediction are used to compute whether the actual prediction is a TP, TN, FP, or FN. So, the accuracy refers to the ability of a smart system to correctly predict both positive and negative samples (TPs and TNs).

The F1 is a metric used to summarise two commonly used metrics: the precision and the recall. The precision (see Eq. 2) of a class measures the percentage of correct predictions done out of the total predictions and, hence, it is desirable to have fewer FPs to increase its value. Intuitively, the recall (see Eq. 3) represents the ability of a system to predict the possible positive samples, penalised by the FNs, i.e., when the system is not able to correctly classify a positive sample. To combine both metrics, instead of the arithmetic mean, the harmonic mean is employed for the F1, illustrated in Eq. 4. Therefore, the F1 will always be between the values of precision and recall. When the F1 per class is averaged using the arithmetic mean, the macro-F1 is obtained.

$$Accuracy = \frac{TP + TN}{TP + TN + FP + FN} \tag{1}$$

$$Precision = \frac{TP}{TP + FP} \tag{2}$$

$$Recall = \frac{TP}{TP + FN} \tag{3}$$

$$F1 = 2 * \frac{precision * recall}{precision + recall} \tag{4}$$

The macro-F1 metric will be an interesting alternative to the accuracy due to the accuracy paradox. That is, when comparing two different models, it may happen that it is better to select the model with the lowest accuracy due to its higher predictive power. This is often the case with imbalanced class distributions such as those of the datasets of the GTEA family, in which the class distribution is far from following a uniform distribution. In these cases, the accuracy of dominating classes (those with the highest amount of samples) can be very high in comparison with other classes, in which the accuracy can be poor. Due to how the accuracy is computed, taking into account the total number of samples without doing an evaluation per class, the accuracy can show a high value due to the high result of the dominating classes. The minor classes do not contribute as much and, thus, their poor performance does not penalise the accuracy that much. This phenomenon does not occur with the macro-F1, in which this imbalanced performance will be reflected.

3.2 Object Detection with the Faster R-CNN

For later sections, object detections are required, i.e., locations and boundaries of objects within single images. Thus, we first present how these are going to be obtained. Specifically, our interest is detecting objects by means of bounding Boxes

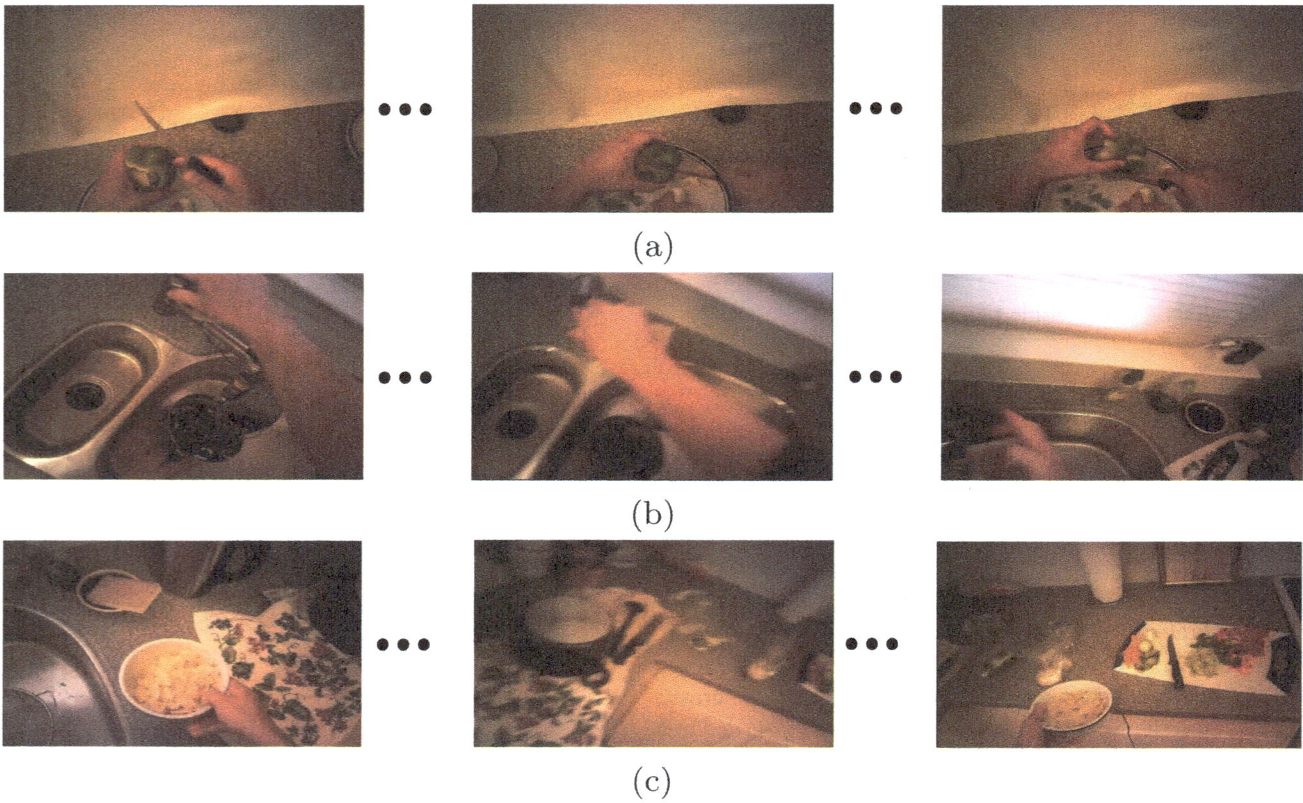

Fig. 2 EGTEA Gaze+ action examples sampled from the dataset: **a** "cut bell pepper" action, **b** "wash pan" action, and **c** "cut tomato" action

(BBs), rectangular areas within images that have an associated probability distribution for a set of objects (see Fig. 3 for an example).

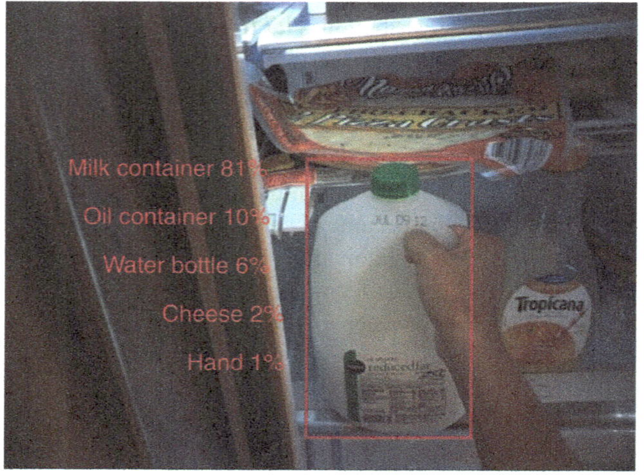

Fig. 3 Sample image from the GTEA Gaze+ dataset with a bounding box inscribing a milk container object. An example of a probability distribution (in percentages) for that bounding box is provided

Object Detection Models

With the increased popularity of DL methods, various authors have proposed methods to apply DL techniques for the object recognition task. A highly addressed method was the R-CNN [19] in 2015. It first leverages the selective search algorithm [58] to create proposals of connected regions (or better said, per-pixel predictions). Each region proposal is resized to an standard shape to match the input size of a CNN and, then, (i) a classifier such as an SVM is used on top to predict the probability distribution of the region and (ii) a linear regressor is used to tighten the BB to the putative object's shape. The second step allows for fine-grained predictions in which rectangular boxes envelop objects with the minimum possible noise (visual information not related to the object of interest in each case). The architecture of the R-CNN is represented in Fig. 4.

A new version of this network was later presented, called Fast R-CNN [18], that aimed at alleviating the computational burden of the first approach. This network takes the whole image as input to the CNN (instead of iterating the forward pass for each proposal). Regions are extracted from the output feature map and the same branched objectives (object classi-

Fig. 4 Region-based Convolutional Network (R-CNN). From the work of [19]

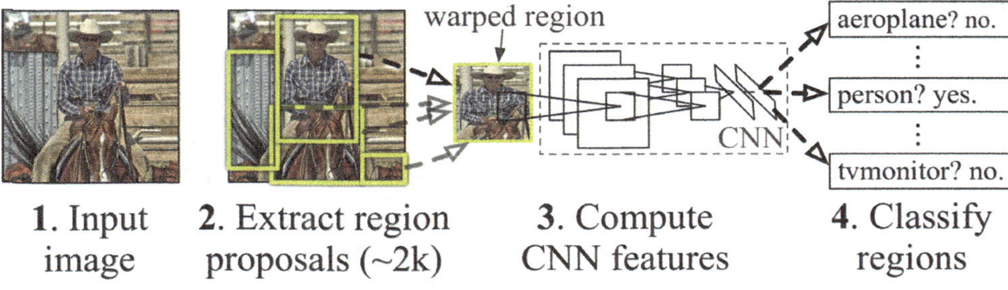

Fig. 5 Fast Region-based Convolutional Neural Network (Fast R-CNN). From the work of [18]

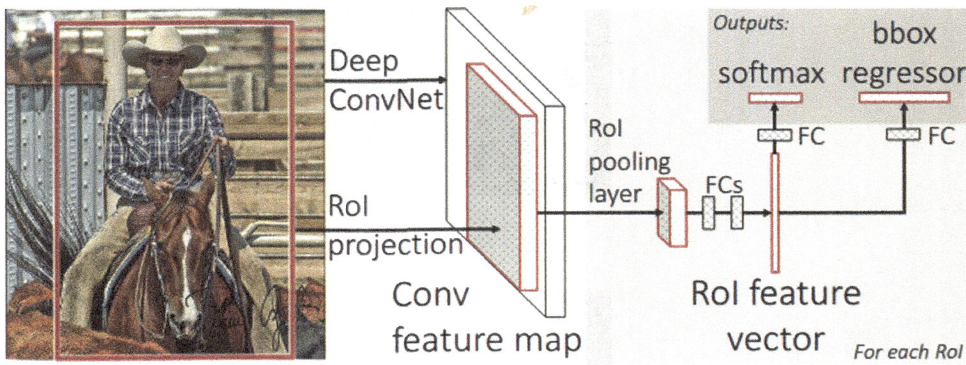

fication and BB adjustment) can be applied again. The architecture is presented in Fig. 5. However, this version was still dependent on the Selective Search method, which was a computationally expensive method. That is why the Faster R-CNN was finally proposed [49]. In this last update, the RPN module was added. The RPN creates BB proposals at the beginning (not needing anymore the selective search) and these are processed by the Fast R-CNN. However, the system cannot be seen as separated modules, as both modules (the RPN and the Fast R-CNN) are jointly trained in an end-to-end fashion. To summarise, the Faster R-CNN is a network that takes an image and is capable of outputting BBs that inscribe objects (and have associated probability distributions). This network will be employed through this section.

Experiments

In order to have a functional object detector, for a given dataset, the detector must be trained for the specific set of objects and their shape. However, pre-trained models can be reused to improve the convergence time and the overall results of fine-tuned detectors, given that the pre-training was done using large datasets such as COCO (Common Objects in Context) [32]. This is a standard procedure with the R-CNN family of networks. Nevertheless, image annotations are still required for the fine-tuning and the evaluation, i.e., for each image, a set of BBs (including the position of the rectangle and the ground truth class). Some datasets already provide these annotations, but the GTEA Gaze+ did not. That is why the authors manually annotated several samples (images) across different classes and subjects [45] to be able to train and

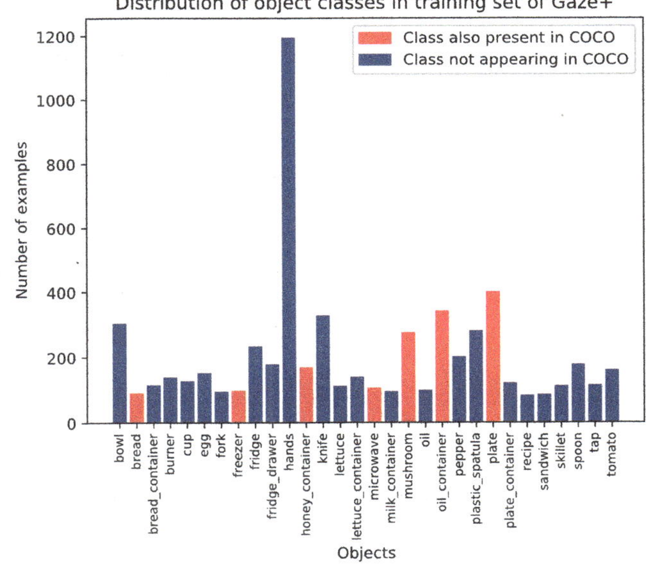

Fig. 6 Object classes annotated for the GTEA Gaze+ dataset. The classes that intersect with the COCO dataset are highlighted in red

evaluate an object detector. A total of 30 objects were annotated, including hands as another object too. Figure 6 shows an example of the distribution of object annotations across several images in Ahmad's fold. It can be observed that the presence of hands dominates the rest of the classes, as they appear in almost all the action classes.

The Faster R-CNN, with a ResNet101 as the backbone feature extractor, was trained for each subject individually.

Fig. 7 Object detections from the Faster R-CNN network on GTEA Gaze+ dataset's images. The black boxes are ground truth annotations

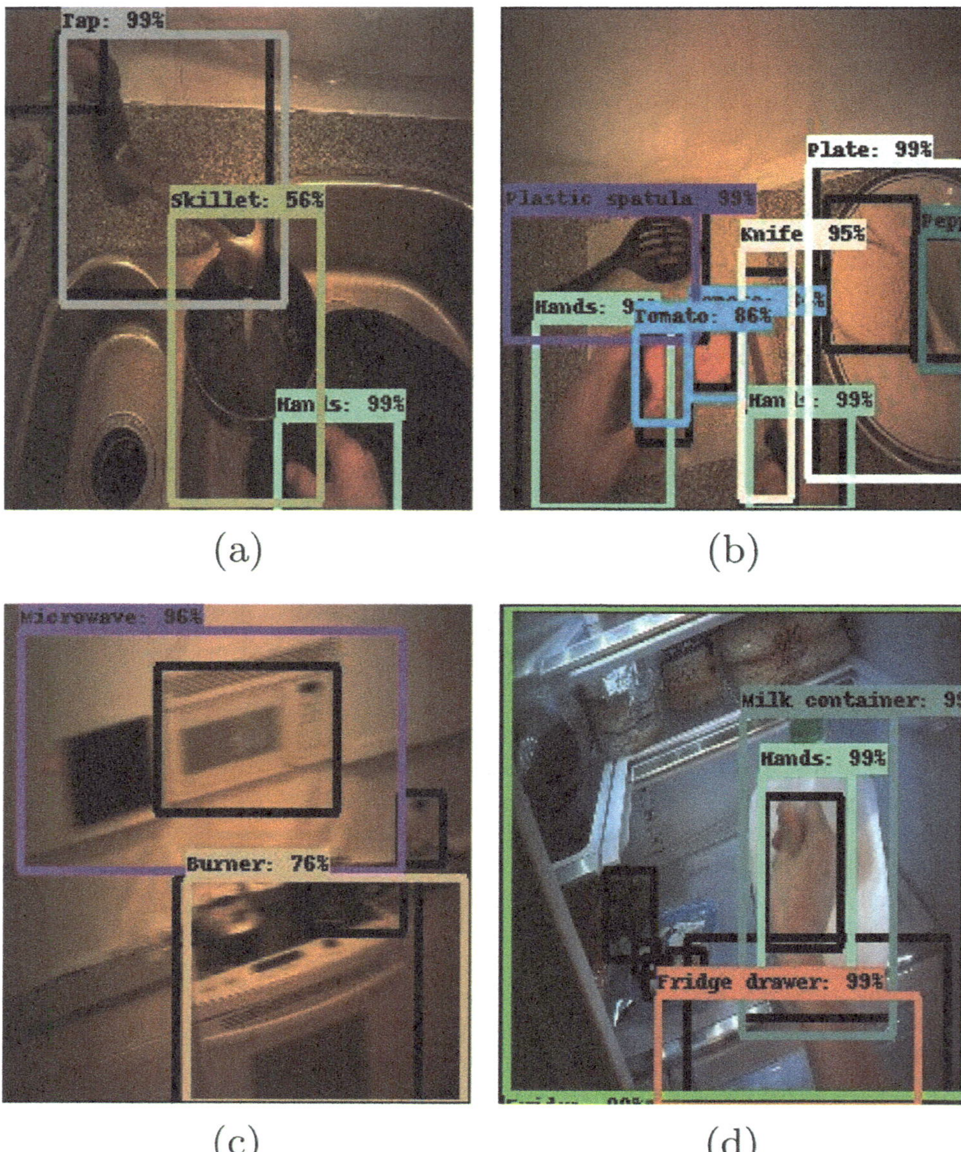

(a) (b)

(c) (d)

The training data of each subject's split was used to fine-tune the network, which was already pre-trained in the COCO dataset. Hence, the convolutional layers were frozen for the fine-tuning. For the RPN's anchors, the stride was set to 8 and five scales $(0.1, 0.25, 0.5, 1, \text{and } 2)$ and three aspect ratios $(0.5, 1, \text{and } 2)$ were used. At the first stage, the Non-Maximum Suppression (NMS) (used to remove some proposals and predictions) score and the Intersection over Union (IoU) threshold (explained later) were set to 0 and 0.7, while for the second stage these were changed to 0.3 and 0.6, respectively. In addition, the first stage considered up to 100 proposals while this was reduced to 10 in the second one (the total number of output predictions). Regarding the hyperparameters used for training, the learning rate was set fixed to $3e^{-4}$, the input size was 224×224 (any image larger or smaller than that was

resized), and a batch size of 1 was used. For data augmentation, the standard random horizontal flipping and random cropping were applied.

After the training, the object detector was able to, given an image, output 10 predicted objects containing the BB position, its class (and the confidence), and a feature vector. The results obtained for each subject's model are summarised in Table 3 and some visualisations of the predicted BBs are provided in Fig. 7. The metrics employed in Table 3 are the COCO evaluation metrics that are based on the Average Precision (AP) and the Average Recall (AR). To explain what AP and AR are, first, the values of TP, FP, FN, and TN for the object detection task must be defined. But, even before these, the concept of the IoU is pivotal to define them. It is a numeric value that determines the amount of overlap between two BBs, i.e., the area where

Table 3 Object detection results on the GTEA Gaze+ dataset's folds using the COCO dataset's evaluation metrics

Subject	Samples	AP@[.5:.95]	AP@.5	AP@.75	AR@1	AR@10	AR@100$_{small}$	AR@100$_{medium}$	AR@100$_{large}$
Ahmad	766	33.0	50.0	37.9	35.9	39.1	5.8	33.8	61.9
Alireza	185	36.2	54.9	39.8	38.3	41.3	13.4	39.6	67.3
Carlos	251	38.1	57.8	41.5	40.7	43.0	9.1	41.3	60.8
Rahul	231	29.3	47.0	31.2	30.3	33.7	8.8	29.3	52.1

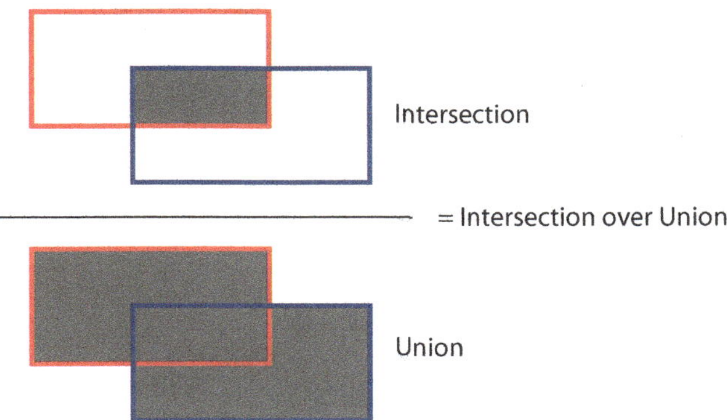

Fig. 8 The Intersection over Union (IoU) between two bounding boxes

both BBs intersect divided by the total area (the union) of both BBs. Figure 8 shows a graphical representation of the idea. The value is represented with a float number in the range [0.0, 1.0]: when both BBs are completely overlapped the IoU is 1.0, but if there is no overlapping it is 0.0. With this concept, the TP, FP, FN, and TN can be formulated as follows:

- TP: A BB has an $IoU > t_{iou}$ with the ground truth BB and both are tagged with the same object class, being t_{iou} a threshold value.
- FP: A BB has an $IoU <= t_{iou}$ with the ground truth BB and both are tagged with the same object class, being t_{iou} a threshold value.
- FN: If an object is present in an image and the object detector failed at detecting it.
- TN: Any part of the image not predicted as an object. However, for the object detection task, this value is not useful and is not employed for computing evaluation metrics.

Using these values, the precision (Eq. 2) and recall (Eq. 3) can be computed. Notice that having BB predictions larger or smaller than the ground truth will harm the precision, as the IoU with the ground truth box can be smaller than the threshold. For the recall, the inability to detect all the ground truth boxes will be penalised.

The evaluation metrics used in COCO can now be defined with all the aforementioned terms. Their main purpose is to provide meaningful metrics for the object detection task, adapting the usual classification scheme to the detection scheme. This includes the previous definition of TP, FP, and FN. Specifically, the metrics used in COCO and included for these experiments are variations of the precision and the recall. The AP is a term that averages the precision across several t_{iou} values. It also averages the results across classes, which would be known as mean AP or mAP, but COCO makes no distinction between them. Specifically, the $AP@[.5 : .95]$, $AP@.5$, and $AP@.75$ metrics are used. The $AP@[.5 : .95]$ averages t_{iou} values ranging from 0.5 to 0.95 with a step of 0.05, with a total of 10 values. It is usually considered the primary challenge metric for the evaluation in the COCO dataset. The $AP@.5$ and $AP@.75$ evaluate the performance using a single t_{iou} value, 0.5 and 0.75, respectively. Then, there is also the AR, which is presented with the $AR@1$, $AR@10$, $AR@100_{small}$, $AR@100_{medium}$, and $AR@100_{large}$ variations and is averaged across all classes and IoU thresholds. The $AR@1$ and the $AR@10$ metrics compute the AR using the top-1 and top-10 predictions (the ones with the highest confidence score). It is common to present the $AR@100$ too, but, in this case, the maximum number of predictions is 10 and, thus, $AR@10 = AR@100$ no matter what. Finally, the $AR@100_{small}$, $AR@100_{medium}$, and $AR@100_{large}$ compute the $AR@100$ for small, medium, and large objects, respectively. COCO defines small objects as those whose area is smaller than 32^2, then medium ones as those whose area is between 32^2 and 96^2, and the large ones as those whose area is larger than 96^2. Notice that $AR@100$ is employed instead of $AR@10$ to follow COCO's conventions, although both values are the same.

In addition to the BB information, feature vectors from the step previous to the classification of proposals are extracted. To get them, the Faster R-CNN gets the feature cube of a region proposal, with shape $N \times M \times C$, being N and M the width and height of the region and C is the number of channels of the last feature cube of the backbone network, being 2048 for the ResNet101. A pooling operation (global average pooling) is applied to it to get a vector of size C, then fed through FC layers. This is the feature vector used

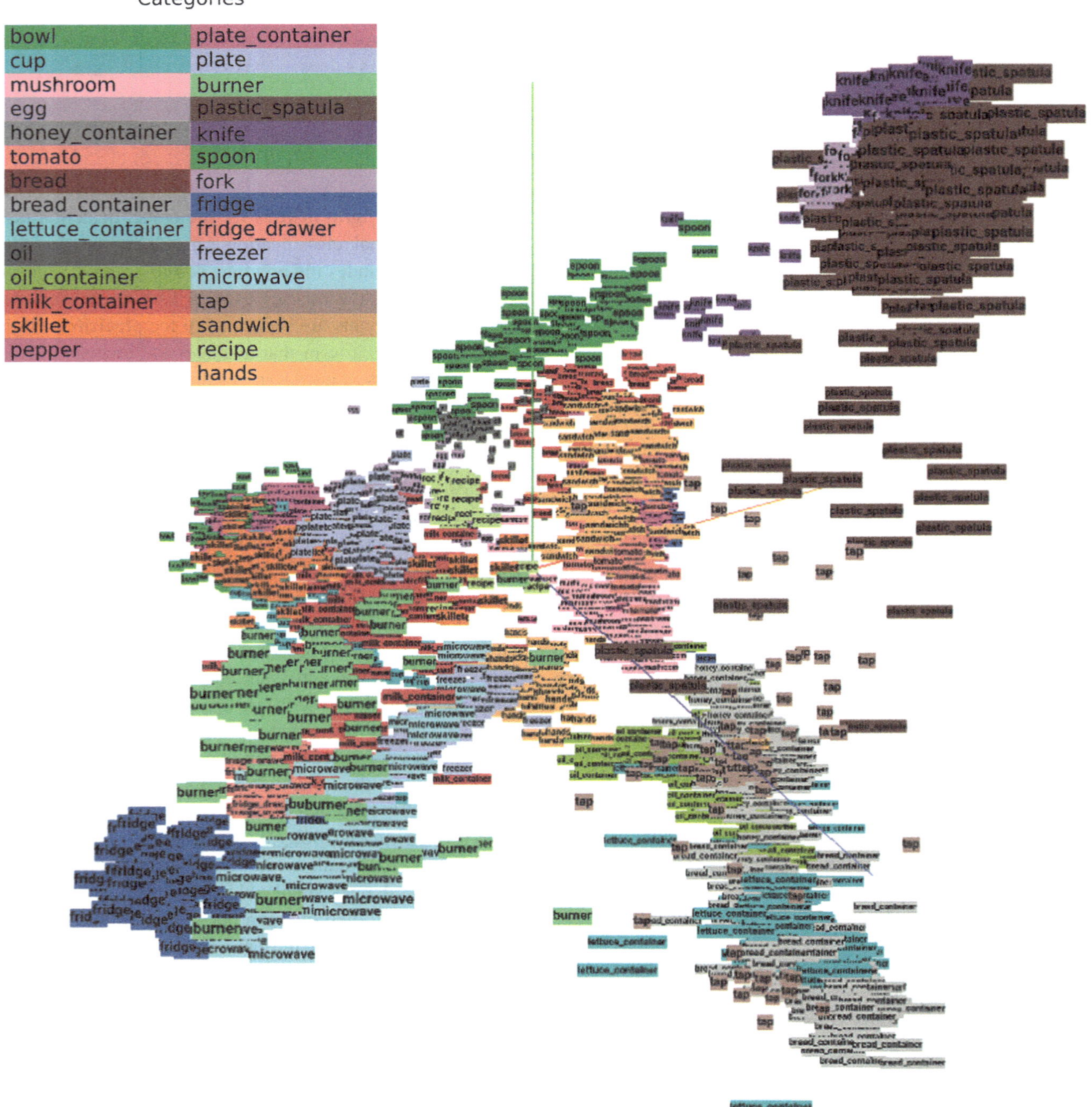

Fig. 9 Feature vectors extracted from the Faster R-CNN represented after a Principal Component Analysis, leaving 3 components. Each class is assigned a colour for a better visualisation

for classification and the one our object detector outputs. It should encode, at least, the position of the BB and its class. We will be using this feature vectors in the following Sect. 5. We visualised a set of feature vectors using PCA, leaving 3 components, in Fig. 9. A colour was assigned to each class alongside its name for a better visualisation. As it can be observed, each class is fairly well clustered.

4 Object Classification Network: The SpatialNet

The *SpatialNet*, a CNN used to learn the appearance of clips of videos, was employed and popularised by the work of [51] in their two-stream approach. Later, it was named *AppearanceNet* [36], although both works referred to the same type of network with the same objective: learning the appearance, the visual content of the videos, i.e., the objects and the scene. Because, apart from the physical place where actions occur, objects are also contained within the visual features of what it is called "the scene". Depending on the task, features focused on objects, the scene, or other cues can be obtained, but in it essence, the visual features are the ones that are exploited.

Our first approach also used a single-stream CNN structure but with a different objective. This time, we aimed at predicting actions and active objects using visual features of videos. That is, the implicit learning of objects and the scene was the main driver of the learning and the classification of actions and active objects.

4.1   Architecture

For the backbone network used to extract RGB features, we followed the work done by [36] and used a CNN-M-2048 network [10]. In contrast to the motion detector, for the visual features, RGB images are not stacked and fed as input to the network. Instead, following the approach of [36], if the appearance stream takes as input single frames of videos, then each of the frames can vote for a label. That is, the architecture takes a sequence of inputs, each one being a frame $X \in \mathbb{R}^{H \times W \times 3}$, where W and H are the width and height of the image and 3 the number of channels; instead of having a single probability distribution as output, each frame of the sequence has its own output distribution. We may see this as if each of the inputs of the sequence would have its own vote. By averaging these votes, a new probability distribution is obtained, representing the vote for the sequence. Figure 10 illustrates this process.

4.2   Experiments

Two sets of experiments are proposed: in the first one, the objective is to classify actions, while, in the second one, active

objects. For both sets, the same architecture and hyperparameters are employed. 10 timesteps are used as input, being each frame normalised by subtracting the Imagenet mean. The networks are trained for 200 epochs with early stopping with a patience of 20 epochs. A learning rate of 0.0001 is used, alongside a mini-batch size of 32. The first three convolutional layers' weights are frozen. Class weights generated from the training set distribution were not employed for the learning phase.

The GTEA Gaze+ dataset is used for the evaluation, applying the leave-one-subject-out evaluation. For this problem, we defined the following TP, FP, TN, and TN for the accuracy and F1 metrics:

- TP: for the class i, if a sequence of images is labelled with class i and the class i is the one with the highest confidence after the average voting.
- FP: for the class i, if a sequence of images is labelled with class j and the class i is the one with the highest confidence after the average voting, being j any class different to i.
- TN: for the class i, if a sequence of images is labelled with class j and the class k is the one with the highest confidence after the average voting, being j and k any classes different to i and being possible that $j = k$.
- FN: for the class i, if a sequence of images is labelled with class i and the class j is the one with the highest confidence after the average voting, being j any class different to i.

The results are shown in Tables 4 (for action classification) and 5 (for active object classification). These are presented per fold (subject) and as the average of all the folds. Each fold is run three times and the average of those three experiments is provided alongside the standard deviation.

These results can be seen as baselines. Other authors such as [36] also followed this type of strategy, i.e., having a CNN extracting visual features from single frames and then averaging the votes. However, they also included motion features as an extra branch. The vote emitted in a single timestep would take into account both the visual appearance of the frame and

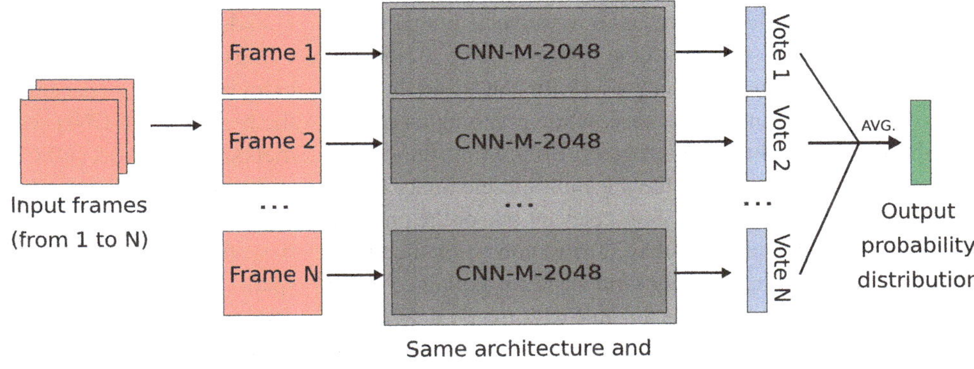

Fig. 10 A CNN-M-2048 network [10] is repeated N times, each of them having the same architecture and weights. Each copy extracts visual features from each frame and outputs a probability distribution (a vote). All the votes are averaged to obtain the final probability distribution. For the training, only a set of weights is trained, as if there would be only a single CNN-M-2048

Table 4 Results of the experiments with our SpatialNet and the GTEA Gaze+ dataset for action classification. The results are given per subject and as the average of all of them. Each of the subject's experiments is run three times and averaged. This mean is provided in the top row, while the standard deviation is shown at the bottom

Action classification									
Average		Ahmad		Alireza		Carlos		Rahul	
Accuracy	F1	Accuracy	F1	Accuracy	F1	Accuracy	F1	Accuracy	F1
46.55% (±7.84)	36.11 (±4.44)	38.89% (±1.27)	32.67 (±2.07)	52.19% (±0.55)	38.88% (±0.55)	41.9 (±0.43)	31.84 (±0.38)	52.63% (±0.60)	38.03 (±2.55)

Table 5 Results of the experiments with our SpatialNet and the GTEA Gaze+ dataset for active object classification. The results are given per subject and as the average of all of them. Each of the subject's experiments is run three times and averaged. This mean is provided in the top row, while the standard deviation is shown at the bottom

Active object classification									
Average		Ahmad		Alireza		Carlos		Rahul	
Accuracy	F1	Accuracy	F1	Accuracy	F1	Accuracy	F1	Accuracy	F1
58.92% (±6.05)	47.95 (±4.14)	53.90% (±0.75)	47.00 (±0.18)	63.97% (±0.82)	54.35 (±0.97)	52.07% (±0.26)	43.16 (±1.02)	65.74% (±0.91)	47.29 (±1.14)

the local motion (taking the previous and next frames to create an OF stack). In fact, we could add multiple streams of information to improve the vote per timestep. For the moment, we will keep using only the visual stream.

Observing the results per subject, it is noticeable that there is a significant difference among splits. The class distribution in each split and the variance introduced by each subject can be crucial on this. For example, if a subject follows a similar pattern cutting vegetables, both in the training set and test set, then it may be easier to recognise the action of cutting vegetables. In contrast, having different poses, patterns, or even tools to cut (e.g., knives of different shapes or colours) increases the difficulty to learn actions. Therefore, the results of the test set are expected to be lower if not all the variance can be explained in the training set or there is not enough data to generalise correctly. For objects, first, the variance of objects can pose a problem. For instance, a whole vegetable compared to a sliced vegetable will look different, even more compared with a minced vegetable, divided into small pieces. In fact, understanding which among all the objects present in a scene is the active one can be difficult without understanding the dominant motion pattern, i.e., how subjects interact with objects, that is also related to the appearance of the object. The second problem is the occlusion with hands and the cluttered background. In the first case, while grabbing an object, hands may be occluding the object, difficulting the recognition. In the second case, having multiple elements in the background, identifying the most relevant one or the one that is being manipulated (the active object) can be challenging. As in the action case, if all this variance is not explained in the training set or if the system is not able to correctly generalise, there can be huge differences between data and subject splits.

Table 6 compares the obtained results with some approaches of the literature in the GTEA Gaze+ dataset. For the active object classification, our results are not that far from approaches such as that of [36]. However, the results reported by them are given by a Spatial CNN using single inputs instead of a sequence of frames using our time-distributed Spatial CNN. In fact, they are superior to us even with this handicap. This may be due to the fact that their Spatial CNN exploits hand information to localise objects within images instead of using the whole frame. Moreover, after jointly training their full system for actions (the spatial and motion CNNs are jointly trained), the object classification result improves to 74.34% of accuracy. Focusing the attention of the learning in specific regions of images may alleviate background clutter issues, as well as removing not desirable information in the learning phase. However, there is a dependence on a hand detection system or a similar method to localise objects.

For the action classification, as expected, we obtained some of the lowest results compared to other approaches. Our baseline, however, obtains such a low result given that (i) we have not adopted any attention mechanism, (ii) the temporal modelling of actions was very naive, (iii) we have not included any extra information (streams of information), and (iv) that using the best possible CNN was out of the scope of these experiments. Meanwhile, [60,61] proposed the Dense Trajectories (DT) and the IDT to model actions. Their method is based on trajectory recognition, i.e., feature points are densely sampled from frames and, then, the tracking is performed within the spam of L frames using a median filtering in a dense OF field. The trajectory is represented by relative point coordinates and various descriptors (HOG, HOF, and MBH) are computed in

Table 6 Comparative table with the state-of-the-art approaches for active object classification and action classification using the GTEA Gaze+ dataset. The best result is highlighted in bold. The results are given as the mean of a leave-one-subject-out cross-validation approach. Furthermore, for our experiments we repeated each fold three times and we provide the mean and the standard deviation

Action classification		
Approach	Accuracy	F1
Dense Trajectories (DT) [60]	42.40%	–
Improved Dense Trajectories (IDT) [61]	49.60%	–
O+E+H [29]	57.40%	–
O+M+E+H [29]	60.50%	–
O+M+E+G [29]	60.30%	–
Motion stream [36]	62.62%	–
Two-stream [36]	**65.05%**	–
Two-stream [66]	59.02%	–
TSN [52]	55.25%	–
Two-stream [52]	60.13%	–
Appearance stream [34]*	57.63%	–
Motion stream [34]*	57.42%	–
Two-stream [34]*	64.74%	–
Time-Distributed Spatial CNN (Ours)	46.55% (±7.84)	36.11 (±4.44)
Active object classification		
Approach	Accuracy	F1
Spatial stream [36]	61.87%	–
Spatial stream (after joint training) [36]	**74.34%**	–
Time-Distributed Spatial CNN (Ours)	58.92% (±6.05)	47.95 (±4.14)

*They took six subjects into account instead of four (see Sect. 3.1 for the evaluation strategy)

$N \times N$ neighbourhoods within each trajectory. See Fig. 11 for an example of dense trajectories for the action "kiss". Wang and Schmid [61] improved DT by matching feature points between frames using SURF descriptors. These points allowed to estimate an homography using RANSAC. This improvement cancels out the motion generated by the camera and removes inconsistent matches. Our baseline improved the result obtained by DT features, probably due to the short-term spam of DT features and the robust features computed by CNNs. Nonetheless, DT methods are very appropriate for action recognition due to the modelling of the dynamics of actions instead of the simple observation of the appearance (as in our baseline approach). However, the approaches followed by [60,61] are quite general, i.e., they were not designed to be EAR methods, but rather a more general way to represent the motion. In contrast, [29] exploited egocentric features (see Sect. 2) as well as DT features, motion features (OF), and object features, augmenting those of the DT by computing histograms of LAB colour and Local Binary Patterns (LBP) along the trajectories. The use of several of these features obtained an accuracy of 60.50%, creating a gap of 13.95 points with our baseline. This hint towards the efficacy of egocentric features is quite significant. In fact, the approach of [36] for active object detection was also based on one of the egocentric cues: the position of hands.

Previously, the result of object classification of [36] was discussed. However, the most significant contribution of their work is that their result for action recognition remains the highest one of the literature for the GTEA Gaze+ dataset. As aforementioned, they exploited hand positions (egocentric cue) to extract an object-centred region. This allowed to remove background information and focus on the learning of objects. This appearance stream and their motion stream are fused by concatenation and a FC layer on top is in charge of the classification of actions. Moreover, they added two more objectives: the learning of objects and motion in each stream. With this setting, their approach obtained state-of-the-art results.

The two-stream network was also used in the work of [66] and in the work of [34]. The latter added various modifications such as attention mechanisms. Each stream is composed of an spatial attention network and a temporal network. The spatial attention networks at the beginning aim to output an attention distribution map using the gaze information (a gaussian bump generated from the gaze) as supervision to train this part. Those attention maps are then multiplied with the original inputs to get gaze-aware inputs. The next part is the temporal network, modelled by a bi-directional LSTM network. Both streams are fused at the end. This method highlights the importance of using attention and a more sophisticated temporal modelling. In contrast, our baseline employed a naive

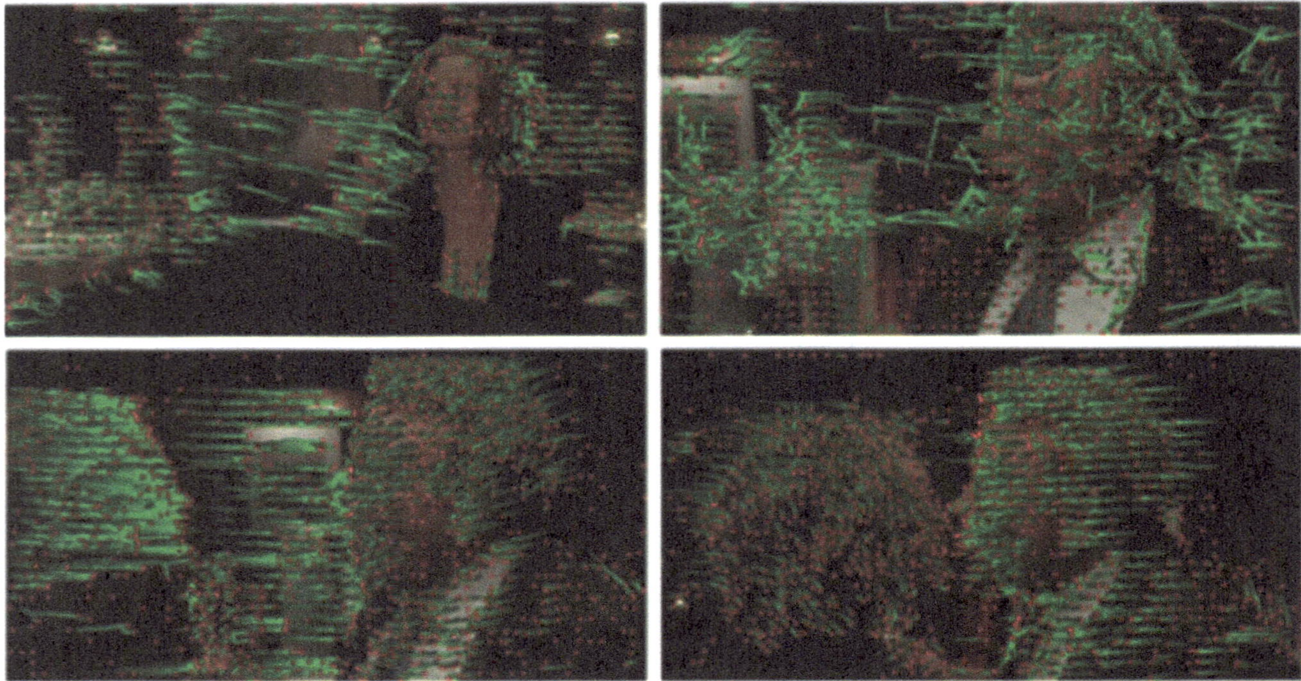

Fig. 11 Visualisation of dense trajectories for the action "kiss". From the work of [60]

approach such as the average of votes and does not include any type of attention.

Many conclusions can be extracted from this baseline and the comparison with other approaches. For active object classification, there is a need to localise objects better. In fact, various objects can appear in each frame, making the task difficult. If the aim is to explicitly recognise the active object, trying to predict it based on several separate frame predictions from CNNs may not be the best idea. There is a need of attention mechanisms to do so. Nevertheless, the visual information from frames can also be exploited without explicitly learning objects, as several methods do, even though the best result was obtained by explicitly predicting object labels alongside actions [36].

5 The Bag-of-Objects Matrix Representation

Section 3.2 explained how objects could be automatically inferred from images without further help (for the inference phase only). With the aim of creating an active object recognition system, the set of detected objects can be leveraged to create a system that is able to process it and, then, predict active objects and actions. That will be the goal of this section. But first, the output obtained from the previous section's Faster R-CNN will be formalised.

A video contains a set of N frames. For each frame fed to the Faster R-CNN, P predictions (set to 10 in our work) are obtained. Therefore, for each frame, the following information is extracted:

- BB coordinates ($P \times 4$ matrix): an element p_i ($0 \leq i \leq P$) within this matrix is a vector of four values (y_1, x_1, y_2, and x_2) corresponding to the ith BB. The pair (y_1, x_1) defines the top-left point of the BB, while the pair (y_2, x_2) defines the bottom-right one.
- Score or confidence (P-sized vector): an element p_i ($0 \leq i \leq P$ and $0 \leq p_i \leq 1$) within this vector corresponds to the confidence in the predicted class of the ith BB.
- Classes (P-sized vector): an element p_i ($0 \leq i \leq P$ and $0 \leq p_i < |O|$) within this vector corresponds to the class identifier of the ith BB, taking $|O|$ possible object class values, where O is a set of objects.
- Number of detections (integer): the number of not null predictions M ($0 \leq M \leq P$). That is, out of P entries, only the first M BBs are valid predictions.
- Feature vector ($P \times C$ matrix): an element p_i ($0 \leq i \leq P$) within this matrix encodes features related to the ith BB. C is fixed to 2048 due to the choice of the ResNet101 as the backbone of the Faster R-CNN (number of channels in the last feature cube).

So far, outputs of single images have been analysed; therefore, the first objective of this section is to produce representations of videos given all these features. That is, a single representation that encodes all the object information from a video. As videos have different lengths, there is a need to collapse or pool the information to a standardised size. Formally, videos have a varying length of L_v (number of frames) and we aim to obtain a representation of size L. This work proposes to pool the information following these rules: (i) if the size matches, no pool is applied; (ii) if $L_v > L$, uniform subsampling is applied; and, (iii) if $L_v < L$, we augment the original video by copying elements. For the latter, if the original video has a set of frames $\{ f_0, f_1, f_2,\ldots f_{L_v} \}$, we duplicate the frames to get an arrangement like $\{ f_0, f_0, f_1, f_1, f_2, f_2,\ldots f_{L_v}, f_{L_v} \}$. If the new length is greater than L_v, the method applied to subsample in (ii) is used. Now each video should have a common length of L. The question now is, how should the information from the Faster R-CNN be arranged? We propose the following two approaches.

5.1   Input Representations

The raw representation. This first encoding of the video, as it can be seen in Fig. 12, has a cube shape of $P \times C \times L$, where the depth dimension represents the time dimension (the evolution of the video frame to frame) and, thus, the depth is set to L (number of frames). A depth slice of shape $P \times C$ encodes the information about a frame, where P and C are the maximum number of predictions and the size of the feature vectors, respectively, as described at the beginning of Sect. 5. That is, the feature vectors from the objects detected in the ith frame are stacked so that they form a matrix of shape $P \times C$ and this matrix is located in the ith depth slice of the final representation of the video.

The segments approach. The second approach aims at collapsing more information. Given a video of size L, we define K segments from where to extract T frames with a stride or separation of S frames. K and T are fixated for all the

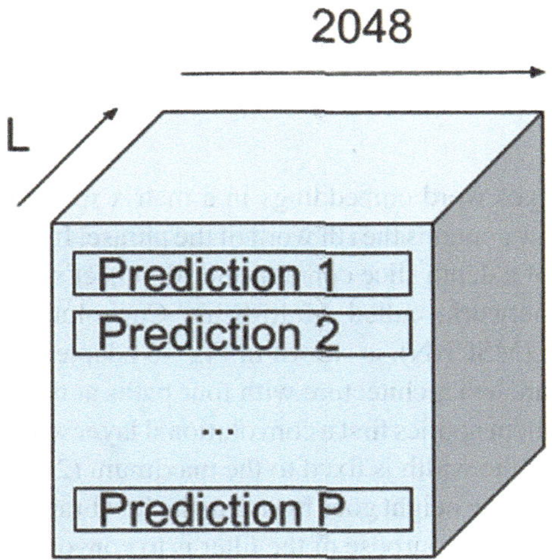

Fig. 12 The raw representation proposed to encode the Faster R-CNN output of all the frames of a video

videos. Figure 13 represents a video as a rectangular block, in which the time dimension is the width (with a size of L slices) and the content of each temporal slice is defined later. It can be seen how K blocks are built, each one constructed with T frames. Depending on the stride S, the blocks can be overlapped, as in the example, in which block 1 and 2 have a little overlap. For instance, in the case of setting K to 5 and T to 10, sampling segments from a video with an L of 50, we would cover the whole video (and use all the frames) with a stride S of 10, creating non-overlapping segments. For these experiments, we uniformly sample blocks by setting S to $\frac{L-T}{K-1}$.

When the blocks are defined, we aim at collapsing each block so that the object information is compressed. For that, we start by defining a matrix of shape $|O| \times C$, where O is the set of objects and C the dimension of their feature vectors, initialised to zero. We call this type of structure, yet to be filled, the Bag-of-Objects Matrix (BOM) of the block. In fact, a BOM is just a matrix collecting objects in a row-wise arrangement, each of the raw representation's slices can also be considered BOMs. Regarding how the BOM in this approach is filled, assume that the first dimension is a dictionary with $|O|$ elements (one per object), with entries of size C that represent the feature of the ith object ($0 \leq i < |O|$). We want to pool the information about every type of object into a feature vector within the time span of T frames of a block.

For that, for each of the T frames within a block, the predictions of the ith object (for all i such that $0 \leq i < |O|$) are added by vector addition, specially for those cases in which the object is repeated within the frame. The null predictions are ignored, so any object not appearing in a frame would have a feature vector of zeros after the addition. With this, the new structure has a shape $|O| \times T \times C$ and there are K of these, one per block. Figure 14 illustrates this process.

In a second step, the frame-wise BOMs are going to end up collapsed in a single BOM (representing the information from a block). For that, we applied a mean pooling operation across the depth dimension (of size T). That is, for the ith object, all the feature vectors of the same object class of the block are mean pooled. From this step, a set of K BOMs of shape $|O| \times C$ are obtained. The final input is obtained by arranging the obtained structure to have a shape $|O| \times C \times K$ (Fig. 15).

5.2   Architecture

In Sect. 5.1, the raw and the segments representations were explained. These allowed for a encoding of the object information of a video. Nonetheless, apart from the representation of the data, a feature extractor (CNN in this case) and a classi-

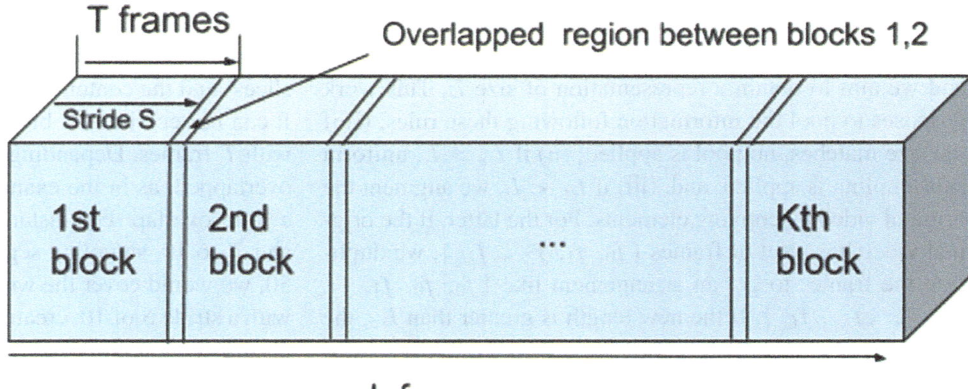

Fig. 13 The segments representation proposed to encode the Faster R-CNN output of all the frames of a video

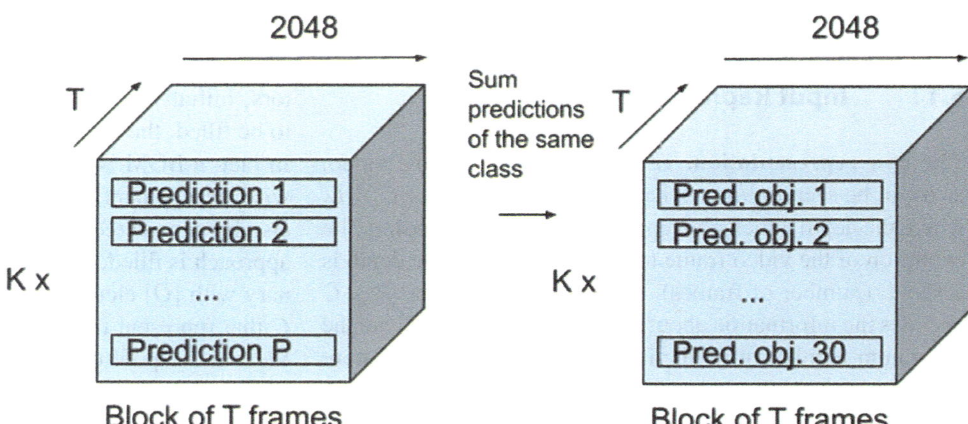

Fig. 14 The feature vectors of each object class are added frame-wise (objects can be repeated within a frame, so their feature vectors are added)

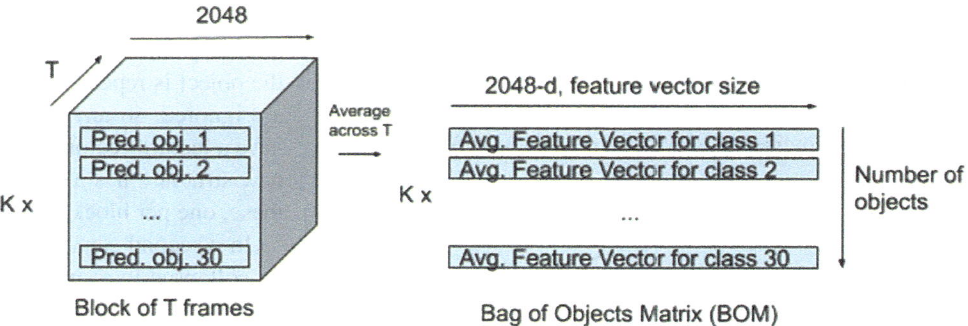

Fig. 15 Within each block, a mean pooling operation across the depth dimension is done. This way, the BOMs of a single block are pooled

fier capable of inferring active objects and actions from those structures are needed.

Due to the structure of the input, not being a space in which the adjacency of pixels is meaningful as in images, the use of pre-trained networks and the standard image processing networks is discarded from the beginning. We draw inspiration from the Natural Language Processing (NLP) field, and, more specifically, from the work of [27], who proposed a CNN architecture for NLP. The connection between the latter task and ours might not be obvious at first. However, the extended use of word embeddings (feature vectors encoding words) used in that work resembles our object feature vectors.

He arranges word embeddings in a matrix row-wise, where the ith row contains the ith word of the phrase. In our case, the ith row of a depth slice contains the ith object's information.

The network, called Multi-Scale Convolutional Neural Network (MSCNN), is shown in Fig. 16 adapted to our task. It is a branched architecture with four paths at the beginning. Each of them applies first a convolutional layer with a variable filter size: the width is fixed to the maximum (2048) in every filter, while the height goes from 2 in the first branch to 5 in the last branch. The purpose of the filter is to convolve together a set of objects, sets of different sizes depending on the height of the filter. The result is a matrix that is max pooled in the sec-

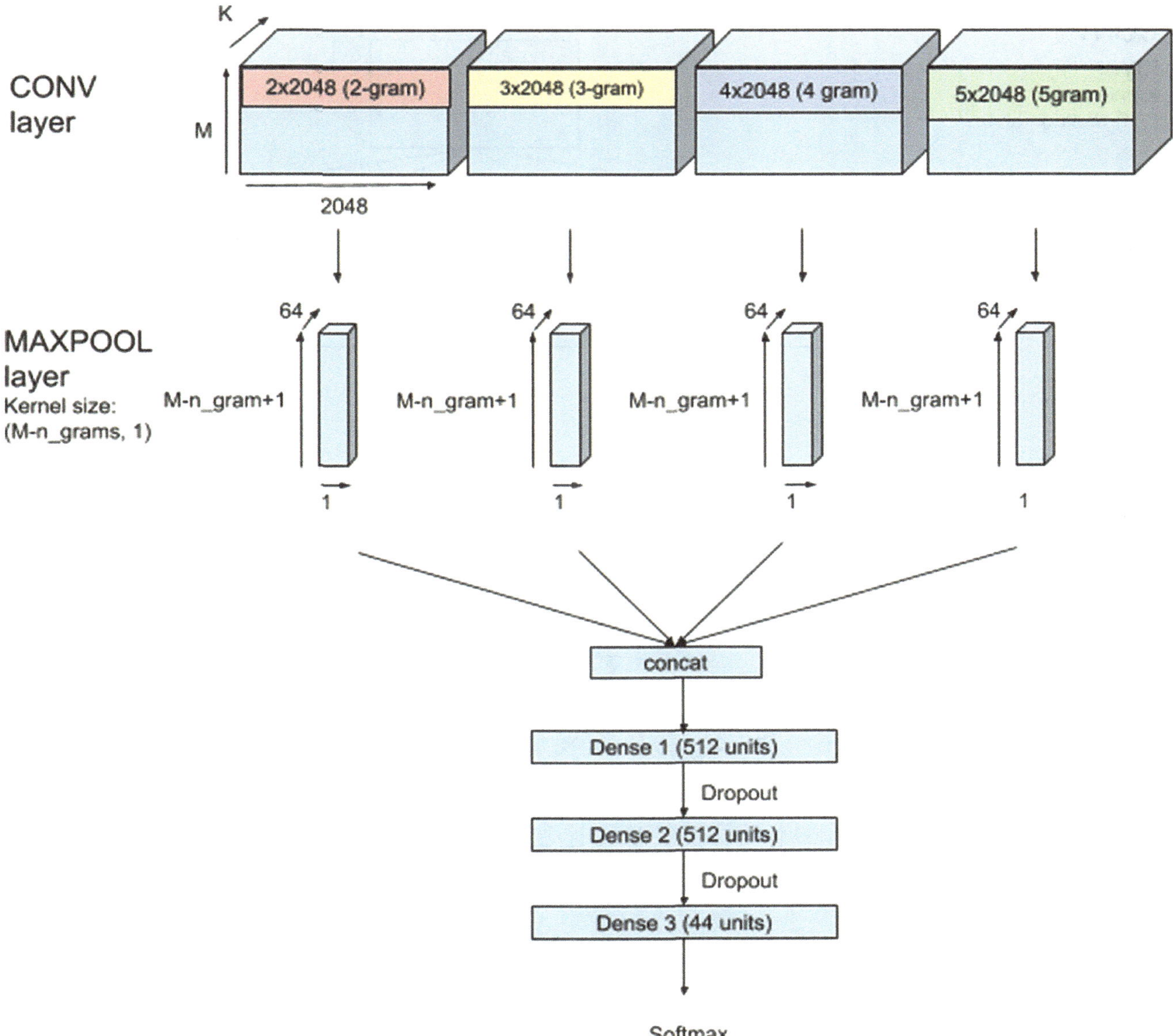

Fig. 16 The CNN architecture used by [27] adapted to the task of active object and action recognition with encoded object detection information as input

ond step. The shape of the max pooling filter is also adapted to the new height of the feature cube (varying from branch to branch); thus, resulting in a feature vector per branch as output. All of them are concatenated to create a single feature vector and this is fed to an MLP classifier to be trained on active objects and action labels.

Nevertheless, we believe the first convolution of each branch collapses too much information at once, in contrast to what happens in the work of [27], i.e., words embeddings often have a lower dimensionality compared with object feature vectors. That is why another variation of the network is proposed by adding another convolution step first, slowly reducing the dimensionality. The new architecture can be seen in Fig. 17.

5.3   Experiments

The GTEA Gaze+ dataset is used for the training and evaluation of the MSCNN model. Hence, a leave-one-subject-out cross-validation is applied. For each fold, a Faster R-CNN model is trained using the BB annotations of the rest of the subjects as explained in Sect. 3.2. For this problem, we defined the following TP, FP, TN, and FN for the accuracy and F1 metrics:

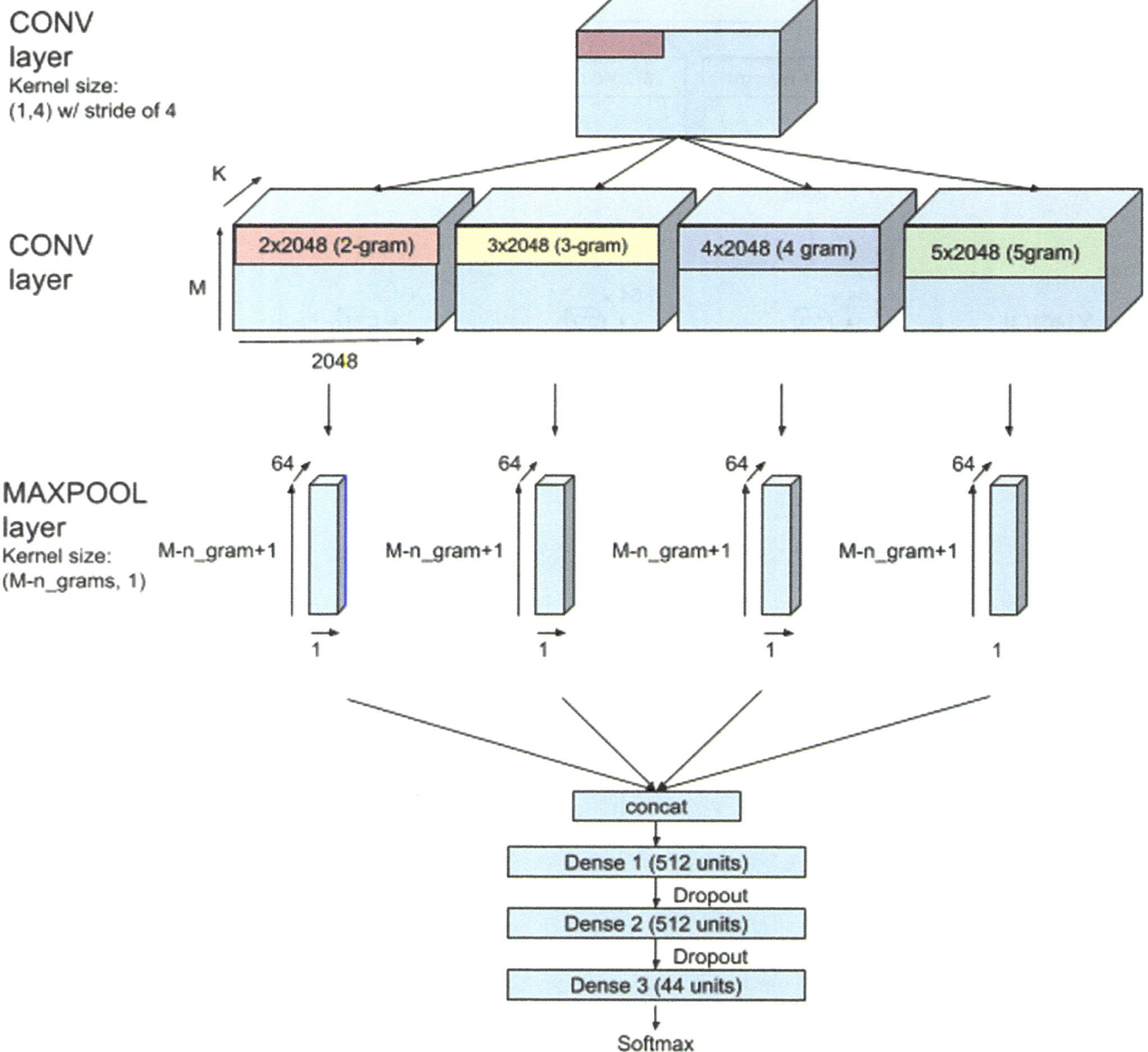

Fig. 17 A variation of the CNN architecture used by [27] adapted to the task of active object and action recognition with encoded object detection information as input. Another convolution has been added at the beginning to reduce the dimensionality of the object feature vectors

- TP: for the class i, if an input stack of BOMs is labelled with class i and the class i is the one with the highest confidence.
- FP: for the class i, if an input stack of BOMs is labelled with class j and the class i is the one with the highest confidence, being j any class different to i.
- TN: for the class i, if an input stack of BOMs is labelled with class j and the class k is the one with the highest confidence, being j and k any classes different to i and being possible that $j = k$.

- FN: for the class i, if an input stack of BOMs is labelled with class i and the class j is the one with the highest confidence, being j any class different to i.

Several experiments to tune the hyperparameters are done using the cross-validation approach. Initially, 500 epochs are set, but the training is stopped using the macro-F1 metric in the validation set, with a patience of 10 epochs. The validation set was created taking a stratified set with the 15% of the training

Table 7 Results of the experiments with the Multi-Scale Convolutional Neural Network and the inputs built using the raw approach for the action classification task. For each row and column, the average result is presented on top and the standard deviation is shown below. The highest column-wise mean is highlighted in bold

L	FC units	Dropout	Learning rate	Batch size	Accuracy	Macro-F1	Accuracy	Macro-F1	Accuracy	Macro-F1	Accuracy	Macro-F1	Accuracy	Macro-F1
Hyperparameters					Average		Ahmad		Alireza		Carlos		Rahul	
50	1024	0.5	0.001	256	38.36% (±5.35)	24.03 (±2.74)	32.47% (±1.62)	19.97 (±0.49)	43.32% (±1.51)	25.72 (±2.69)	33.96% (±0.69)	25.47 (±0.21)	43.67% (±1.51)	24.95 (±0.45)
50	1024	0.5	0.0001	256	**41.25%** (±4.42)	**27.20** (±2.27)	**37.37%** (±0.73)	**25.16** (±1.53)	43.21% (±1.24)	**27.35** (±1.01)	**37.05%** (±1.36)	29.76 (±2.46)	**47.37%** (±0.60)	26.54 (±0.23)
30	1024	0.5	0.001	256	37.80% (±6.12)	24.17 (±2.51)	30.36% (±0.28)	20.36 (±0.91)	42.31% (±0.97)	25.02 (±2.12)	33.47% (±1.03)	25.66 (±0.56)	45.06% (±0.79)	25.62 (±0.24)
30	1024	0.5	0.0001	256	39.65% (±4.58)	27.11 (±2.87)	34.66% (±0.37)	23.59 (±0.23)	**43.66%** (±0.16)	26.58 (±0.40)	35.58% (±0.62)	**31.39** (±1.03)	44.69% (±0.47)	**26.88** (±0.81)

Table 8 Results of the experiments with the Multi-Scale Convolutional Neural Network and the inputs built using the segments approach for the action classification task. For each row and column, the average result is presented on top and the standard deviation is shown below. The highest column-wise mean is highlighted in bold

L	K	T	FC units	Dropout	Learning rate	Batch size	Accuracy	Macro-F1	Accuracy	Macro-F1	Accuracy	Macro-F1	Accuracy	Macro-F1	Accuracy	Macro-F1
Hyperparameters							Average		Ahmad		Alireza		Carlos		Rahul	
50	5	5	1024	0.5	0.001	256	44.57% (±5.91)	34.71 (±3.02)	40.28% (±0.58)	29.99 (±0.34)	**46.91%** (±0.57)	36.22 (±0.72)	38.11% (±0.30)	34.96 (±0.49)	53.00% (±1.45)	37.66 (±1.56)
50	5	10	1024	0.5	0.001	256	44.00% (±5.87)	33.73 (±1.87)	**41.93%** (±0.25)	**31.60** (±0.68)	43.66% (±1.66)	32.77 (±0.37)	37.40% (±0.20)	36.05 (±0.43)	53.00% (±2.42)	34.49 (±1.32)
50	5	2	1024	0.5	0.001	256	42.77% (±4.05)	32.58 (±3.16)	38.69% (±0.16)	27.72 (±1.19)	44.89% (±0.88)	32.63 (±0.88)	39.30% (±1.11)	35.39 (±0.99)	48.20% (±0.90)	34.60 (±1.08)
50	10	5	1024	0.5	0.001	256	43.62% (±5.99)	32.15 (±3.88)	38.43% (±1.60)	26.53 (±0.78)	45.12% (±0.73)	32.15 (±0.25)	38.32% (±1.05)	34.91 (±1.80) (±1.80)	52.63% (±0.82)	35.00− (±3.00)
50	10	10	1024	0.5	0.001	256	42.84% (±5.58)	32.14 (±2.87)	**41.93%** (±0.89)	30.18 (±0.68)	40.40% (±0.99)	29.69 (±2.15)	37.12% (±0.43)	35.32 (±1.84)	51.89% (±1.02)	33.38 (±1.75)
50	10	2	1024	0.5	0.001	256	44.00% (±6.45)	34.08 (±5.89)	39.35% (±2.11)	28.14 (±2.68)	42.09% (±2.62)	29.72 (±0.97)	40.00% (±0.17)	36.11 (±0.91)	**54.57%** (±1.38)	**42.37** (±1.58)
50	5	5	1024	0.5	0.0001	256	**45.47%** (±5.02)	**35.25** (±3.47)	41.40% (±0.52)	30.33 (±0.70)	**46.91%** (±0.16)	34.04 (±0.74)	40.56% (±0.53)	37.62 (±0.51)	53.00% (±0.68)	39.01 (±0.19)
50	5	10	1024	0.5	0.0001	256	44.93% (±5.19)	33.99 (±4.59)	39.75% (±0.34)	26.84 (±0.40)	46.58% (±1.36)	33.90 (±0.94)	**40.84%** (±0.75)	**38.05** (±0.68)	52.54% (±1.02)	37.19 (±2.23)
30	5	5	1024	0.5	0.001	256	41.96% (±5.07)	33.77 (±3.78)	36.71% (±0.32)	27.98 (±1.49)	44.78% (±0.99)	35.57 (±0.90)	37.61% (±1.05)	34.67 (±2.44)	48.75% (±0.45)	36.87 (±1.05)
30	5	10	1024	0.5	0.001	256	42.20% (±5.29)	32.58 (±3.57)	37.50% (±0.43)	27.13 (±1.12)	45.45% (±0.48)	35.02 (±1.61)	36.91% (±2.24)	33.33 (±1.84)	48.94% (±0.69)	34.83 (±1.54)
30	5	2	1024	0.5	0.001	256	42.17% (±5.01)	32.45 (±3.44)	38.23% (±0.09)	27.57 (±0.95)	45.01% (±2.34)	33.34 (±1.49)	36.98% (±0.95)	33.61 (±0.99)	48.48% (±1.93)	35.29 (±3.05)
30	10	5	1024	0.5	0.001	256	41.68% (±5.75)	32.69 (±5.92)	36.18% (±0.73)	22.90 (±1.96)	45.45% (±2.23)	35.77 (±2.23)	36.07% (±0.87)	36.17 (±1.57)	49.03% (±0.60)	35.91 (±1.17)
30	10	10	1024	0.5	0.001	256	41.00% (±5.78)	31.32 (±4.44)	36.57% (±1.04)	26.30 (±2.13)	44.67% (±2.77)	35.45 (±3.22)	34.74% (±1.66)	32.07 (±4.24)	48.01% (±0.73)	31.46 (±1.76)
30	10	2	1024	0.5	0.001	256	43.66% (±5.85)	35.01 (±5.50)	37.37% (±0.73)	25.69 (±0.50)	46.24% (±1.11)	**37.88** (±0.90)	39.23% (±1.60)	37.27 (±1.42)	51.80% (±0.68)	39.19 (±0.19)

samples. Two validation sets were created: one stratifying the object label (for the active object classification task) and the other one stratifying the action label (for the action classification task). For the results, the accuracy and macro-F1 metrics are provided, both as the average of all the subjects and per subject. For each subject, three runs are executed and averaged. The best accuracy and macro-F1 results are considered those with the highest average result, not taking into account the standard deviation due to the higher variability it supposes. That is, two results with the same value may have different standard deviations: the one with the highest deviation may

obtain higher results sometimes, but it may also obtain much lower results in other occasions. Thus, we believe the average is a better tool to compare two results.

For the action classification task, the results can be found in Tables 7 (using the raw representation) and 8 (using the segments representation). For the active object classification task, the results are shown in Tables 10 (using the raw representation) and 11 (using the segments representation) (Table 9).

The segments representation seems to get slightly better results than the raw one. We can observe in both cases that sampling fewer frames (30 in comparison with 50) leads to

Table 9 Comparative table with the state-of-the-art approaches for action classification and active object using the GTEA Gaze+ dataset. The best results are highlighted in bold. The results are given as the mean of a leave-one-subject-out cross-validation approach. Furthermore, for our experiments we repeated each fold three times and we provide the mean and the standard deviation

Action classification		
Approach	Accuracy	F1
Dense Trajectories (DT) [60]	42.40%	–
Improved Dense Trajectories (IDT) [61]	49.60%	–
O+E+H [29]	57.40%	–
O+M+E+H [29]	60.50%	–
O+M+E+G [29]	60.30%	–
Motion stream [36]	62.62%	–
Two-stream [36]	**65.05%**	–
Two-stream [66]	59.02%	–
TSN [52]	55.25%	–
Two-stream [52]	60.13%	–
Appearance stream [34]*	57.63%	–
Motion stream [34]*	57.42%	–
Two-stream [34]*	64.74%	–
Time-Distributed Spatial CNN (Ours)	46.55% (±7.84)	36.11 (±4.44)
MSCNN Raw (Ours)	41.25% (±4.42)	27.70 (±2.27)
MSCNN Segments (Ours)	45.57% (±5.02)	33.99 (±4.59)
Active object classification		
Approach	Accuracy	F1
Spatial stream [36]	61.87%	–
Spatial stream (after joint training) [36]	**74.34%**	–
Time-Distributed Spatial CNN	58.92% (±6.05)	47.95 (±4.14)
MSCNN Raw (Ours)	52.47% (±4.08)	35.39 (±4.65)
MSCNN Segments (Ours)	57.40% (±6.05)	43.70 (±6.58)

*They took six subjects into account instead of four (see Sect. 3.1 for the evaluation strategy)

Table 10 Results of the experiments with the Multi-Scale Convolutional Neural Network and the inputs built using the raw approach for the active object classification task. For each row and column, the average result is presented on top and the standard deviation is shown below. The highest column-wise mean is highlighted in bold

L	FC units	Dropout	Learning rate	Batch size	Accuracy	Macro-F1	Accuracy	Macro-F1	Accuracy	Macro-F1	Accuracy	Macro-F1	Accuracy	Macro-F1
Hyperparameters					Average		Ahmad		Alireza		Carlos		Rahul	
50	1024	0.5	0.001	256	50.08% (±2.86)	31.25 (±2.73)	47.02% (±0.28)	27.75 (±1.77)	50.62% (±1.14)	30.85 (±0.73)	48.56% (±1.04)	32.46 (±4.27)	54.11% (±1.47)	33.96 (±2.21)
50	1024	0.5	0.0001	256	**52.47%** (±4.08)	35.39 (±4.65)	46.36% (±0.25)	27.90 (±0.76)	54.88% (±0.73)	36.06 (±1.51)	**51.65%** (±0.88)	39.26 (±1.49)	**56.97%** (±1.12)	**38.36** (±1.03)
30	1024	0.5	0.001	256	50.94% (±3.84)	32.38 (±4.47)	47.02% (±1.27)	28.67 (±2.22)	**55.11%** (±0.42)	**36.19** (±4.38)	47.72% (±1.14)	34.94 (±2.74)	53.92% (±1.95)	29.71 (±2.50)
30	1024	0.5	0.0001	256	51.83% (±3.75)	**35.40** (±5.41)	**47.16%** (±0.41)	**31.32** (±2.99)	53.87% (±1.20)	34.46 (±4.26)	49.61% (±0.10)	**42.46** (±4.27)	56.69% (±0.35)	33.34 (±0.20)

lower results. The median of frames for the GTEA Gaze+ dataset is 31, so one could have expected a good result for a value close to that. However, in this case, it is better to bias that towards longer videos, i.e., prioritise a value of L larger than the median of the length that half of the dataset's videos have. In fact, there are very long videos in the dataset, specially those related to cutting vegetables. It would make sense that, after undersampling them, the performance of the system on those classes would not be hurt due to the low variance long videos have across frames, as the objects should not vary much. Regarding the other parameters to build the segments approach, K and T, it is difficult to extract conclusions from these experiments. This may be due to the low effect they have in the performance. The best results with the raw and the segments representations are compared with the state-of-the-art approaches and with our baseline SpatialNet in Table 9.

Table 11 Results of the experiments with the Multi-Scale Convolutional Neural Network and the inputs built using the segments approach for the active object classification task. For each row and column, the average result is presented on top and the standard deviation is shown below. The highest column-wise mean is highlighted in bold

L	K	T	FC units	Dropout	Learning rate	Batch size	Accuracy	Macro-F1	Accuracy	Macro-F1	Accuracy	Macro-F1	Accuracy	Macro-F1	Accuracy	Macro-F1
Hyperparameters							Average		Ahmad		Alireza		Carlos		Rahul	
50	5	5	1024	0.5	0.001	256	54.84% (±4.07)	43.15 (±4.21)	51.32% (±0.94)	37.40 (±2.54)	57.35% (±0.57)	48.20 (±0.24)	50.67% (±1.21)	43.65 (±2.32)	60.02% (±0.86)	43.34 (±0.21)
50	5	10	1024	0.5	0.001	256	53.34% (±4.02)	42.11 (±5.11)	50.40% (±0.43)	34.53 (±0.76)	55.78% (±0.69)	45.02 (±1.97)	49.47% (±1.47)	45.51 (±2.36)	57.71% (±3.62) (±3.62)	43.36 (±3.91)
50	5	2	1024	0.5	0.001	256	53.53% (±2.68)	43.01 (±4.32)	51.52% (±1.17)	38.63 (±3.60)	55.78% (±1.04)	47.49 (±1.39)	50.67% (±0.78)	45.22 (±1.70)	56.14% (±1.29)	40.71 (±2.74)
30	5	5	1024	0.5	0.001	256	53.83% (±6.05)	41.55 (±7.15)	47.62% (±1.13)	32.29 (±1.57)	57.69% (±1.14)	47.58 (±3.30)	48.42% (±0.45)	37.59 (±0.38)	61.59% (±0.91)	48.75 (±1.09)
50	10	5	1024	0.5	0.001	256	55.29% (±3.84)	43.83 (±3.26)	**52.31%** (±0.52)	39.04 (±3.26)	56.34% (±0.69)	45.43 (±1.03)	51.58% (±1.03)	45.72 (±2.57)	60.94% (±1.26)	45.15 (±1.99)
50	10	10	1024	0.5	0.001	256	55.09% (±3.96)	43.57 (±3.69)	51.26% (±0.89)	**39.40** (±2.59)	56.90% (±1.67)	45.84 (±3.94)	51.72% (±0.26)	43.85 (±1.92)	60.48% (±0.73)	45.18 (±1.84)
50	10	2	1024	0.5	0.001	256	54.81% (±3.57)	43.31 (±4.30)	51.98% (±0.33)	37.33 (±2.75)	57.58% (±0.00)	48.09 (±1.01)	50.88% (±0.65)	43.06 (±1.17)	58.82% (±1.33)	44.75 (±1.78)
50	5	5	1024	0.5	0.0001	256	**57.40%** (±6.05)	43.70 (±6.58)	50.20% (±1.33)	36.27 (±1.46)	**60.94%** (±0.27)	**53.82** (±0.74)	**53.19%** (±0.53)	40.98 (±0.58)	**65.28%** (±0.35)	43.75 (±2.24)
50	5	10	1024	0.5	0.0001	256	56.72% (±5.46)	43.06 (±5.71)	52.12% (±0.19)	34.92 (±0.53)	57.80% (±0.69)	48.32 (±1.11)	51.79% (±0.17)	40.73 (±0.88)	65.19% (±0.65)	48.26 (±1.34)
30	5	5	1024	0.5	0.001	256	53.83% (±6.05)	41.55 (±7.15)	47.62% (±1.13)	32.29 (±1.57)	57.69% (±1.14)	47.58 (±3.30)	48.42% (±0.45)	37.59 (±0.38)	61.59% (±0.91)	48.75 (±1.09)
30	5	10	1024	0.5	0.001	256	55.80% (±5.54)	44.70 (±7.59)	50.73% (±1.17)	34.39 (±1.13)	59.26% (±1.26)	49.42 (±1.60)	50.53% (±2.48)	43.53 (±6.08)	62.70% (±0.79)	**51.45** (±3.73)
30	5	2	1024	0.5	0.001	256	53.69% (±4.11)	41.48 (±5.30)	50.26% (±0.77)	33.40 (±1.56)	56.34% (±0.84)	44.61 (±1.16)	49.26% (±0.52)	40.78 (±0.46)	58.91% (±0.65)	47.12 (±1.08)
30	10	5	1024	0.5	0.001	256	54.91% (±4.72)	44.60 (±7.24)	50.13% (±0.52)	33.95 (±0.40)	59.37% (±1.38)	52.12 (±0.52)	50.60% (±1.01)	42.87 (±3.02)	59.56% (±1.71)	49.46 (±1.78)
30	10	10	1024	0.5	0.001	256	54.88% (±5.42)	43.25 (±5.86)	49.14% (±0.92)	33.63 (±1.22)	57.58% (±0.99)	47.10 (±1.01)	50.67% (±1.74)	45.11 (±1.33)	62.14% (±1.38)	47.18 (±2.62)
30	10	2	1024	0.5	0.001	256	55.25% (±3.90)	**45.42** (±5.25)	51.46% (±1.56)	37.93 (±3.93)	58.02% (±0.42)	49.39 (±0.75)	51.86% (±0.60)	**49.25** (±1.08)	59.65% (±2.23)	45.12 (±2.55)

Despite the promising approach used to represent videos, the results are not as high as expected, being even lower than the baseline proposed in Sect. 4. There may be various reasons for this. For example, the part of the Faster R-CNN from which the features are extracted may be one of the keys. For instance, [37] exploited object features from an object detector and explained that they did not extract these features from the R-CNN part (as we did), but rather from the object proposal network (RPN) itself. Taking the feature vectors from the R-CNN leads to a cross-domain problem, which may be one of the reasons for having low results. In their setting, they also mention that by taking pruned results from the R-CNN (only considering annotated objects) there is a possibility of missing objects that are not recognised as objects. This means objects are taken without labelling, just exploiting the information of the feature vectors. This is a reasonable approach to represent the objects of the scene. In fact, [37] also leveraged attention mechanisms to represent the interactions between objects, leading to competitive results comparable to those of I3D [8] and TSN [62] in the Kinetics dataset [8]. This work may provide a hint on the importance of using feature vectors from the RPN and the contribution of attention mechanisms towards compressing all the features. In a similar fashion, [50]

extracted features of specific regions using the RPN's detections instead of those of the R-CNN. We believe this was one of the main shortcomings of our experiments. However, it was not the unique one. The way the feature vectors are used in the previous works or in recent ones such as the one carried out by [64] lead to the conclusion that the features must be pooled or attended so that all the information they contain is better represented for the following task (such as action classification or active object, as in this case).

6   Hand-Based Attention Masks

The Faster R-CNN's feature vectors contain many details about objects, although that information is encoded, requiring a system to extract patterns from them. Nevertheless, object detectors also provide human-understandable information such as BBs, which can be easily visualised. In fact, these boxes can be seen as a type of hard attention, in which specific regions of images are surrounded by "attention masks". Given the importance that hands have in egocentric settings, a BB around a hand or both hands can be seen as a way of attending the manipulation of objects or the interaction with them, as objects are supposed to be close to hands when they become active objects [70]. In fact, this idea has already been explored in the literature in other forms. Ma et al. [36] trained a network to segment hands, then a gaussian bump was created around hands, where objects should have lain. A gaussian bump can be interpreted as a soft BB around the location of hands. This part was cropped for object classification, removing any other spatial information. Lu et al. [34] aimed at creating attention masks using gaussian bumps as supervision. This may not be directly correlated to the previous approach, but both have something in common. In this approach, instead of the position of hands, they used the gaze position to create the gaussian bump. The main idea behind both works is that there are points in the space that are being attended by a human and so each one applied their own methodology to focus the attention on those regions.

In this part, an attention mechanism to exploit the attention point created by the position of hands is developed. For that, we leveraged the Faster R-CNN's predictions of Sect. 3.2 that included the prediction of hands. Looking back at Fig. 6, the "hand" class predominated among others, which led to a high-recall hand detector.

6.1 Attention Masks

An attention mask $A \in \mathbb{R}^{H \times W}$, with $A_{ij} \in [0, 1]$, is a matrix with the spatial shape of the input of a neural network $X \in \mathbb{R}^{H \times W \times C}$, being H, W, and C the height, width, and the number of channels, respectively. Positions (i, j) with high values in this attention matrix A (close to 1) are positions that should be attended in the equivalent (i, j) positions of the original image X. When creating A, the BB coordinates of hands detected in X are taken into account. These coordinates (y_1, x_1) and (y_2, x_2) are two points in the space of X that can be used to draw a BB that includes a single hand (from the wrist to the fingers, not including the arm), being (y_1, x_1) the top-left corner point and (y_2, x_2) the bottom-right corner. In the case of the detection of two hands in a single frame, the BB that needs to be created would include the BBs of both hands. That is, a new BB with coordinates (y_1, x_1) and (y_2, x_2) must be created, using the coordinates (y_1', x_1') and (y_2', x_2'), and (y_1'', x_1'') and (y_2'', x_2'') of the first and second hand BBs, respectively. To compute the coordinates of the new BB, the following formulas are used:

$$x_1 = min(x_1', x_1'') \tag{5}$$
$$y_1 = min(y_1', y_1'') \tag{6}$$
$$x_2 = max(x_2', x_2'') \tag{7}$$
$$y_2 = max(y_2', y_2'') \tag{8}$$

With this idea, a naive approach to create A would be to create a binary mask, in which all the pixel values of A within the BB would be set to 1 and any value outside of it to 0. However, we propose a softened version of the binary mask. It implies creating a 2D anisotropic gaussian bump centred in the BB with a sigma equal to the height and width of the BB. Those height and width are multiplied by a scaling factor of 0.5 in our experiments. In contrast to a binary mask, the attention mask is expanded through the whole image instead of just having null values out of the hand area. However, positions outside of the BB will have very small values, smaller as the distance to the centre of the BB (or the gaussian bump) increases. Sample masks can be seen applied to images of the EGTEA Gaze+ dataset in Fig. 18. To obtain these representations, an element-wise product between A and X is done, for visualisation purposes.

If a single input contains several frames (as in the case of a stack of OF), then the mask that needs to be created for that input would be based on a BB that includes all the BBs of the frames of the stack. This can be seen as an extension of Eqs. 5, 6, 7, and 8 to more than two terms, as many as frames are stacked. If the mask is applied to an input that consists of a single frame, then the mask is directly computed with the BB of that frame.

6.2 Architecture

So far, the CNN-M-2048 has been employed as an off-the-shelf DL architecture for the feature extraction part, apart from the specialised architectures of Sect. 5.2 (due to the type of data they used). However, the former only extracts short-term patterns and can only provide predictions for individual timesteps of clips, leaving another function (such as the majority voting) the task of deciding the prediction for the whole clip. To go one step further and inspired by the work of [52], the architecture used for the experiments of this section will include a long-term modelling of clips. The type of structure suggested for that in the literature is a CNN-RNN similar to that of [52]. Figure 19 illustrates the general scheme followed by CNN-RNN architectures. Given a sequence of frames $\{F_1, F_2, \ldots F_N\}$ (being N the number of frames), a feature extractor g (implemented with a CNN) extracts features for each frame F_i ($0 \leq i \leq N$), obtaining a sequence of features $\{g(F_1), g(F_2), \ldots g(F_N)\}$. These are passed to the RNN to get a sequence of temporal or spatio-temporal features $\{h_1, h_2, \ldots h_N\}$, in which h_i represents the information of the clip until the ith step. Usually, the last one, h_N, is sent to the classifier, which outputs a probability distribution.

Going into details, the chosen CNN architecture is a ResNet50 network [23], a standard architecture in the lit-

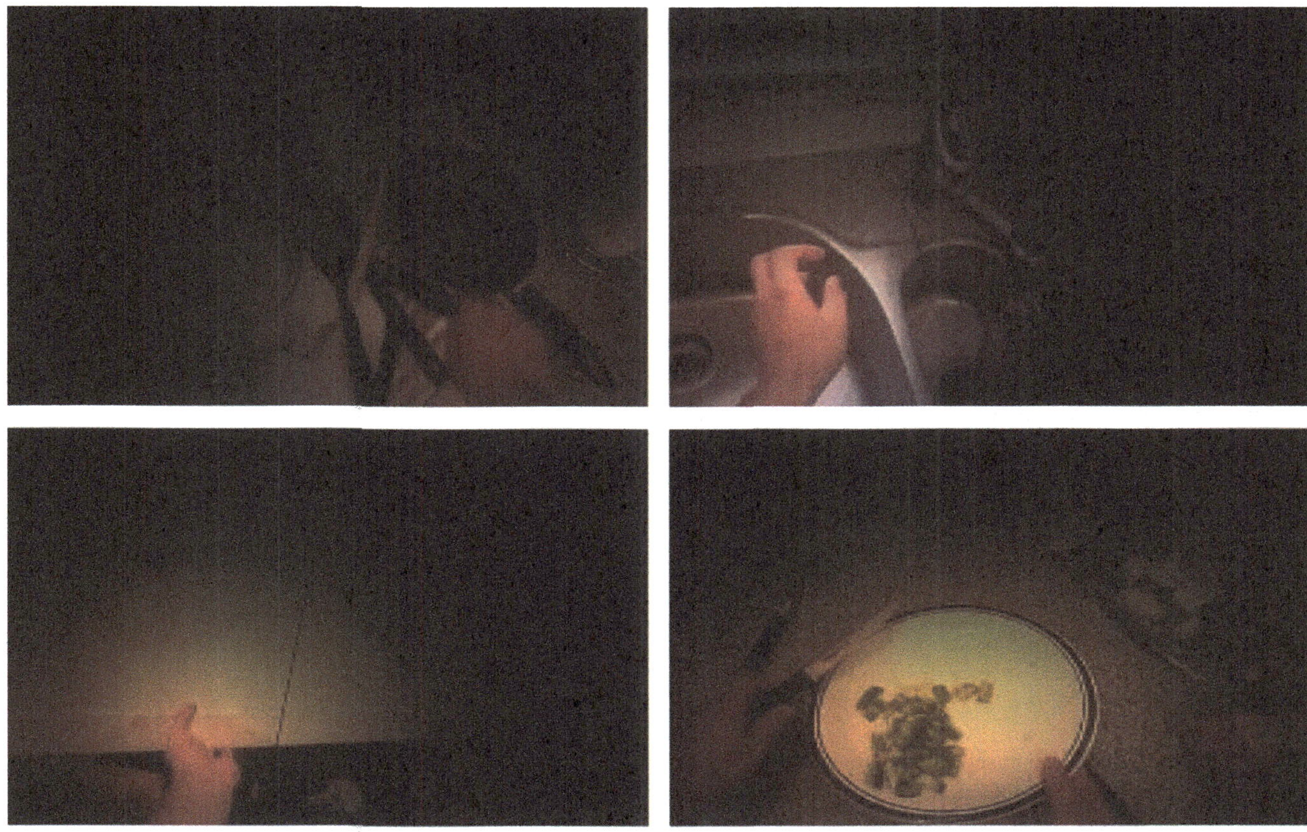

Fig. 18 Gaussian masks applied to images of the EGTEA Gaze+ dataset

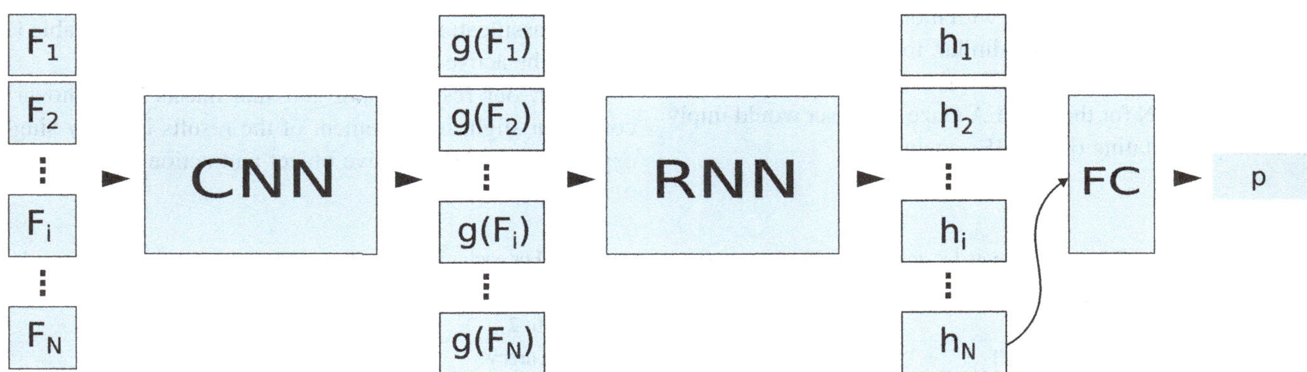

Fig. 19 The Convolutional Neural Network (CNN)—Recurrent Neural Network (RNN) paradigm has two main parts: the feature extractor g, implemented as a CNN, and the long-term modelling RNN. The system is fed with a sequence of frames $\{F_1, F_2, \ldots F_N\}$ sampled from a video, being N the amount of frames. Each frame is transformed by g, extracting the features $g(F_i)$ for each frame F_i. A RNN learns long-term temporal patterns, predicting the $\{h_1, h_2, \ldots h_N\}$ hidden states. The last hidden state, h_N, is sent to the FC layer (the classifier) and a prediction is given, a probability distribution p over a set of classes

erature. The feature cube $g(F_i)$ obtained from the network has a high dimensionality in the depth dimension due to the network applying many kernels. To alleviate the task for the RNN module, a 1×1 convolution with 256 kernels is applied so that the depth dimension reduces to 256. The RNN that takes this sequence is a ConvLSTM [67], whose hidden states h_i are 3D structures containing spatio-temporal patterns. The FC layer has a number of units that match the number of classes of the problem and applies a softmax activation to obtain a normalised distribution. Formally, the output is $p = \{p_1, p_2, \ldots, p_M\}$, where $p_i \in [0, 1]$ is the probability of the class i, $\sum_{i=1}^{M} p_i = 1$, and M is the number of classes. The predicted class is computed as $max_i\{p_i\}$, where i is the index of a class.

To apply the masking operation, we set the mask at each timestep as another input to the system. Each mask will be multiplied element-wise with its corresponding feature cube, applying the same spatial mask to each channel. For that, the mask is resized to match the spatial dimensionality of the feature cube. Moreover, to disturb as little as possible the pre-training of the feature extractor, the ResNet50, the multiplication is performed with the last feature cube of the network, $g(F_i)$, in the final convolution (prior to the 1×1 convolution). More formally, given a feature cube $g(F_i)$ of shape $H' \times W' \times C'$ from the last convolution and a mask M of shape $H \times W$, a resizing r and a depth-wise broadcasting b is applied to the mask to match the dimensionality of $g(F_i)$, i.e., $r(M) \in \mathbb{R}^{H' \times W'}$ and $b(r(M)) \in \mathbb{R}^{H' \times W' \times C'}$. Then, the Hadamard product is applied between $g(F_i)$ and $b(r(M))$ to get $g(F_i)'$, a masked feature cube of shape $H' \times W' \times C'$. This will be fed to the 1×1 convolution as the next step in the architecture, and so on.

6.3 Experiments

So far the GTEA Gaze+ dataset has been used for the experiments. However, with the launch of the EGTEA Gaze+ dataset, a larger version of the previous dataset, this was adopted for the last set of experiments. As EGTEA Gaze+ contains GTEA Gaze+, the statements done so far hold, as the former just extends the latter with more classes and samples. In fact, as both datasets are similar, the hand object detector trained for GTEA Gaze+ can be reused. Otherwise, training a Faster R-CNN for the EGTEA Gaze+ dataset would imply manually annotating object BBs again.

The following sets of experiments are carried out in this part: one set of experiments aiming at classifying actions and the other one active objects. For this problem, we defined the following TP, FP, TN, and FN for the accuracy and F1 metrics:

- TP: for the class i, if a sequence of images is labelled with class i and the class i is the one with the highest confidence.
- FP: for the class i, if a sequence of images is labelled with class j and the class i is the one with the highest confidence, being j any class different to i.
- TN: for the class i, if a sequence of images is labelled with class j and the class k is the one with the highest confidence, being j and k any classes different to i and being possible that $j = k$.
- FN: for the class i, if a sequence of images is labelled with class i and the class j is the one with the highest confidence, being j any class different to i.

For the training, 500 epochs are set with early stopping with a patience of 10 epochs using the Macro-F1 metric in the validation set. The latter is built using a stratified set containing 10% of the training samples. For the object classification task, the validation set is built stratifying according to the object label and, for the action classification task, using the action tag. The Adam optimiser is used with a learning rate of 10^{-5}, a batch size of 16 and 25 timesteps per sample. The results are given per split and as the average of the three splits. For each split, three consecutive experiments are averaged. For the action classification, the results are summarised in Table 12, and, for the active object classification, in Table 13.

So far, our results using gaussian masks have shown a consistent slight improvement of the results in every single experiment, both for active object and action classification.

Table 12 Results of the experiments for action classification with gaussian masks. For each row and column, the average result is presented on top and the standard deviation is shown below

	Average		Split 1		Split 2		Split 3	
Experiment	Accuracy	F1	Accuracy	F1	Accuracy	F1	Accuracy	F1
Baseline	55.32% ($\pm$2.60)	44.78 ($\pm$2.52)	58.21% ($\pm$0.69)	47.99 ($\pm$0.16)	55.56% ($\pm$1.26)	44.12 ($\pm$0.81)	52.20% ($\pm$0.35)	42.24 ($\pm$1.06)
Gaussian mask	55.98% ($\pm$2.26)	45.12 ($\pm$2.20)	58.37% ($\pm$0.56)	47.49 ($\pm$0.62)	56.46% ($\pm$0.31)	44.96 ($\pm$0.16)	53.11% ($\pm$0.87)	42.91 ($\pm$1.90)

Table 13 Results of the experiments for object classification with gaussian masks. For each row and column, the average result is presented on top and the standard deviation is shown below

	Average		Split 1		Split 2		Split 3	
Experiment	Accuracy	F1	Accuracy	F1	Accuracy	F1	Accuracy	F1
Baseline	66.66% ($\pm$2.25)	59.57 ($\pm$3.32)	69.39% ($\pm$0.84)	63.99 ($\pm$1.30)	66.11% ($\pm$0.87)	57.18 ($\pm$0.64)	64.49% ($\pm$1.16)	57.53 ($\pm$1.28)
Gaussian mask	67.49% ($\pm$2.52)	60.74 ($\pm$3.82)	70.85% ($\pm$0.77)	65.75 ($\pm$1.43)	66.50% ($\pm$0.69)	57.34 ($\pm$1.31)	65.10% ($\pm$0.23)	59.14 ($\pm$0.84)

Table 14 Comparative table with the state-of-the-art approaches for action classification using the EGTEA Gaze+ dataset. The best results are highlighted in bold. For our experiments we repeated each fold three times and we provide the mean and the standard deviation

Action classification		
Approach	Accuracy	F1
Single-stream, RGB and flow inputs [30]	53.30%	—
Two-stream [59]	66.00%	—
Original two-stream [52]	41.84%	—
I3D [52]	51.68%	—
TSN [52]	55.93%	—
Two-stream [52]	60.76%	—
LSTA [53]	61.86%	—
Multi-tasking network [25]*	**68.99%**	—
Two-stream with STAM [35]	68.60%	—
Multi-stream with SAP [65]	62.70%	—
CNN-ConvLSTM with hands-aware attention (Ours)	55.98% (±2.26)	45.12 (±2.20)

*Reports results only for the split 1

Specially for the former, the accuracy increased by 1%, similar to new state-of-the-art results in other Computer Vision tasks [31,57,69]. The use of gaussian bumps as an attention mechanism has already been explored in the literature [30,71] as a supervision signal to generate a mask that is later applied to the features, as in our case. Ma et al. [36] generated gaussian bumps to crop RoIs of images instead. Nonetheless, to the best of our knowledge, we were the first ones implementing it using an object detector to recognise hands and applying the attention mask generated from the position of the hands.

Nevertheless, the results are not as high as expected. The possible reasons for not obtaining higher results can be attributed to (i) the performance of the hand detector, (ii) the quality of some videos of the dataset (due to the lighting, hands are not correctly detected), or (iii) the implementation of the mask in the network, although the reason is not clear. Regarding the latter issue, the specific hyperparameters to build the mask and apply it may not be the most appropriate ones (although there has been an exploration of some configurations) or it may be that not using masks when no hands are detected or changing the features mid-way could destabilise the training. Other authors applied a mask generated by the network itself, probably avoiding this issue. Another possible reason for the latter approach to perform better is that guiding the training of the feature extractor for the objective of recognising active objects or actions alongside predicting attention masks may be the key to improve this type of attention mechanism.

For the sake of comparison, Table 14 compares the best result obtained on actions using gaussian masks with other state-of-the-art approaches on the EGTEA Gaze+ dataset. To the best of our knowledge, there were no reported results of active object classification for the EGTEA Gaze+ dataset

and, thus, we only show the comparison for action classification. We did improve or equal the result of some off-the-shelf state-of-the-art networks such as I3D and TSN, while other approaches employing more information obtained up to 5-6 points of accuracy more than us. One of the best results, obtained by [25], just employing RGB images like us, went up to 68.99% of accuracy (although just in the first split of the dataset). They argue that a multi-tasking approach forces the network to generalise better, learning verbs, objects, coordinates for hand locations, and the gaze-based visual saliency at the same time. Similarly, for the Gaze+ dataset, [36] learnt verbs, objects, and actions and obtained the best result so far for that dataset. This could point towards the use of multi-tasking approaches as a promising approach for the EAR and, possibly, for the active object detection. Other approaches made use of two-stream architectures including flow information or even object detection features [65] and/or architectures that include attention, such as the LSTA [53] or the two-stream network of [35].

7 Conclusions

In this chapter several proposals for action classification and active object recognition have been proposed. Starting from the baseline SpatialNet to infer actions and active objects, then the BOM representation and the proposed MSCNN architecture to exploit it, and, finally, the use of spatial gaussian masks to focus the attention in regions where hands' presence is detected. After all the experiments, we concluded that the recognition of active objects is not trivial and that more research is required on this topic. However, some valuable observations can be extracted from this chapter.

- The **temporal modelling of videos** must be done carefully. In Sect. 4, our first approach included a mean pooling of the predictions of single inputs to provide an average prediction for the video. However, the latter highly depended on the local patterns extracted, with no correlation between the subsequent timesteps apart from the mean pooling. We believe the addition of the ConvLSTM to the network proposed in Sect. 6 was a step in the correct direction.
- The **object feature vectors from RPN networks seem to be a promising complementary information** that can be used alongside RGB and OF features in the usual multistream approach. Furthermore, going one step further and combining object feature vectors with features extracted from other streams may lead to competitive results [64].
- **Attention mechanisms** have increasingly become more popular as a way to improve results without scaling networks to become bigger and adding little computation and memory overhead in general. The type of attention included in Sect. 6 was our first attempt in introducing a type of attention that does not require specific annotations in the dataset such as gaze points. Although a hand detector is still required for this, it could be obtained from other bigger datasets without requiring any fine-tuning.
- **Multi-tasking approaches may lead to improved generalisation**, as demonstrated by the state-of-the-art results obtained by [25,36] in the GTEA Gaze+ and EGTEA Gaze+ datasets, respectively. In fact, aiming at learning egocentric features, verbs, objects, and actions labels at the same time, following the literature of the EAR field, may be the key to improve active object recognition and EAR even further.

Acknowledgements We gratefully acknowledge the support of the Basque Government's Department of Education for the predoctoral funding of the first author. This work has been supported by the Spanish Government under the FuturAAL-Ego project (RTI2018-101045-A-C22) and the FuturAAL-Context project (RTI2018-101045-B-C21) and by the Basque Government under the Deustek project (IT-1078-16-D).

References

[1] Nachwa Aboubakr, James L Crowley, and Rémi Ronfard. Recognizing manipulation actions from state-transformations. *arXiv preprint* arXiv:1906.05147, 2019.

[2] Ahmad Akl, Jasper Snoek, and Alex Mihailidis. Unobtrusive detection of mild cognitive impairment in older adults through home monitoring. *IEEE Journal of Biomedical and Health Informatics*, 21(2):339–348, 2015.

[3] Maryam Asadi-Aghbolaghi, Albert Clapes, Marco Bellantonio, Hugo Jair Escalante, Víctor Ponce-López, Xavier Baró, Isabelle Guyon, Shohreh Kasaei, and Sergio Escalera. A survey on deep learning based approaches for action and gesture recognition in image sequences. In *2017 12th IEEE International Conference on Automatic Face & Gesture Recognition (FG 2017)*, pages 476–483. IEEE, 2017.

[4] Sven Bambach, Stefan Lee, David J Crandall, and Chen Yu. Lending a hand: Detecting hands and recognizing activities in complex egocentric interactions. In *Proceedings of the IEEE International Conference on Computer Vision*, pages 1949–1957, 2015.

[5] Ardhendu Behera, Matthew Chapman, Anthony G Cohn, and David C Hogg. Egocentric activity recognition using histograms of oriented pairwise relations. In *2014 International Conference on Computer Vision Theory and Applications (VISAPP)*, volume 2, pages 22–30. IEEE, 2014.

[6] Ardhendu Behera, David C Hogg, and Anthony G Cohn. Egocentric activity monitoring and recovery. In *Asian Conference on Computer Vision*, pages 519–532. Springer, 2012.

[7] Allah Bux, Plamen Angelov, and Zulfiqar Habib. Vision based human activity recognition: a review. In *Advances in Computational Intelligence Systems*, pages 341–371. Springer, 2017.

[8] Joao Carreira and Andrew Zisserman. Quo vadis, action recognition? a new model and the kinetics dataset. In *proceedings of the IEEE Conference on Computer Vision and Pattern Recognition*, pages 6299–6308, 2017.

[9] Alejandro Cartas, Petia Radeva, and Mariella Dimiccoli. Contextually driven first-person action recognition from videos.

[10] Ken Chatfield, Karen Simonyan, Andrea Vedaldi, and Andrew Zisserman. Return of the devil in the details: Delving deep into convolutional nets. *arXiv preprint* arXiv:1405.3531, 2014.

[11] Liming Chen, Jesse Hoey, Chris D Nugent, Diane J Cook, and Zhiwen Yu. Sensor-based activity recognition. *IEEE Transactions on Systems, Man, and Cybernetics, Part C (Applications and Reviews)*, 42(6):790–808, 2012.

[12] Dima Damen, Teesid Leelasawassuk, Osian Haines, Andrew Calway, and Walterio W Mayol-Cuevas. You-do, i-learn: Discovering task relevant objects and their modes of interaction from multi-user egocentric video. In *BMVC*, volume 2, page 3, 2014.

[13] Alireza Fathi and James M Rehg. Modeling actions through state changes. In *Proceedings of the IEEE Conference on Computer Vision and Pattern Recognition*, pages 2579–2586, 2013.

[14] Alireza Fathi, Ali Farhadi, and James M Rehg. Understanding egocentric activities. In *2011 International Conference on Computer Vision*, pages 407–414. IEEE, 2011.

[15] Alireza Fathi, Xiaofeng Ren, and James M Rehg. Learning to recognize objects in egocentric activities. In *CVPR 2011*, pages 3281–3288. IEEE, 2011.

[16] Alireza Fathi, Yin Li, and James M Rehg. Learning to recognize daily actions using gaze. In *European Conference on Computer Vision*, pages 314–327. Springer, 2012.

[17] Amy Fire and Song-Chun Zhu. Learning perceptual causality from video. *ACM Transactions on Intelligent Systems and Technology (TIST)*, 7(2):1–22, 2015.

[18] Ross Girshick. Fast r-cnn. In *Proceedings of the IEEE International Conference on Computer Vision*, pages 1440–1448, 2015.

[19] Ross Girshick, Jeff Donahue, Trevor Darrell, and Jitendra Malik. Region-based convolutional networks for accurate object detection and segmentation. *IEEE Transactions on Pattern Analysis and Machine Intelligence*, 38(1):142–158, 2015.

[20] Georgia Gkioxari, Ross Girshick, and Jitendra Malik. Contextual action recognition with r* cnn. In *Proceedings of the IEEE International Conference on Computer Vision*, pages 1080–1088, 2015.

[21] Nadee Goonawardene, Hwee-Pink Tan, and Lee Buay Tan. Unobtrusive detection of frailty in older adults. In *International Conference on Human Aspects of IT for the Aged Population*, pages 290–302. Springer, 2018.

[22] Mary Hayhoe. Vision using routines: A functional account of vision. *Visual Cognition*, 7(1-3):43–64, 2000.

[23] Kaiming He, Xiangyu Zhang, Shaoqing Ren, and Jian Sun. Deep residual learning for image recognition. In *Proceedings of the IEEE Conference on Computer Vision and Pattern Recognition*, pages 770–778, 2016.

[24] Hongwen Kang, Martial Hebert, and Takeo Kanade. Discovering object instances from scenes of daily living. In *2011 International Conference on Computer Vision*, pages 762–769. IEEE, 2011.

[25] Georgios Kapidis, Ronald Poppe, Elsbeth van Dam, Lucas Noldus, and Remco Veltkamp. Multitask learning to improve egocentric action recognition. In *Proceedings of the IEEE International Conference on Computer Vision Workshops*, pages 0–0, 2019.

[26] Georgios Kapidis, Ronald Poppe, Elsbeth van Dam, Lucas PJJ Noldus, and Remco C Veltkamp. Object detection-based location and activity classification from egocentric videos: A systematic analysis. In *Smart Assisted Living*, pages 119–145. Springer, 2020.

[27] Yoon Kim. Convolutional neural networks for sentence classification. *arXiv preprint* arXiv:1408.5882, 2014.

[28] Michael Land, Neil Mennie, and Jennifer Rusted. The roles of vision and eye movements in the control of activities of daily living. *Perception*, 28(11):1311–1328, 1999.

[29] Yin Li, Zhefan Ye, and James M Rehg. Delving into egocentric actions. In *Proceedings of the IEEE Conference on Computer Vision and Pattern Recognition*, pages 287–295, 2015.

[30] Yin Li, Miao Liu, and James M Rehg. In the eye of beholder: Joint learning of gaze and actions in first person video. In *Proceedings of the European Conference on Computer Vision (ECCV)*, pages 619–635, 2018.

[31] Jun Li, Xianglong Liu, Wenxuan Zhang, Mingyuan Zhang, Jingkuan Song, and Nicu Sebe. Spatio-temporal attention networks for action recognition and detection. *IEEE Transactions on Multimedia*, 2020.

[32] Tsung-Yi Lin, Michael Maire, Serge Belongie, James Hays, Pietro Perona, Deva Ramanan, Piotr Dollár, and C Lawrence Zitnick. Microsoft coco: Common objects in context. In *European Conference on Computer Vision*, pages 740–755. Springer, 2014.

[33] Yang Liu, Ping Wei, and Song-Chun Zhu. Jointly recognizing object fluents and tasks in egocentric videos. In *Proceedings of the IEEE International Conference on Computer Vision*, pages 2924–2932, 2017.

[34] Minlong Lu, Ze-Nian Li, Yueming Wang, and Gang Pan. Deep attention network for egocentric action recognition. *IEEE Transactions on Image Processing*, 28(8):3703–3713, 2019.

[35] Minlong Lu, Danping Liao, and Ze-Nian Li. Learning spatiotemporal attention for egocentric action recognition. In *Proceedings of the IEEE International Conference on Computer Vision Workshops*, pages 0–0, 2019.

[36] Minghuang Ma, Haoqi Fan, and Kris M Kitani. Going deeper into first-person activity recognition. In *Proceedings of the IEEE Conference on Computer Vision and Pattern Recognition*, pages 1894–1903, 2016.

[37] Chih-Yao Ma, Asim Kadav, Iain Melvin, Zsolt Kira, Ghassan AlRegib, and Hans Peter Graf. Attend and interact: Higher-order object interactions for video understanding. In *Proceedings of the IEEE Conference on Computer Vision and Pattern Recognition*, pages 6790–6800, 2018.

[38] Steve Mann. 'wearcam'(the wearable camera): personal imaging systems for long-term use in wearable tetherless computer-mediated reality and personal photo/videographic memory prosthesis. In *Digest of Papers. Second International Symposium on Wearable Computers (Cat. No. 98EX215)*, pages 124–131. IEEE, 1998.

[39] Kenji Matsuo, Kentaro Yamada, Satoshi Ueno, and Sei Naito. An attention-based activity recognition for egocentric video. In *Proceedings of the IEEE Conference on Computer Vision and Pattern Recognition Workshops*, pages 551–556, 2014.

[40] Tomas McCandless and Kristen Grauman. Object-centric spatio-temporal pyramids for egocentric activity recognition. In *BMVC*, volume 2, page 3. Citeseer, 2013.

[41] Ajay K Mishra, Yiannis Aloimonos, Loong Fah Cheong, and Ashraf Kassim. Active visual segmentation. *IEEE Transactions on Pattern Analysis and Machine Intelligence*, 34(4):639–653, 2011.

[42] Erik T Mueller. *Commonsense reasoning: an event calculus based approach*. Morgan Kaufmann, 2014.

[43] Tomoya Nakatani, Ryohei Kuga, and Takuya Maekawa. Preliminary investigation of object-based activity recognition using egocentric video based on web knowledge. In *Proceedings of the 17th International Conference on Mobile and Ubiquitous Multimedia*, pages 375–381, 2018.

[44] Thi-Hoa-Cuc Nguyen, Jean-Christophe Nebel, Francisco Florez-Revuelta, et al. Recognition of activities of daily living with egocentric vision: A review. *Sensors*, 16(1):72, 2016.

[45] Adrián Núñez-Marcos, Gorka Azkune, and Ignacio Arganda-Carreras. Object bounding box annotations for the GTEA Gaze+ dataset, July 2020.

[46] Hamed Pirsiavash and Deva Ramanan. Detecting activities of daily living in first-person camera views. In *2012 IEEE Conference on Computer Vision and Pattern Recognition*, pages 2847–2854. IEEE, 2012.

[47] Iris Rawtaer, Rathi Mahendran, Ee Heok Kua, Hwee Pink Tan, Hwee Xian Tan, Tih-Shih Lee, and Tze Pin Ng. Early detection of mild cognitive impairment with in-home sensors to monitor behavior patterns in community-dwelling senior citizens in singapore: Cross-sectional feasibility study. *Journal of Medical Internet Research*, 22(5):e16854, 2020.

[48] Joseph Redmon, Santosh Divvala, Ross Girshick, and Ali Farhadi. You only look once: Unified, real-time object detection. In *Proceedings of the IEEE Conference on Computer Vision and Pattern Recognition*, pages 779–788, 2016.

[49] Shaoqing Ren, Kaiming He, Ross Girshick, and Jian Sun. Faster r-cnn: Towards real-time object detection with region proposal networks. In *Advances in Neural Information Processing Systems*, pages 91–99, 2015.

[50] Liyue Shen, Serena Yeung, Judy Hoffman, Greg Mori, and Li Fei-Fei. Scaling human-object interaction recognition through zero-shot learning. In *2018 IEEE Winter Conference on Applications of Computer Vision (WACV)*, pages 1568–1576. IEEE, 2018.

[51] Karen Simonyan and Andrew Zisserman. Two-stream convolutional networks for action recognition in videos. In *Advances in Neural Information Processing Systems*, pages 568–576, 2014.

[52] Swathikiran Sudhakaran and Oswald Lanz. Attention is all we need: Nailing down object-centric attention for egocentric activity recognition. *arXiv preprint* arXiv:1807.11794, 2018.

[53] Swathikiran Sudhakaran, Sergio Escalera, and Oswald Lanz. Lsta: Long short-term attention for egocentric action recognition. In *Proceedings of the IEEE Conference on Computer Vision and Pattern Recognition*, pages 9954–9963, 2019.

[54] Li Sun, Ulrich Klank, and Michael Beetz. Eyewatchme—3d hand and object tracking for inside out activity analysis. In *2009 IEEE Computer Society Conference on Computer Vision and Pattern Recognition Workshops*, pages 9–16. IEEE, 2009.

[55] Dipak Surie, Thomas Pederson, Fabien Lagriffoul, Lars-Erik Janlert, and Daniel Sjölie. Activity recognition using an egocentric perspective of everyday objects. In *International Conference on Ubiquitous Intelligence and Computing*, pages 246–257. Springer, 2007.

[56] Bugra Tekin, Federica Bogo, and Marc Pollefeys. H+ o: Unified egocentric recognition of 3d hand-object poses and interactions. In *Proceedings of the IEEE Conference on Computer Vision and Pattern Recognition*, pages 4511–4520, 2019.

[57] An Tran and Loong-Fah Cheong. Two-stream flow-guided convolutional attention networks for action recognition. In *Proceedings of the IEEE International Conference on Computer Vision Workshops*, pages 3110–3119, 2017.

[58] Jasper RR Uijlings, Koen EA Van De Sande, Theo Gevers, and Arnold WM Smeulders. Selective search for object recognition. *International Journal of Computer Vision*, 104(2):154–171, 2013.

[59] Sagar Verma, Pravin Nagar, Divam Gupta, and Chetan Arora. Making third person techniques recognize first-person actions in egocentric videos. In *2018 25th IEEE International Conference on Image Processing (ICIP)*, pages 2301–2305. IEEE, 2018.

[60] Heng Wang, Alexander Kläser, Cordelia Schmid, and Cheng-Lin Liu. Dense trajectories and motion boundary descriptors for action recognition. *International journal of computer vision*, 103(1):60–79, 2013.

[61] Heng Wang and Cordelia Schmid. Action recognition with improved trajectories. In *Proceedings of the IEEE International Conference on Computer Vision*, pages 3551–3558, 2013.

[62] Limin Wang, Yuanjun Xiong, Zhe Wang, Yu Qiao, Dahua Lin, Xiaoou Tang, and Luc Van Gool. Temporal segment networks: Towards good practices for deep action recognition. In *European Conference on Computer Vision*, pages 20–36. Springer, 2016.

[63] Jindong Wang, Yiqiang Chen, Shuji Hao, Xiaohui Peng, and Lisha Hu. Deep learning for sensor-based activity recognition: A survey. *Pattern Recognition Letters*, 119:3–11, 2019.

[64] Xiaohan Wang, Yu Wu, Linchao Zhu, and Yi Yang. Baidu-uts submission to the epic-kitchens action recognition challenge 2019. *arXiv preprint* arXiv:1906.09383, 2019.

[65] Xiaohan Wang, Yu Wu, Linchao Zhu, and Yi Yang. Symbiotic attention with privileged information for egocentric action recognition. *arXiv preprint* arXiv:2002.03137, 2020.

[66] Michael Wray, Davide Moltisanti, and Dima Damen. Towards an unequivocal representation of actions. In *Proceedings of the IEEE Conference on Computer Vision and Pattern Recognition Workshops*, pages 1127–1131, 2018.

[67] SHI Xingjian, Zhourong Chen, Hao Wang, Dit-Yan Yeung, Wai-Kin Wong, and Wang-chun Woo. Convolutional lstm network: A machine learning approach for precipitation nowcasting. In *Advances in Neural Information Processing Systems*, pages 802–810, 2015.

[68] Hong-Bo Zhang, Yi-Xiang Zhang, Bineng Zhong, Qing Lei, Lijie Yang, Ji-Xiang Du, and Duan-Sheng Chen. A comprehensive survey of vision-based human action recognition methods. *Sensors*, 19(5):1005, 2019.

[69] Hang Zhang, Chongruo Wu, Zhongyue Zhang, Yi Zhu, Zhi Zhang, Haibin Lin, Yue Sun, Tong He, Jonas Mueller, R Manmatha, et al. Resnest: Split-attention networks. *arXiv preprint* arXiv:2004.08955, 2020.

[70] Yang Zhou, Bingbing Ni, Richang Hong, Xiaokang Yang, and Qi Tian. Cascaded interactional targeting network for egocentric video analysis. In *Proceedings of the IEEE Conference on Computer Vision and Pattern Recognition*, pages 1904–1913, 2016.

[71] Zheming Zuo, Longzhi Yang, Yonghong Peng, Fei Chao, and Yanpeng Qu. Gaze-informed egocentric action recognition for memory aid systems. *IEEE Access*, 6:12894–12904, 2018.

Pulmonary Fibrosis Progression Prediction Using Image Processing and Machine Learning

Amr Essam Aboeleneen, Massoud Khan Patel, and Somaya Al-maadeed

Abstract

The onset of COVID-19 has focused the attention of the research community on lung diseases and conditions. Idiopathic pulmonary fibrosis (IPF), in which internal scarring of the lung takes place, has gone undetected among the various populace. This condition has no known cure. So far, computer vision researchers, along with radiologists, have been successfully able to identify the IPF through lung CT-scans but have had difficulty in identifying the severity of IPF. In this research, we will investigate the use of image processing and machine learning techniques to identify the progression of the disease. For that, we will build two machine learning models and compare them. The first model uses patients' biological indications and some histogram features of the CT scans. The second model uses the ensemble method of a convolution neural network (CNN) of patients CT scans and quantile regression of the patient's biological data for predicting the Forced Vital Capacity (FVC, an indicator of IPF severity). The results showed that by using the second model, we got a higher r^2 value of 0.93 versus 0.89 using the first model and that the biological data had more importance than the CT scans for predicting the lung declination.

A. E. Aboeleneen (✉) · M. K. Patel · S. Al-maadeed
Qatar University, Doha, Qatar
e-mail: aa1405465@qu.edu.qa

M. K. Patel
e-mail: mp1912826@qu.edu.qa

S. Al-maadeed
e-mail: s_alali@qu.edu.qa

1 Introduction

1.1 Pulmonary Fibrosis

The lungs is made up of millions of tiny air sacs called Alveolus, these sacs are responsible for absorbing oxygen into the blood stream through its outer membrane (alveolus walls). These walls are very thin which allows oxygen to get in and carbon dioxide out of the blood stream. In medicine, the alevous walls dieases is under the family of interstitial lung diseases [1]. This family includes alevous walls dieases of proliferation, inflammation and fibrosis. Among these dieases is pulmonary fibrosis, which happen as a result of alveolar wall scare and inflammation. Idiopathic pulmonary fibrosis is considered one type of Pulmonary Fibrosis diseases. Idiopathic pulmonary fibrosis is considered to be the most severe among the pulmonary fibrosis family. In general pulmonary fibrosis causes some inflammation to the alevous wall, which creates a build up over that wall that makes it difficult for air to enter the blood stream (difficulty in the inhaling process). Thus the patients suffer from short breath. According to [2, 3], the mean and median life expectancy for IPF patients is 3.5 and 2.5 years respectively which is very short period of time.

Pulmonary Fibrosis can happen from multiple reasons such as: The prior or current exposure to dusts, welding fume, vapors or fibers (e.g. coal, silica and others) [4]. Another reason of PF is Hypersensitivity pneumonitis which is the high sensitivity of lungs to airborne particles due to some exposure to animals and mold. Moreover, The use and exposure of drugs that affects the lungs such as amiodarone and chemotherapy can also cause PF. Furthermore, The repetitive chest scans radiations can also damage the alveolus walls causing Pulmonary Fibrosis. PF can also happen without any known reason such conditions can be called idiopathic, Non-specific, Interstitial and pneumonia PF [5, 6].

© Springer Nature Switzerland AG 2021
J. Aljaâ am et al. (eds.), *Emerging Technologies in Biomedical Engineering and Sustainable TeleMedicine*, Advances in Science, Technology & Innovation, https://doi.org/10.1007/978-3-030-14647-4_11

In the past years, the treatment of interstitial lung diseases in general has changed as the research started to focus more on the lung dieases. FDA approved medicine such as pirfenidone [7] and nintedanib [8], were proven to slow down the declination of the FVC [3] but with huge side effects. Some research works in [9] believe that a lung implant would be one of the best options to treat pulmonary fibrosis patients specially the idiopathic pulmonary fibrosis patients.

The identification of pulmonary fibrosis is done by either of the two ways imaging or biopsy. The first way is by using imaging devices such as X-ray, CT-scanners which is a combination of multiple X-ray slices taken from multiple directions and Echocardiogram which unlike previous methods, uses sound waves to take an image of the heart and visualize the pressure occurring in the right side of the heart. These methods will detect the existence of UIP pattern in the lung. However, sometimes, the UIP pattern is not revealed so an invasive biopsy will be done to patients, where the medical doctors takes some small tissues from the lung for analysis [10, 11]. Moreover, some doctors would also require the patients to do other tests as Forced vital capacity (FVC) test, where the patient has to exhale rapidly through a tube that is connected to a measurement machine The output of this device will be the amount of air the lung can hold and how quick is the exhaling process [12]. Many studies has been done to test the reliability of the FVC measurement and it was proven to be reliable measurement in [13]. An overview of the methods used in PF identification is presented in Fig. 1. Figure 2 shows the effect of PE on alevous wall.

1.2 Machine Learning and Lung Diseases

Yann LeCun's work in 1998 showed the possibility of several neurons stacked as different layers, as a multi-layer perceptron (MLP), can help recognize the alphabets or numbers from an image. But later the field went into a silent decade as the availability of data was scarce and computation power by machines was expensive. The advent of powerful graphical processing units (GPU) which were primarily manufactured for gaming purposes in the 2000s decade, enabled various scientists to renew interest in this possibility. Even the problem of scarcity of data was resolved with the advent and efficiency of the internet. Thereby, making large scale research in the computationally expensive and data-intensive field of deep learning possible. Deep learning is a short word to describe deep neural networks. Each layer is a set of mathematical functions with in-built values known as weights. When a network is trained, i.e., the weights are adjusted so that the output is as much correct as possible with the maximum accuracy. Image recognition was still a difficult task computationally, slowly progressing towards handwritten digits recognition, using other classical image processing techniques.

According to LeCun [14, 15], by early 2000s, many banks were using the same technique to check the authenticity of signatures on cheques.

In 2012 ImageNet Large-Scale Visual Recognition Challenge (ILSVRC) [16], a grand competition for image recognition challenges, large deep convolutional neural

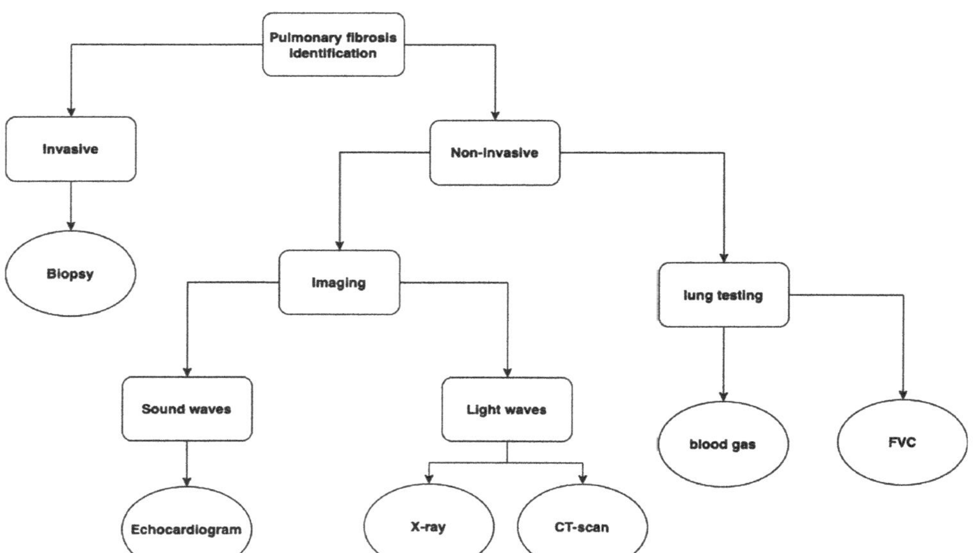

Fig. 1 Diffrent methods used to in the identification of pulmonary fibrosis

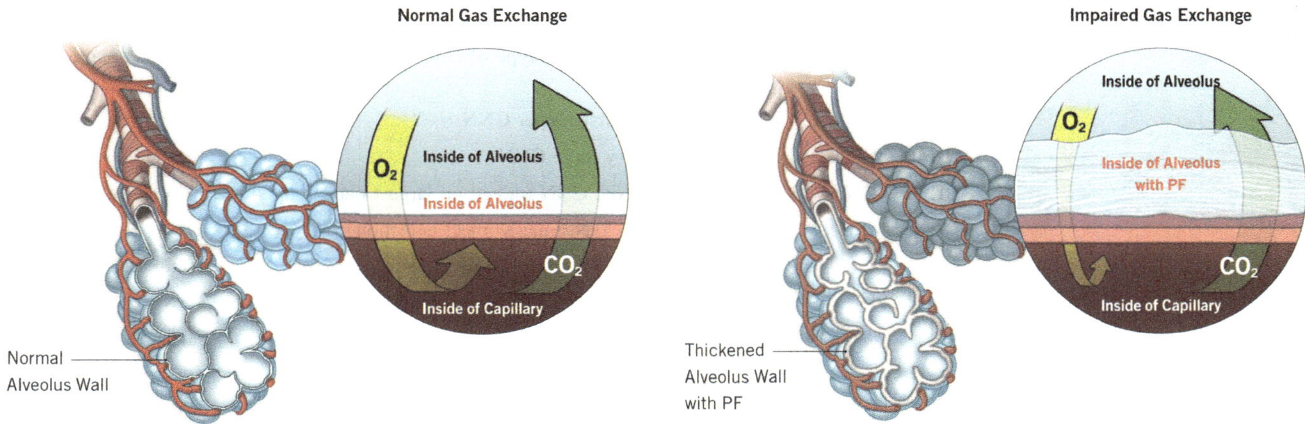

Fig. 2 Alevous wall with and without Pulmonary fibrosis

networks architecture emerged as an unexpected winner. Since then, the focus of image recognition tasks has been convolutional network networks, where convolution is a mathematical image processing operation. Since then, various large CNNs trained on bigger datasets have been released which have been correctly able to identify almost every object on the internet, culminating with GoogLeNet [17] CNN released in 2015 by Google trained on every image that they have in their database.

Later enhancements in object detection and segmentation techniques, such as R-CNN [18], enabled the successful multi-class multilabel detection and classification. The researchers then came up with a technique known as transfer learning, where a pretrained model, for example, GoogLe-Net can be directly downloaded, and with little modification to the massive downloaded CNN, the trained model can be applied to any task and good results can be obtained. This technique eliminated the need for many researchers to create a model from scratch, train the model, which is computationally expensive and long duration task. Any trained model can then be downloaded and then used on any image classification task by anyone, even with little complexity.

Radiologists such as Levin et al., utilized the power of transfer learning, taking the pre-trained ResNet-v2 [19] model and applying it to lung CT-scans to effectively classify the patients who suffer from idiopathic pulmonary fibrosis. This was mere classification with good accuracy and results but could not tell the severity of the disease and how long the patient can live more. This is where the scope of our research lies, predicting the severity of pulmonary fibrosis and giving the FVC value and how long the patient can live more. Table 1 gives a timeline of major Convolutional Neural Networks advancements and specific remarks about them in relation to our research.

Quantile regression is an advanced version of the most commonly used standard linear regression. It is used when we also need to have confidence on our regression output. Unlike normal linear regression models, which calculates the conditional mean using the method of least squares, in quantile regression, we are looking for the conditional mean.

We are not limited to finding the median for quantile regression, but we quantify every quantile—(percentage) in the function variables for a given value. For example, if we were to find the 25th quantile for a particular home's price, it would mean that there is a 25% risk that the real house price is below the projection, and there is a 75% probability that the price is higher.

It is a highly scalable statistical modeling technique because it uses a linear model to match conditional quantities of the response without assuming a parametric distribution. It estimates the whole conditional distribution of the response and allows predictors to rely on the form of the distribution. The plots show the effects of predictors on various parts of the distribution of response. When correcting for the effects of covariates, it may estimate the quantile levels of observations.

Since the identification process of pulmonary fibrosis involves the usage of CT images and/or FVC measurement, researchers has taken this opportunity to explore the usage of machine and deep learning techniques such as Convolution neural network (CNN) to identify the existence of pulmonary fibrosis using the CT scan images. However, none of the past researches has discussed the usage of machine and deep learning techniques in predicting the severity of the lung declination (in terms of amount of FVC or lung volume) in pulmonary fibrosis.

In this work, we will create two machine learning models to predict the declination of lung performance through predicting the lung FVC value for patients that were diagnosed with pulmonary fibrosis. The first model will utilize some biological data about patients such as their sex and age in addition to some CT image processed features such as the

Table 1 Timeline of CNN and their milestones

Year	Method	Applications/Remarks	References
1998	Small CNN	Lenet-5, first prototype of CNN	Lederer and Martinez [1]
2012	CNN	AlexNet, first proper CNN	King et al. [7]
2014	CNN	VGG, very large CNN	Richeldi et al. [8]
2015	CNN	GoogLeNet, CNN trained on largest dataset	Cosgrove [4]
2015	R-CNN	Faster R-CNN, image object detection	King et al. [5]
2017	Transfer learning	First demonstration of transfer learning	Yu et al. [9]
2018	Transfer learning	Inception-ResNet-v2, transfer learning on pulmonary fibrosis CT-scan, just classification	Vasarmidi et al. [6]
2019	Efficient CNN	EfficientNet, Enhanced CNN architecture	Cottin et al. [10]

Table 2 Glossary of all medical terms used

Term	Description
CT	A computerized tomography (CT) scan created by specialized devices for pulmonary diagnosis
IPF	Idiopathic pulmonary fibrosis is a type of lung disease that results in scarring (fibrosis) of the lungs for an unknown reason
UIP	Usual interstitial pneumonia (UIP) is a form of lung disease characterized by progressive scarring of both lungs.
COPD	Chronic obstructive pulmonary disease (COPD) is a type of obstructive lung disease characterized by long-term breathing problems and poor airflow
ARD	Acute respiratory disease events (i.e. Severe shortness of breath or breathlessness. Rapid and labored breathing.)
RNA-seq	RNA-seq (RNA-sequencing) is a technique that can examine the quantity and sequences of RNA in a sample using next-generation sequencing (NGS).
concordance statistic	Measure of goodness of fit for binary outcomes in a logistic regression model
Biposy	Sample of tissue taken from the body in order to examine it more closely.
AUC	Area under curve
CADe	Computer-aided detection (CADe) and diagnosis

hounsfield histogram of the pixels. The other model will use an ensemble method of CNN of CT scans and quantile regression of the biological data (Table 2).

2 Dataset

In 2020, Open Source Image Consortium (OSIC) [20], released the dataset containing 176 cases of idiopathic pulmonary fibrosis (IPF). This dataset contains two types of data, the first is the CT scans of the patient's lungs. The second data type is the patient's biological indicators such as age, sex, smoking data and forced vital capacity (FVC) and is in a CSV format. The tabular data description is as follows:

(1) Patient: a unique Id for each patient (also the name of the patient's DICOM folder)

(2) Weeks: the relative number of weeks pre/post the baseline CT (may be negative)

(3) FVC: the recorded lung capacity in ml

(4) Percent: a computed field which approximates the patient's FVC as a percent of the typical FVC for a person of similar characteristics

(5) Age: The age of the patient (mostly older than 60 years old)

(6) Sex

(7) Smoking Status: Smoker, ex-smoker or non-smoker

3 Literature Review

The difficulty of lung disease diagnosis for usual interstitial pneumonia (UIP) or Pulmonary fibrosis, has motivated some researchers in finding solutions that are faster, cost-efficient, and accurate instead of the manual radiologist's diagnosis [21]. Overall, the approaches explored can be categorized into three main categories: firstly, the usage of Deep learning along with CT scans, secondly the usage of deep learning with genomes, and finally, the use of computer-aided software that utilizes machine learning intelligence.

3.1 IPF and CT Scans Using Deep Learning

Authors in [22] have created a deep convolution neural network (CNN) algorithm that uses high resolution CT scans to categorize the patient's CT images into three categories: positive PF, possible to have PF, and negative PF. The authors have divided these categories twice. Firstly, based on the 2011 ATS/ERS/JRS/ALAT criteria [11] and secondly based on Fleischner Society criteria [21]. The authors' retrieved the data from two specialized health centers for lung diseases. The data consisted of 1157 high-resolution CT scans that were divided into three categories training, testing, and validation; after that, the lung area was segmented, then data was augmented to increase the size before being trained using the CNN. When testing with unseen data of 150 High-resolution CT scans. The algorithm has shown great testing results that outperformed 91 sub radiologists by a mean accuracy of 73.3% versus 70.7% respectively, in less than 3s. Although the paper showed that deep learning could have the same performance as the radiologists. The amount of data used for training was only 929 CT scans, which is usually lower than what is provided for deep learning tasks. That problem was partially addressed using data augmentation. Moreover, the writers did neither mention the structure of CNN nor how they have chosen the optimal parameters. Furthermore, only one expert has done the labeling for the main training set, which might have caused some incorrect or biased algorithm decision.

Since IPF is considered as a single disease in a family of chronic obstructive pulmonary diseases (COPD) Authors in [23] have shown CNN usage in staging, predicting both the mortality and acute respiratory disease events (ARD) of COPD in smokers dataset. The training CT scan dataset was acquired from COPDGene and had 7983 participants. The testing dataset was composed of around 2672 CTs, 1000 of them were acquired from COPDGene patients, and 1672 was from ECLIPSE patients. Logistic regression was used for both COPD diagnosis and ARD prediction. Cox regression has been used to estimate mortality. In COPDGene, the concordance-index for COPD detection was 0.856. Participants were accurately staged(i.e., the patient was known to be in which phase of the COPD) with a probability > 50%, meaning that nearly half of the participants were phased correctly. Around 75% were within one or an adjacent COPD stage. On the other hand, the algorithm predicted

much lower results in identifying the correct phase of ECLIPSE patients with a percentage of 29% and 75% for being in one stage or an adjacent COPD stage respectively. Another CNN model built by the same authors predicting ARD fatality of patients had concordance-index of 0.64 and 0.55 for COPDGene and ECLIPSE patients respectively. Moreover, CNN predicted patients mortality with moderate distinction (c-indices 0.72 and 0.60, respectively). Overall, the authors provided multiple experiments and good results; however, the number of CT scans used was not enough; a data augmentation would have been needed. Moreover, accuracy results for predicting the patients' COPD phases were low (51.1%). Furthermore, the authors have not discussed ECLIPSE patient data having a lower accuracy percentage in nearly all tests.

3.2 IPF and Genomes Using Deep Learning

Researchers in [24] have explored the usage of genes to identify IPF. The researchers used samples of genes of individuals suffering from IPF extracting the effective part of the genome in a process called RNA-sequencing. The RNA-sequencing helped to identify which genomes are active and which are not. In particular, this information has been used along with a machine learning algorithm to discriminate between individuals with IPF and non-IPF based on the genome activity's heterogeneity. The data used was collected from 113 patients with multiple samples per patient as an RNA sequence of 26 K genomes taken using the patient's lung biopsy. The authors stratified the dataset to avoid overfitting before doing cross-validation during the training and testing phases. Moreover, researchers tested multiple classifiers such as random forest, support vector machine, neural network, and the penalized logistic regression had the best results of Area under curve (AUC),specificity, and sensitivity with 0.90, 0.92, and 0.73 respectively. Overall, the paper showed exciting results and a unique way of classifying patients. However, acquiring RNA from a patient using a lung biopsy is not preferable to medical doctors since many patients might be medically fragile to withstand a surgical biopsy.

3.3 IPF and Computer-Aided Software

Other contributions in IPF identification were examined in [25] to find the best CT scans parameters that identify the progression of IPF. The authors evaluated CALIPER's use (Computer-Aided Lung Informatics for Pathology Evaluation and Rating) for analyzing the severity and progression of some pulmonary abnormalities. The CALIPER was able to detect and extract features that were not visually identifiable in CT scans. Researchers have assessed the CALIPER performance with high-resolution CTs for over two years. They have found that predicting pulmonary vessel volume (PVV) from CALIPER was an accurate feature to diagnose the progression of the IPF. Although the testing duration of the CADe is long, the number of patients samples(283 patients) tested was low.

Most of the reviewed papers have concentrated on identifying idiopathic pulmonary fibrosis or COPD cases, among other lung conditions, using some approaches as genomes, CT scans, and CADe. However, none of the papers have discussed machine learning usage to predict the progression of the IPF specifically. This is needed nowadays because of the effect of COVID19 and its side effects even after recovery that may lead to pulmonary fibrosis as mentioned in [6, 26]. We will investigate the usage of two different machine learning models based on high-resolution CT scans and some biological patient features to predict PF progression.

4 Methodology

We have created two different approaches to tackle the problem of predicting lung capacity declination. The two Approaches we proposed can be seen in Table 3. Both Approaches uses the two data types described earlier in the dataset section (i.e., tabular + CT scans). However, The two models differ in the processing of the biological data and the extraction of the CT scans' features. The first model uses state of the art regression model of the biological data and uses CT slices Hounsfield histogram values such as the mean, skewness, and kurtosis. Extracting Hounsfield histogram values of CT scans has been used in previous work [27], and it has been proven that the Hounsfield histogram changes according to the condition of the lungs, Fig. 3 represents the changes in Hounsfield unit (HU) for healthy and non-healthy lung [27]. On the other hand, The second approach uses a Quantile regression neural network based on patients biological dataset to predict their FVC along with extracting the patterns in the CT scan images using the EfficientNet convolution neural network (CNN).

4.1 Analysis

Since this is real medical data, each patient has their number of CT scans as presented in Fig. 6. The data includes about 1549

row of biological data, 33026 CT scans, 880 of them is used for testing, some sample CT slices are shown in Fig. 4, it is important to note that some of the CT slices were having different resolutions as depicted in Fig. 5c and some CT images needed color correction. Moreover, the dataset provides unbalanced categories of data where the number of males exceeds the number of females, and the number of ex-smokers exceeds the smokers and non-smokers as seen in Fig. 5a. Most of the used data is for older adults. The age distribution is shown in Fig. 7. The lung FVC declination of three random samples per week is shown in Fig. 8.

4.2 Pre Processing

Starting out with the data analysis, we did not find any missing data. Some data had outliers, but we have decided not to remove these outliers since the number of records in the tabular data is small and corresponds to large amount of CT scan. Moreover, we had many observations about the current data, as seen in the previous section. In the pre-processing phase, we solved the problems we had earlier, such as different image sizes, which were solved by cropping or scaling up the images. Black images were solved by exposure correction, as it gave us the best experimental results. Moreover, to be able to understand the components of the CT scans, a windowing operation has been applied to linearly transform the ct slices pixel values to Hounsfield unit (HU); once this is done, the components scanned by CT scanners can be identified as presented in Table 4. Furthermore, the CT scans included the lung, the bones and blood vessels around the lung, so we had to segment out the lungs only. For lung segmentation, we have used k-mean clustering to cluster hu values and multiple erosion and morphological dilation operations to remove vessels and holes in the lung to make it one piece. This method has been used because it was easier to implement. Other methods for lung segmentation which could have been chosen, can be found in [28]. After that, the extraction of the CT scans Hounsfield histogram properties was quickly done. The successive steps included the creation of a machine learning model for both approaches that we used. In the first approach, we have selected the extra tree regressor after many experiments. On the other hand, The second approach included quantile regression, which has proven its advantages over other regression methods, and CNN, which is one of the most famous techniques used for CT scan analysis. A full overview of the taken steps is presented in Fig. 9.

Table 3 Different approaches used to solve the problem

Approach	1st approach (Tabular + hu histogram)	2nd approach (Ensemble, Tabular + CT)
Input (after feature engineering)	– Base FVC – Age – Sex – Smoking Status – Baseline week – Lung Percent – CT Hounsfield histogram features (Mean, Skewness, Kurthosis) – Lung volume	– Base FVC – Age – Sex – Smoking Status – Baseline week – Lung Percent
Output	FVC	
Framework	NA	PyTorch
Model techniques	Extra Tree regressor Decision Tree other State of art	75% quantile regression+ 25% CNN

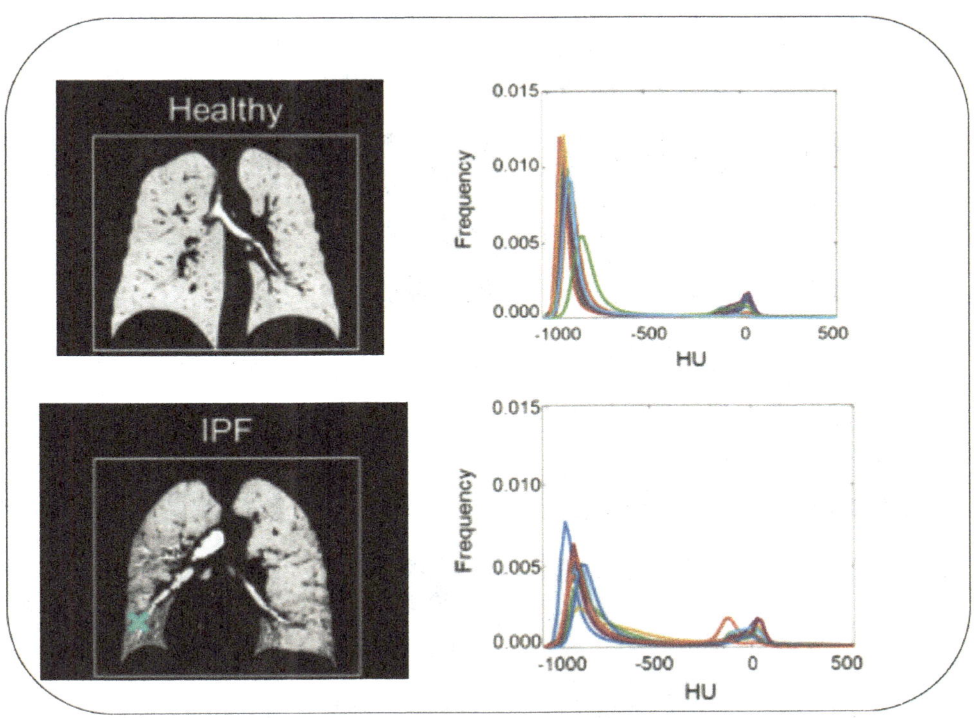

Fig. 3 Hounsfield histogram for Healthy and IPF individuals

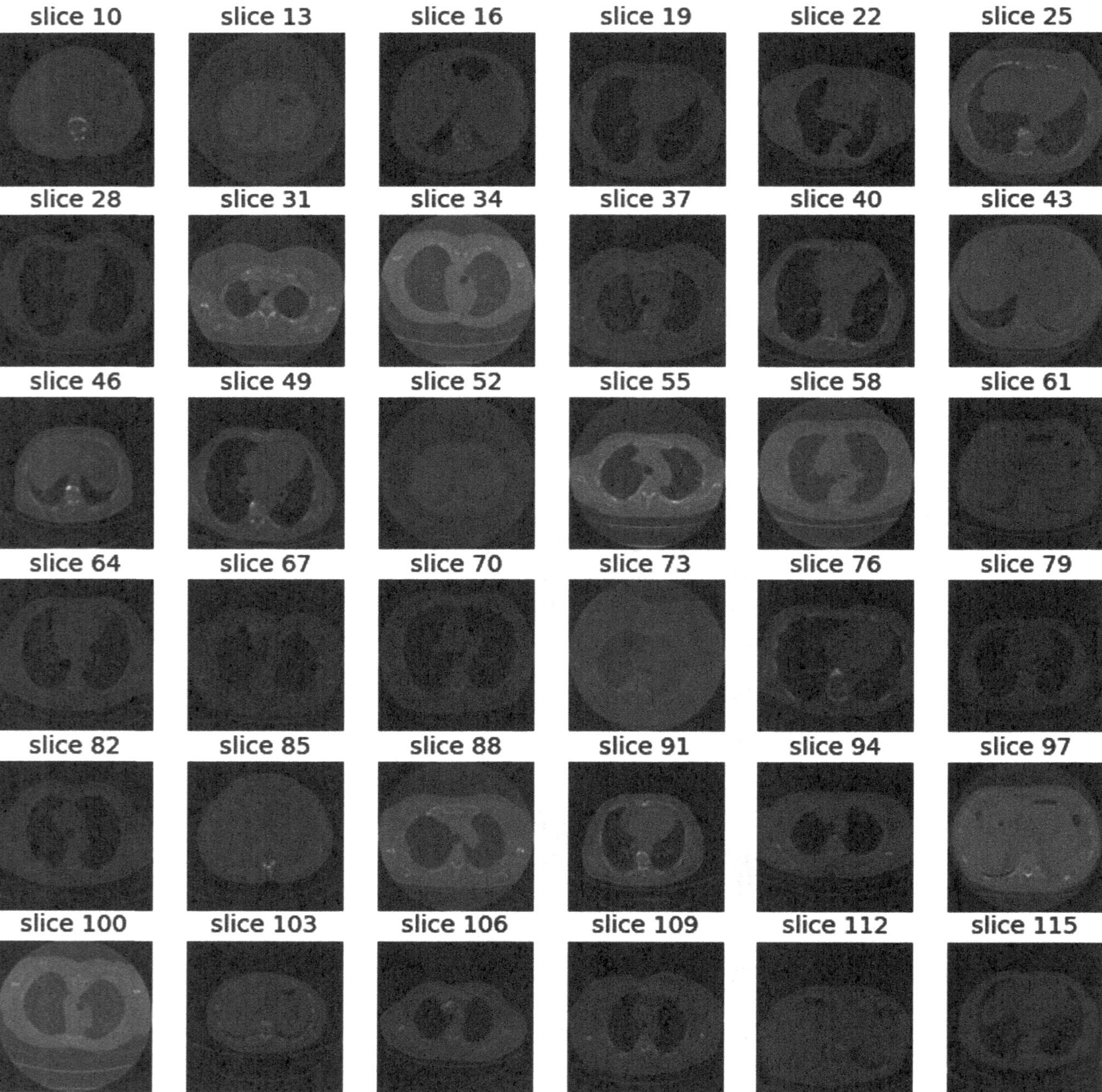

Fig. 4 Sample CT slices

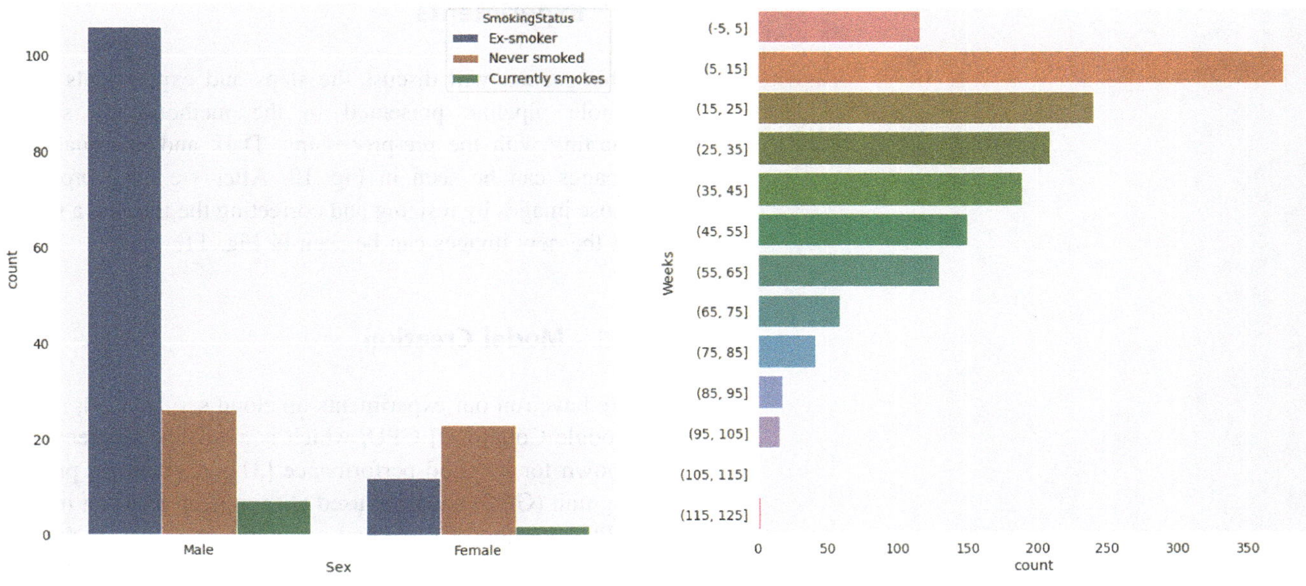

(a) Unbalanced dataset, for gender and Smoking   (b) Unbalanced dataset, different number of followup weeks per patient

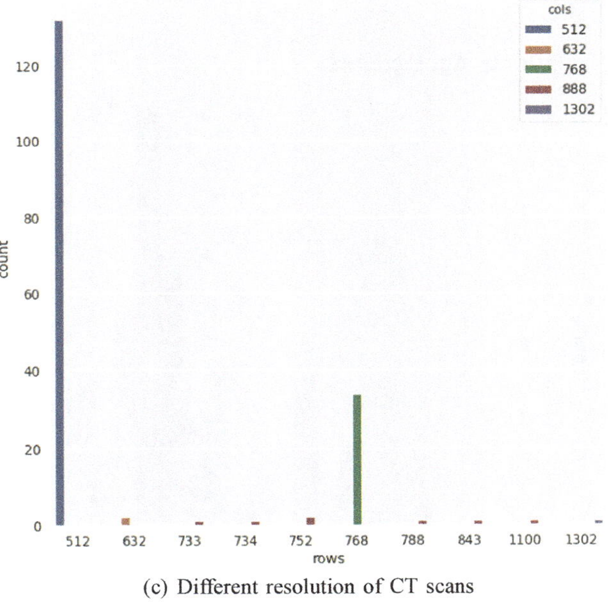

(c) Different resolution of CT scans

Fig. 5 UnBalanced dataset problems

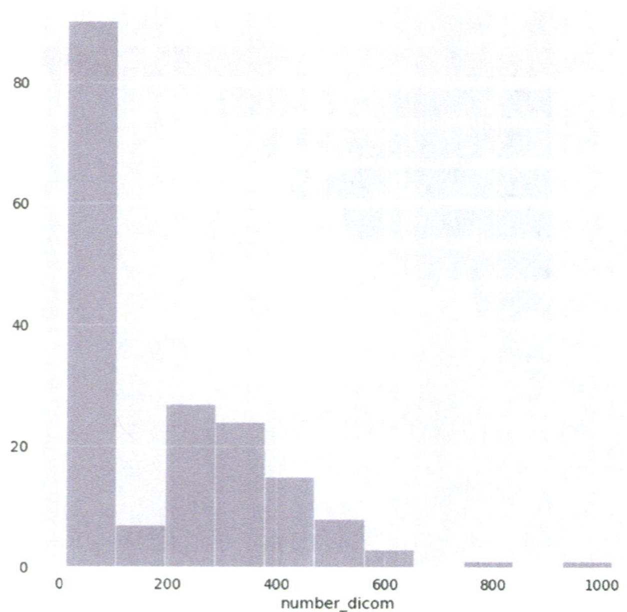

Fig. 6 Different number of CT scans per patient

Fig. 7 Age distribution of patients

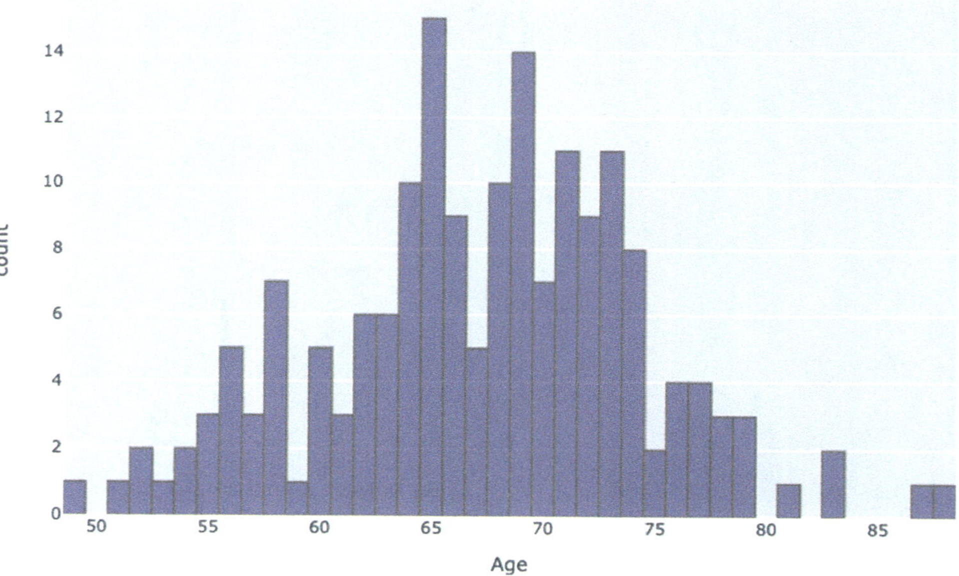

5 Experiments

This section will discuss the steps and experiments in the whole pipeline presented in the methodology section. Starting with the pre-processing, Dark and un-equal sized images can be seen in Fig. 10. After we have processed those images by resizing and correcting the images, a sample of the new images can be seen in Fig. 11.

5.1 Model Creation

We have run our experiments on cloud service [29], namely Google Colab [30] GPU, which is available for free and is known for its good performance [31]. A graphical processing unit (GPU) has been used to train deep learning models. GPUs are good for parallel computation, which is done by various deep learning libraries [32, 33]. We have trained our deep learning model (second approach) using PyTorch [34] deep learning framework.

Fig. 8 Lung FVC declination for samples of different groups

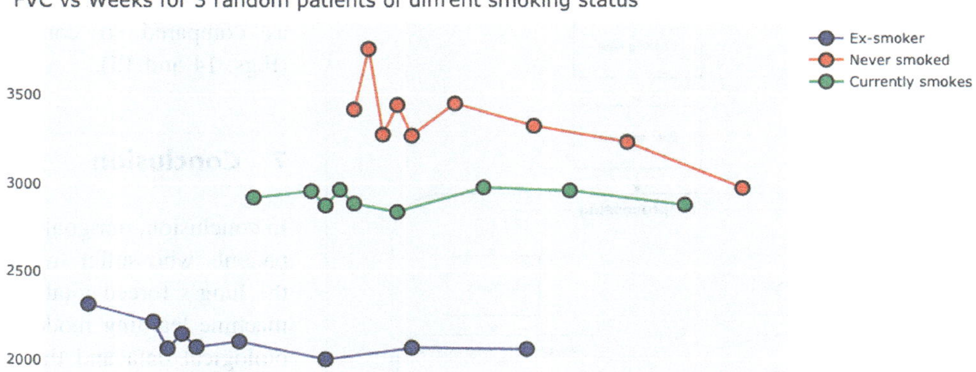

Table 4 Hounsfield values corresponding to different substances

Substance	Hounsfield Unit value (HU)
Bone	From +700 to +3000
Soft tissue	From +100 to +300
Blood	From +30 to +80
Muscle	From +10 to +40
Water	0
Fat	From −100 to −50
Lung	−500
Air	−1000

(1) *First model:* For the first model, we have used PyCaret library [35], which is a library that helps with experimenting with different machine learning state of art algorithms with k-fold validation method. We have used the hold-out method to split our data into 80% training and 20% to be used for validation. The results of the training set for most of the regression algorithms after parameter tuning with error measures such as mean absolute error (MEA), mean square error (MSE), root mean squared error (RMSE), R^2 error, root mean squared logarithmic error (RMSLE), mean absolute percentage error (MAPE) given by various models can be seen in Table 5, the prediction plot is also available in Fig. 14. Testing the models on the testing set is presented in Table 6.

(2) *Second Model:* For the second model, we have trained the deep learning networks in batches, using batch normalization [36]. Adam optimizer [37] has been used as optimization function. The most used activation function in our neural networks was the Swish [38] activation function, which have proven its advantage over ReLU activation function in complex datasets. We created a simple ensemble blend of 2 models, with best folds from EfficientNet and Quantile Regression Dense Neural Network (QRDNN), quantile regression

prediction can be seen in 15. Figure 12 shows us the best epoch marked by green during the training of QRDNN along with the uncertainty in prediction, also known as a confidence value.

6 Results and Discussion

The first model approach that has used the patients' biological data and the hounsifield histogram features has resulted in a r^2 value of 0.98 and 0.89 in the training and testing set respectively. On the other hand, the second approach has improved this results with small amount by getting Laplace Log Likelihood error of approximately −6.8 and an r^2 value of 0.93. Figure 13 shows the log likelihood error over optimized predicted FVC and confidence values. Astonishingly, from the first model features Fig. 16 we saw that biological data have more importance than CT scans features. This might be because of the individuals' genomes structure or their cell structure, which needs to be further investigated. In the second model, we had the same observation where the quantile regression model based on the biological data had more accurate results than CT scans alone. CT scan analysis only provided partial improvement

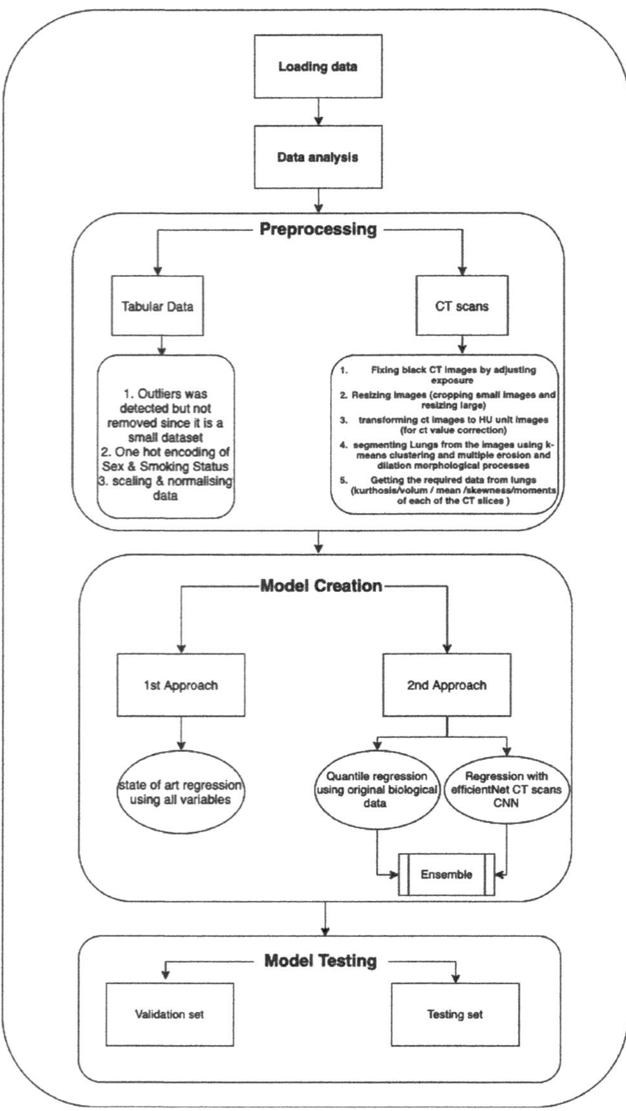

Fig. 9 Methodology overview

over the quantile regression model. Also, most preprocessing techniques such as data augmentation and normalization did not help make better predictions. In some cases, it has been found that biological data alone gives good enough results, as compared to combined CT-scan based predictions (Figs. 14 and 15).

7 Conclusion

In conclusion, our goal was to predict the lung declination of patients who suffer from pulmonary fibrosis by predicting the lung's forced vital capacity (FVC). We have built two machine learning models one that uses image features and biological data and the other model uses an ensemble of EfficientNet and quantile neural network. Our results showed that ensemble learning works better for these medical condition progression detection with r^2 value of 0.93 versus r^2 of 0.89 from the first model. We have also found out CT-scans give only partial information about the progression of PF and that the most useful information was the patient's biological indicators which may need to be further explored. Moreover, most pre-processing techniques such as data augmentation and normalization did not help make better predictions. In some cases, it has been found that biological data alone gives good enough results, as compared to combined CT-scan based predictions.

8 Impact

The following are potential beneficiaries of the research:

- Radiologists who would be able to cut down diagnosis time and prevent exhaustion
- Hospitals that can rapidly process patient data and reduce costs or maximize profits
- Patients and their families would be able to better understand their prognosis, and this will also enable them so psychologically prepare themselves with this incurable lung disease
- Drug manufacturers can enhance their research and development of drug design and its trial, with accelerated

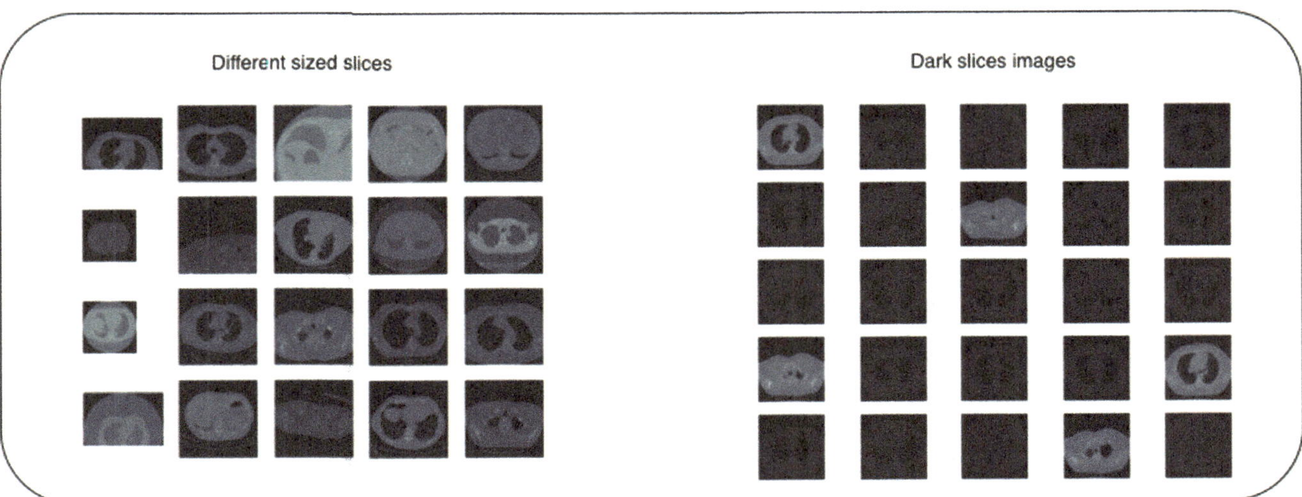

Fig. 10 CT scans problems

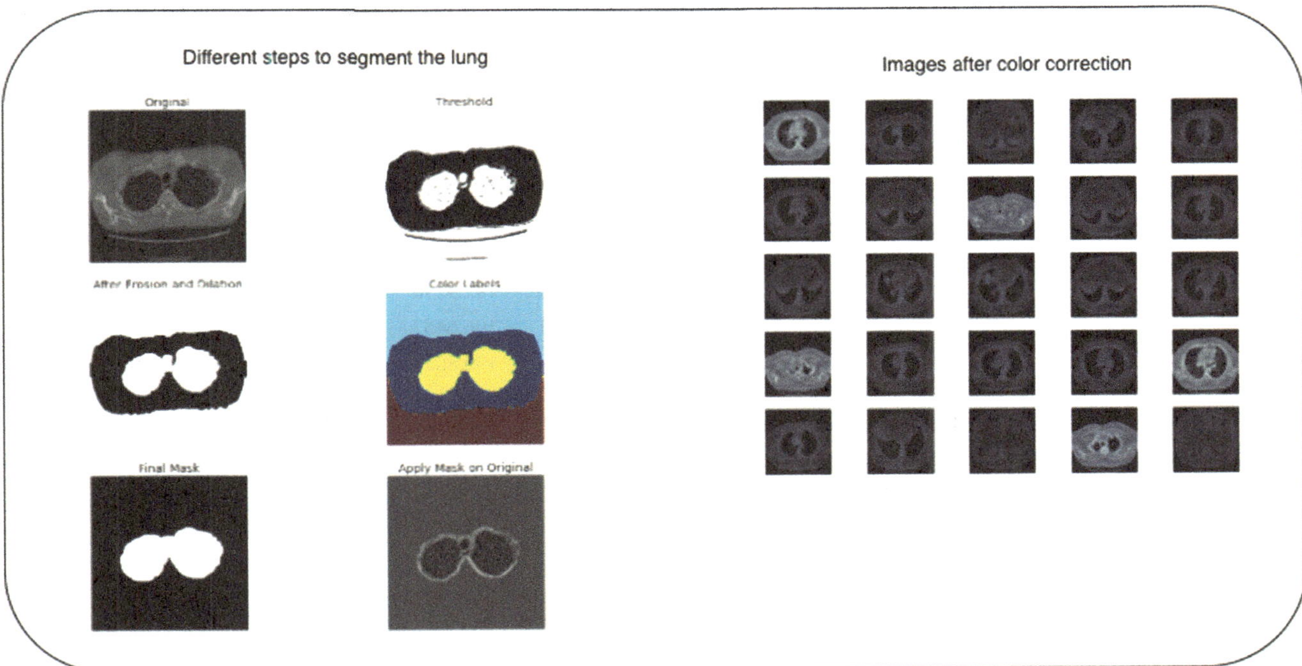

Fig. 11 Lung segmentation and color correction after processing

Table 5 Training results for first approach model

Model	MAE	MSE	RMSE	R2	RMSLE	MAPE	TT (Sec)
Extra trees regressor	57.6229	9722.5702	93.5579	0.9843	0.0382	0.0236	0.2750
CatBoost regressor	66.6890	10306.6491	97.6805	0.9835	0.0394	0.0270	1.1310
Extreme gradient boosting	75.5414	15322.8708	120.6576	0.9746	0.0489	0.0308	0.3380
Light gradient boosting machine	77.1412	16247.9517	122.6801	0.9745	0.0463	0.0307	0.0460
Random forest regressor	82.6138	16556.5800	123.6587	0.9732	0.0520	0.0342	0.3310
Gradient boosting regressor	99.8086	20264.5928	139.3933	0.9672	0.0555	0.0402	0.0660
Decision tree regressor	101.1458	26437.5815	158.7819	0.9570	0.0674	0.0414	0.0110
Lasso regression	134.2200	32225.0555	178.0294	0.9497	0.0738	0.0547	0.0100
Least angle regression	134.9532	32311.3717	178.2815	0.9496	0.0741	0.0551	0.0110
Ridge regression	134.7114	32309.4939	178.2653	0.9496	0.0740	0.0549	0.0090
Linear regression	134.9532	32311.3867	178.2815	0.9496	0.0741	0.0551	0.0100
Lasso least angle regression	141.8080	36683.7819	189.8829	0.9425	0.0780	0.0572	0.0100
Elastic net	144.1506	37889.7180	192.9290	0.9404	0.0797	0.0586	0.0100
Bayesian ridge	147.0046	39342.2331	196.6467	0.9381	0.0817	0.0600	0.0090
AdaBoost regressor	157.8523	40539.7317	199.8037	0.9360	0.0839	0.0639	0.0690
Huber regressor	141.9048	42074.3836	203.2188	0.9337	0.0836	0.0583	0.0230
K Neighbors regressor	143.2599	48199.6139	215.1032	0.9266	0.0850	0.0582	0.0360
Orthogonal matching pursuit	162.4504	51541.6821	225.3735	0.9190	0.0928	0.0661	0.0090
Passive aggressive regressor	237.6534	99813.5897	305.9086	0.8454	0.1288	0.0936	0.0110

Table 6 TOP 5 testing results for first approach model

Model	MAE	MSE	RMSE	R2	RMSLE	MAPE	TT (s)
Extra trees regressor	162.4504	67030.6821	270	0.8943	0.1288	0.0661	0.2240
CatBoost regressor	178.4593	87002.2423	312	0.8635	0.0394	0.0270	1.1310
Extreme gradient boosting	216.2342	99813.5897	343	0.8446	0.0489	0.0308	0.3380
Random forest regressor	223.7832	100233.4355	367	0.8232	0.0520	0.0342	0.3310
Passive aggressive regressor	237.6534	100423.4523	402	0.8135	0.1288	0.0936	0.0110

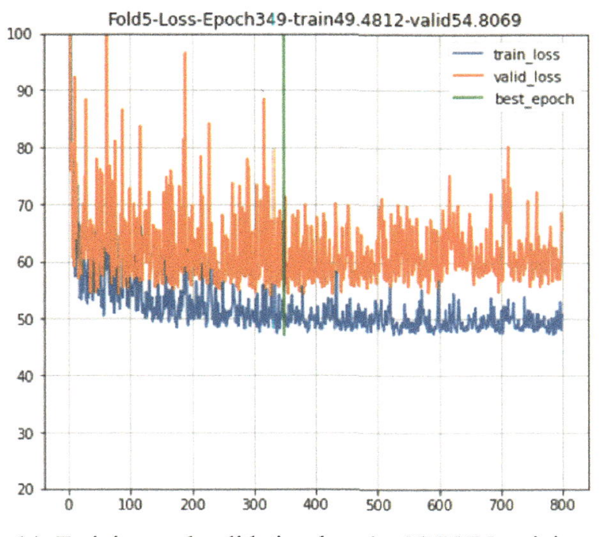

(a) Training and validation loss in QRDNN training

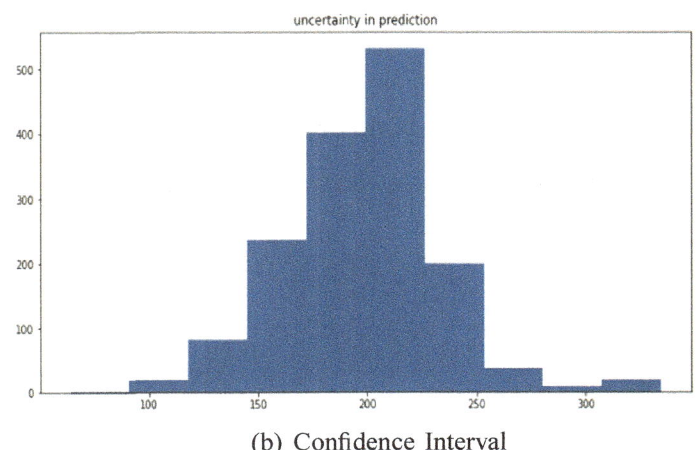

(b) Confidence Interval

Fig. 12 Quantile regression loss and confidence interval

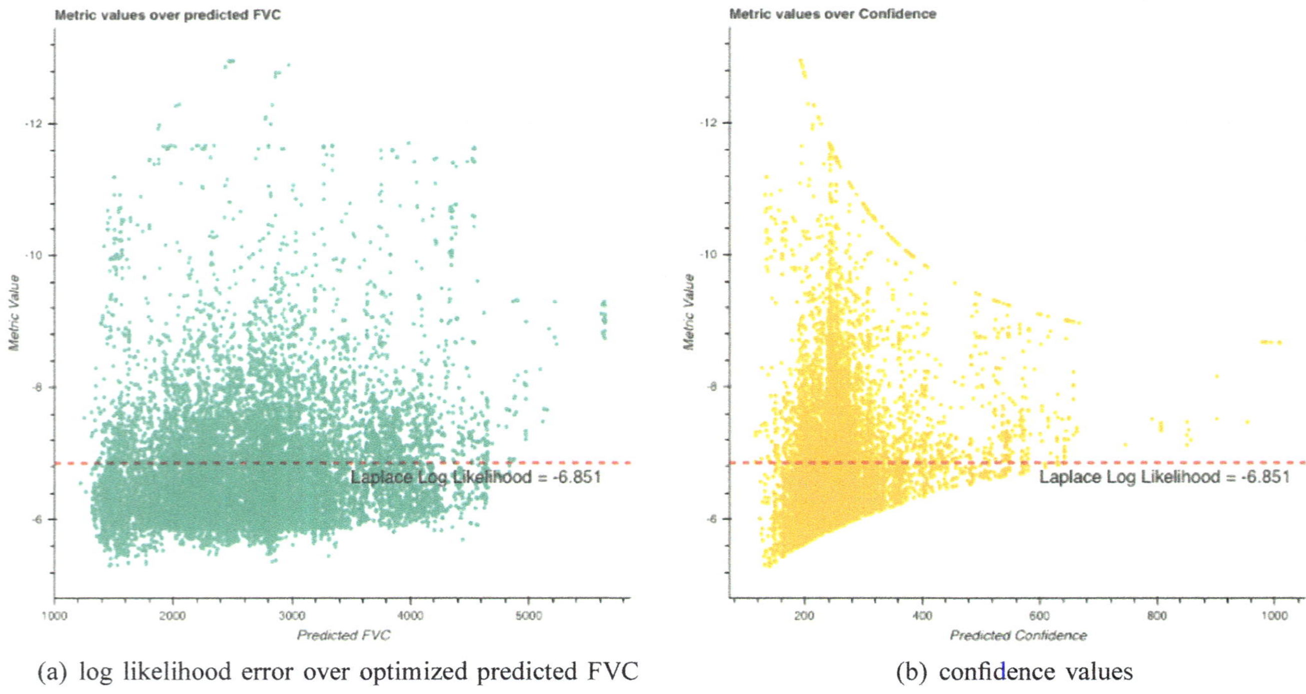

(a) log likelihood error over optimized predicted FVC (b) confidence values

Fig. 13 Error measure over predicted Forced Vital Capacity (FVC) and Confidence value

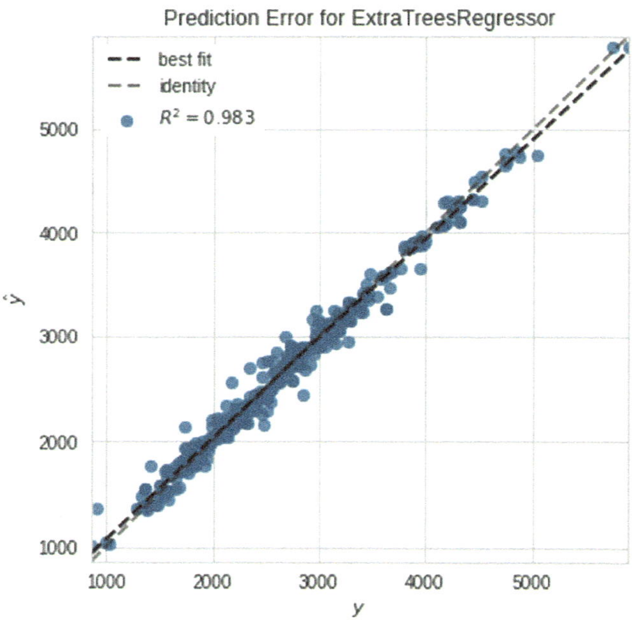

Fig. 14 Prediction error of Extra tree regression after tuning

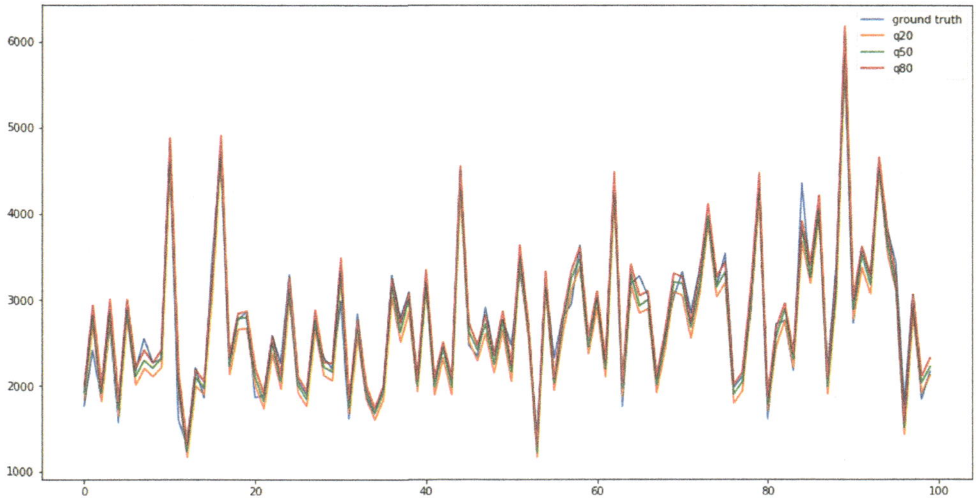

Fig. 15 Quantile regression prediction versus ground truth

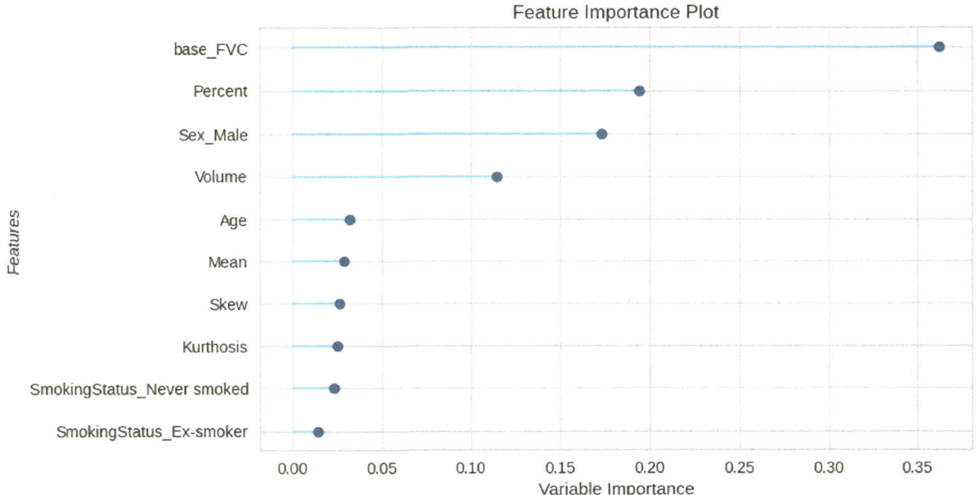

Fig. 16 Feature importance of the first model

development since they will have access to more accurate patient data

- Potential to diagnose and develop novel treatments for other incurable lung diseases

Acknowledgements This publication was made possible by Qatar University Emergency Response Grant (QUERG-CENG-2020-1) from the Qatar University. The statements made herein are solely the responsibility of the authors.

References

1. D. J. Lederer and F. J. Martinez, "Idiopathic Pulmonary Fibrosis," *New England Journal of Medicine*, vol. 378, no. 19, D. L. Longo, Ed., pp. 1811–1823, May 2018, ISSN: 0028-4793. https://doi.org/10.1056/nejmra1705751. [Online]. Available: http://www.nejm.org/doi/10.1056/NEJMra1705751.

2. M. Fisher, S. D. Nathan, C. Hill, J. Marshall, F. Dejonckheere, P.-O. Thuresson, and T. M. Maher, "Predicting Life Expectancy for Pirfenidone in Idiopathic Pulmonary Fibrosis," *Journal of Managed Care & Specialty Pharmacy*, vol. 23, no. 3-b Suppl, S17–S24, Mar. 2017, ISSN: 2376-0540. https://doi.org/10.18553/jmcp.2017.23.3-b.s17. [Online]. Available: https://www.jmcp.org/doi/10.18553/jmcp.2017.23.3-b.s17.

3. J. A. Kropski and T. S. Blackwell, "Progress in Understanding and Treating Idiopathic Pulmonary Fibrosis," *Annual Review of Medicine*, vol. 70, no. 1, pp. 211–224, Jan. 2019, ISSN: 0066-4219. https://doi.org/10.1146/annurev-med-041317102715. [Online]. Available: https://www.annualreviews.org/doi/10.1146/annurev-med-041317-102715.

4. M. P. Cosgrove, *Pulmonary fibrosis and exposure to steel welding fume*, Dec. 2015. https://doi.org/10.1093/occmed/kqv093. [Online]. Available: https://academic.oup.com/occmed/article/65/9/706/1441697.

5. T. E. King, A. Pardo, and M. Selman, "Idiopathic pulmonary fibrosis," in *The Lancet*, vol. 378, Elsevier, Dec. 2011, pp. 1949–1961. https://doi.org/10.1016/s0140-6736(11)60052-4.

6. E. Vasarmidi, E. Tsitoura, D. A. Spandidos, N. Tzanakis, and K. M. Antoniou, "Pulmonary fibrosis in the aftermath of the COVID-19 era (Review)," *Experimental and therapeutic*

medicine, vol. 20, no. 3, pp. 2557–2560, Sep. 2020, ISSN: 1792-0981. https://doi.org/10.3892/etm.2020.8980. [Online]. Available: https://pubmed.ncbi.nlm.nih.gov/32765748%20https://www.ncbi.nlm.nih.gov/pmc/articles/PMC7401793/.

7. T. E. King, W. Z. Bradford, S. Castro-Bernardini, E. A. Fagan, I. Glaspole, M. K. Glassberg, E. Gorina, P. M. Hopkins, D. Kardatzke, L. Lancaster, D. J. Lederer, S. D. Nathan, C. A. Pereira, S. A. Sahn, R. Sussman, J. J. Swigris, and P. W. Noble, "A Phase 3 Trial of Pirfenidone in Patients with Idiopathic Pulmonary Fibrosis," *New England Journal of Medicine*, vol. 370, no. 22, pp. 2083–2092, May 2014, ISSN: 0028-4793. https://doi.org/10.1056/nejmoa1402582. [Online]. Available: https://pubmed.ncbi.nlm.nih.gov/24836312/.

8. L. Richeldi, R. M. du Bois, G. Raghu, A. Azuma, K. K. Brown, U. Costabel, V. Cottin, K. R. Flaherty, D. M. Hansell, Y. Inoue, D. S. Kim, M. Kolb, A. G. Nicholson, P. W. Noble, M. Selman, H. Taniguchi, M. Brun, F. Le Maulf, M. Girard, S. Stowasser, R. Schlenker-Herceg, B. Disse, and H. R. Collard, "Efficacy and Safety of Nintedanib in Idiopathic Pulmonary Fibrosis," *New England Journal of Medicine*, vol. 370, no. 22, pp. 2071–2082, May 2014, ISSN: 0028-4793. https://doi.org/10.1056/nejmoa1402584. [Online]. Available: https://www.nejm.org/doi/full/10.1056/nejmoa1402584.

9. H. Yu, T. Bian, Z. Yu, Y. Wei, J. Xu, J. Zhu, and W. Zhang, "Bilateral Lung Transplantation Provides Better Longterm Survival and Pulmonary Function Than Single Lung Transplantation: A Systematic Review and Meta-analysis," *Transplantation*, vol. 103, no. 12, pp. 2634–2644, Dec. 2019, ISSN: 00411337. https://doi.org/10.1097/tp.0000000000002841. [Online]. Available: https://pubmed.ncbi.nlm.nih.gov/31283687/.

10. V. Cottin, B. Crestani, D. Valeyre, B. Wallaert, J. Cadranel, J. C. Dalphin, P. Delaval, D. Israel-Biet, R. Kessler, M. Reynaud-Gaubert, B. Aguilaniu, B. Bouquillon, P. Carre, C. Danel, J. B. Faivre, G. Ferretti, N. Just, S. Kouzan,´ F. Lebargy, S. Marchand-Adam, B. Philippe, G. Prevot, B. Stach, F. Thivolet-B´ ejui, and J. F. Cordier,´ *Diagnosis and management of idiopathic pulmonary fibrosis: French practical guidelines*, Jun. 2014. https://doi.org/10.1183/09059180.00001814. [Online]. Available: http://ow.ly/uUhKh.

11. G. Raghu, H. R. Collard, J. J. Egan, F. J. Martinez, J. Behr, K. K. Brown, T. V. Colby, J. F. Cordier, K. R. Flaherty, J. A. Lasky, D. A. Lynch, J. H. Ryu, J. J. Swigris, A. U. Wells, J. Ancochea, D. Bouros, C. Carvalho, U. Costabel, M. Ebina, D. M. Hansell, T. Johkoh, D. S. Kim, T. E. King, Y. Kondoh, J. Myers, N. L. Muller, A. G. Nicholson, L.¨ Richeldi, M. Selman, R. F. Dudden, B. S. Griss, S. L. Protzko, and H. J. Schunemann, "An Official ATS/ERS/JRS/ALAT¨ Statement: Idiopathic pulmonary fibrosis: Evidence-based guidelines for diagnosis and management," *American Journal of Respiratory and Critical Care Medicine*, vol. 183, no. 6, pp. 788–824, Mar. 2011, ISSN: 1073449X. DOI:10.1164/ rccm.2009-040GL. [Online]. Available: http://www.atsjournals.org/doi/abs/10.1164/rccm.2009-040GL.

12. *Pulmonary fibrosis - Diagnosis and treatment - Mayo Clinic*. [Online]. Available: https://www.mayoclinic.org/diseasesconditions/pulmonary-fibrosis/diagnosis-treatment/drc-20353695.

13. S. Kafaja, P. J. Clements, H. Wilhalme, C. h. Tseng, D. E. Furst, G. H. Kim, J. Goldin, E. R. Volkmann, M. D. Roth, D. P. Tashkin, and D. Khanna, "Reliability and minimal clinically important differences of FVC results from the scleroderma lung studies (SLS-I and SLS-II)," *American Journal of Respiratory and Critical Care Medicine*, vol. 197, no. 5, pp. 644–652, Mar. 2018, ISSN: 15354970. https://doi.org/10.1164/rccm.201709-1845OC. [Online]. Available: http://www.atsjournals.org/doi/10.1164/rccm.201709-1845OC.

14. Y. LeCun, L. Bottou, Y. Bengio, and P. Haffner, "Gradient-based learning applied to document recognition," *Proceedings of the IEEE*, 1998, ISSN: 00189219. https://doi.org/10.1109/5.726791.

15. Y. LeCun, B. Boser, J. S. Denker, D. Henderson, R. E. Howard, W. Hubbard, and L. D. Jackel, "Backpropagation Applied to Handwritten Zip Code Recognition," *Neural Computation*, vol. 1, no. 4, pp. 541–551, Dec. 1989, ISSN: 0899-7667. https://doi.org/10.1162/neco.1989.1.4.541.

16. O. Russakovsky, J. Deng, H. Su, J. Krause, S. Satheesh, S. Ma, Z. Huang, A. Karpathy, A. Khosla, M. Bernstein, A. C. Berg, and L. Fei-Fei, "ImageNet Large Scale Visual Recognition Challenge," *International Journal of Computer Vision*, vol. 115, no. 3, pp. 211–252, Dec. 2015, ISSN: 15731405. https://doi.org/10.1007/s11263-015-0816-y.

17. C. Szegedy, W. Liu, Y. Jia, P. Sermanet, S. Reed, D. Anguelov, and D. Erhan, "Going Deeper with Convolutions (GoogleLeNet)," *Journal of Chemical Technology and Biotechnology*, 2016, ISSN: 10974660.

18. R. Girshick, "Fast R-CNN," in *Proceedings of the IEEE International Conference on Computer Vision*, 2015, ISBN: 9781467383912. https://doi.org/10.1109/iccv.2015.169.

19. D. L. Levin, *Deep learning and the evaluation of pulmonary fibrosis*, Nov. 2018. https://doi.org/10.1016/s2213-2600(18)30371-0. [Online]. Available: http://dx.doi.org/10.1016/.

20. *OSICild.org • Open Source Imaging Consortium*. [Online]. Available: https://www.osicild.org/.

21. "Updated Fleischner Society Guide-lines for Managing Incidental Pul-monary Nodules: Common Questions and Challenging Scenarios," https://doi.org/10.1148/rg.2018180017. [Online]. Available: https://doi.org/10.1148/rg.2018180017.

22. S. L. Walsh, L. Calandriello, M. Silva, and N. Sverzellati, "Deep learning for classifying fibrotic lung disease on highresolution computed tomography: a case-cohort study," *The Lancet Respiratory Medicine*, vol. 6, no. 11, pp. 837–845, Nov. 2018, ISSN: 22132619. https://doi.org/10.1016/s2213-2600(18)30286-8.

23. G. Gonzalez, S. Y. Ash, G. Vegas-Sanchez-Ferrero, J. O. Onieva, F. N. Rahaghi, J. C. Ross, A. D´ az, R. S. J. Est´ epar, and´ G. R. Washko, *Disease staging and prognosis in smokers using deep learning in chest computed tomography*, Jan. 2018. https://doi.org/10.1164/rccm.201705-0860oc. [Online]. Available: http://www.atsjournals.org/doi/10.1164/rccm.201705-0860OC.

24. Y. Choi, T. T. Liu, D. G. Pankratz, T. V. Colby, N. M. Barth, D. A. Lynch, P. S. Walsh, G. Raghu, G. C. Kennedy, and J. Huang, "Identification of usual interstitial pneumonia pattern using RNA-Seq and machine learning: Challenges and solutions," *BMC Genomics*, vol. 19, no. Suppl 2, 2018, ISSN: 14712164. https://doi.org/10.1186/s12864-018-4467-6.

25. J. Jacob, B. J. Bartholmai, S. Rajagopalan, M. Kokosi, A. Nair, R. Karwoski, S. L. Walsh, A. U. Wells, and D. M. Hansell, "Mortality prediction in idiopathic pulmonary fibrosis: evaluation of computer-based CT analysis with conventional severity measures," *European Respiratory Journal*, vol. 49, no. 1, 2017, ISSN: 13993003. https://doi.org/10.1183/13993003.010112016. [Online]. Available: http://dx.doi.org/10.1183/13993003.01011-2016.

26. F. Gentile, A. Aimo, F. Forfori, G. E. Catapano, A. Clemente, F. Cademartiri, M. Emdin, and A. Giannoni, "COVID-19 and risk of pulmonary fibrosis: the importance of planning ahead," https://doi.org/10.1177/2047487320932695.

27. B. Sul, L. Flors, J. Cassani, M. J. Morris, J. Reifman, T. Altes, and A. Wallqvist, "Volumetric characteristics of idiopathic pulmonary fibrosis lungs: Computational analyses of high-resolution computed tomography images of lung lobes," *Respiratory Research*, vol. 20, no. 1, p. 216, Oct. 2019. ISSN: 1465993X. https://doi.org/10.1186/s12931-019-1189-5. [Online]. Available: https://

respiratory-research.biomedcentral.com/articles/10.1186/s12931-019-1189-5.

28. A. Mansoor, U. Bagci, B. Foster, Z. Xu, G. Z. Papadakis, L. R. Folio, J. K. Udupa, and D. J. Mollura, "Segmentation and image analysis of abnormal lungs at CT: Current approaches, challenges, and future trends," *Radiographics*, vol. 35, no. 4, pp. 1056–1076, Jul. 2015, ISSN: 15271323. https://doi.org/10.1148/rg.2015140232. [Online]. Available: /pmc/articles/ PMC4521615/?report = abstract%20https://www.ncbi.nlm.nih.gov/pmc/articles/PMC4521615/.

29. Y. Wu, L. Liu, C. Pu, W. Cao, S. Sahin, W. Wei, and Q. Zhang, "A Comparative Measurement Study of Deep Learning as a Service Framework," https://doi.org/10.1109/tsc.2019.2928551.

30. E. Bisong and E. Bisong, "Google Colaboratory," in *Building Machine Learning and Deep Learning Models on Google Cloud Platform*, Apress, 2019, pp. 59–64. https://doi.org/10.1007/978- 1- 4842- 4470- 8{\}7. [Online]. Available: https://link.springer.com/chapter/https://doi.org/10.1007/978-1-4842-4470-8 7.

31. T. Carneiro, R. V. M. Da Nobrega, T. Nepomuceno, G. B. Bian, V. H. C. De Albuquerque, and P. P. R. Filho, "Performance Analysis of Google Colaboratory as a Tool for Accelerating Deep Learning Applications," *IEEE Access*, vol. 6, pp. 61677–61685, 2018, ISSN: 21693536. https://doi.org/10.1109/access.2018.2874767.

32. Y. E. Wang, G.-Y. Wei, and D. Brooks, "Benchmarking TPU, GPU, and CPU Platforms for Deep Learning," Jul. 2019. [Online]. Available: http://arxiv.org/abs/1907.10701.

33. "GPU-Based Deep Learning Inference: A Performance and Power Analysis," Tech. Rep., 2015.

34. A. Paszke, S. Gross, F. Massa, A. Lerer, J. Bradbury, G. Chanan, T. Killeen, Z. Lin, N. Gimelshein, L. Antiga, A. Desmaison, A. Kopf, E. Yang, Z. DeVito, M. Raison, A. Tejani, S. Chilamkurthy, B. Steiner, L. Fang, J. Bai, and˜ S. Chintala, "PyTorch: An Imperative Style, High-Performance Deep Learning Library," Dec. 2019. [Online]. Available: http://arxiv.org/abs/1912.01703.

35. *PyCaret Library*. [Online]. Available: https://pycaret.org/.

36. S. Ioffe and C. Szegedy, "Batch normalization: Accelerating deep network training by reducing internal covariate shift," in *32nd International Conference on Machine Learning, ICML 2015*, vol. 1, International Machine Learning Society (IMLS), Feb. 2015, pp. 448–456, ISBN: 9781510810587. [Online]. Available: https://arxiv.org/abs/1502.03167v3.

37. D. P. Kingma and J. L. Ba, "Adam: A method for stochastic optimization," in *3rd International Conference on Learning Representations, ICLR 2015 - Conference Track Proceedings*, International Conference on Learning Representations, ICLR, Dec. 2015. [Online]. Available: https://arxiv.org/abs/1412.6980v9.

38. P. Ramachandran, B. Zoph, and Q. V. Le Google Brain, "SWISH: A SELF-GATED ACTIVATION FUNCTION," Tech. Rep.

A Simulation-Based Method to Study the LQT1 Syndrome Remotely Using the EMI Model

Sebastián Domínguez, Joyce Reimer, Kevin R. Green, Reza Zolfaghari, and Raymond J. Spiteri

Abstract

The COVID-19 pandemic has spurred the development and application of new technologies in telemedicine to overcome limitations on in-person interactions between patients and doctors. In particular, increased use of computer simulations can help us identify underlying mechanisms for pathologies and which treatments may be best suited for them when in-person appointments are not feasible. For example, long QT syndrome (LQTS) is a cardiac condition that can lead to potentially fatal arrhythmias. One of the most common long QT syndromes, LQT1, causes structural abnormalities of potassium ion channels that in turn reduce certain potassium currents at the cellular level in the heart. In this paper, we use the extracellular-membrane-intracellular (EMI) model to simulate the effects of LQTS. The EMI model resolves the detailed characteristics of individual cell membranes, which is where the affected ion channels are localized, thus making it uniquely suitable for studying such effects. We compare simulations from data from healthy cells, cells that exhibit LQT1 syndrome, and cells that have been treated with a drug to restore healthy heart function. These simulations demonstrate that advances in biomedical engineering combined with computer simulation can enhance the power and applicability of telemedicine well beyond the current state.

S. Domínguez
Department of Mathematics and Statistics, University of Saskatchewan, Saskatoon, Saskatchewan S7N 5C9, Canada
e-mail: s.dominguez@usask.ca

J. Reimer
Division of Biomedical Engineering, University of Saskatchewan, Saskatoon, Saskatchewan S7N 5C9, Canada
e-mail: jav630@usask.ca

K. R. Green · R. Zolfaghari · R. J. Spiteri (✉)
Department of Computer Science, University of Saskatchewan, Saskatoon, Saskatchewan S7N 5C9, Canada
e-mail: spiteri@cs.usask.ca

K. R. Green
e-mail: kevin.green@usask.ca

R. Zolfaghari
e-mail: rez299@usask.ca

1 Introduction

The use of telemedicine has risen steadily over the past decade [4, 10]. The benefits it offers to health care are undeniable: shorter wait times for appointments, elimination of in-clinic wait times and travel time, greater access for patients in rural or otherwise remote areas, and lower costs [10, 37]. Until recently, these benefits were still at odds with the status quo of in-person medical treatment, restricting telemedicine to an exception rather than a rule. Since the emergence of COVID-19, however, a healthcare model that is reliant on in-person medical treatment has proven to be inadequate because this model places undue risk on both patients and healthcare providers. In response, there has been a sharp increase in interest from both patients and healthcare providers in using telemedicine services [5]. Fields such as medicine, engineering, computer science, and information technology are continuing to rise to the challenge of developing the technology that is needed to meet this demand.

Computer simulations used to model various systems in the body have a significant role to play in the movement toward telemedicine. Cardiac simulations are one such technology that will add to ways in which physicians can practise medicine in a remote manner. In order for patients to optimally benefit from such technologies, there is a need for cardiac models to be both customizable and accurate. These characteristics will allow the model to take in input that is specific to a patient—disease parameters, medication, implanted devices, etc.—and produce output that is accurate enough to reduce or even eliminate the need for a patient to come in to the clinic for testing. And, as personalized cardiac medicine becomes more prevalent over time [21, 23, 27], cardiac models based on a patient's unique genetic information will have

© Springer Nature Switzerland AG 2021
J. Alja'am et al. (eds.), *Emerging Technologies in Biomedical Engineering and Sustainable TeleMedicine*,
Advances in Science, Technology & Innovation, https://doi.org/10.1007/978-3-030-14647-4_12

the dual benefit of allowing high specificity in diagnosis and treatment of heart conditions along with it being robust to limitations on physical proximity.

In this study, we explore the potential for one particular type of model to contribute to the field of cardiac telemedicine. The extracellular-membrane-intracellular (EMI) model [35] (see also [2,32]) is a recently developed mathematical model that allows for resolution of simulated heart tissue at the cellular level. In order to test the usefulness of the EMI model in cardiac telemedicine, we look at its customizability and fidelity in the context of Long QT Syndrome (LQTS).

LQTS is a heart condition characterized by a prolonged interval between the Q and T waves on an electrocardiogram (ECG) that indicates a delay in ventricular repolarization [7], a necessary step for the next action potential in a heart cell to occur and thus for cardiac contractions to be smooth and coordinated. Individuals with LQTS are prone to cardiac arrhythmias, arrhythmia-induced syncope, and sudden cardiac arrest [1]. LQTS is classified as a channelopathy [27] because it is caused by structural abnormalities in the ion channels that are responsible for conducting cardiac action potentials.

LQTS may be congenital or acquired [28]. If it is congenital, it is caused by an inherited mutation in the genes that encode the various components of different ion channels. The most common type of LQTS is LQT1, caused by a mutation in the KCNQ1 gene [28]. This gene is responsible for the alpha subunit of the KCNQ1/KCNE1 voltage-gated channel, a potassium channel that conducts the slowly activating potassium current, I_{Ks} [7]. I_{Ks} is one of two essential currents implicated in ventricular repolarization [7], and in LQT1, the I_{Ks} current is attenuated [3].

LQT1 syndrome was chosen as the focus in this study because its pathophysiology originates on the membrane, a domain that is omitted in the more homogenized bidomain and monodomain cardiac models [35]. LQT1 was also selected because of its basis in genetics, making it suitable for future applications to personalized cardiac medicine. Although this study focuses on LQT1, it is but one example of possible conditions that may be represented with the EMI model and explored within a telemedicine context.

To demonstrate potential impact on telemedicine, we report the results of three different simulations. First, we simulate a healthy heart using parameters from the cardiac action potential mathematical model of Ten Tusscher and Panfilov [33]. Then, we model LQT1 by adjusting the I_{Ks} conductance (G_{Ks}) to match experimentally determined disease parameters from [20]. Because β-adrenergic stimulation through exercise is known to be arrhythmogenic in individuals with LQT1 syndrome [17], we subsequently add sympathetic activation to our LQT1 simulation to demonstrate the pronounced arrhythmia. And finally, we show the effects of treating this variant of LQT1 with

β-blockers because they are typically the first line of action for prophylactic management of LQT Syndrome [24].

The remainder of this paper is organized as follows. In Sect. 2, we describe the mathematical details behind the simulations, including the simulation domain, the EMI model, and the numerical methods used to solve it. In Sect. 3, we describe the results from the simulations performed. In Sect. 4, we discuss the implications of the results in the context of telemedicine. Finally, in Sect. 5, we offer some conclusions based on this study and potential future directions.

2 Methods

In this section, we present the details behind the simulations, including the simulation domain, the EMI model, and the numerical methods used to solve the system of equations associated with the simulations.

2.1 Simulation Domain

The EMI model is a mathematical description for representing the behavior of excitable cells in living tissue. This model considers three physical domains: the extracellular space, the cell membrane, and the intracellular space. The tissue is described as the collection of cells interacting with each other through their membranes and distributed across the extracellular space. The EMI model represents a more detailed description of the structure of excitable tissue at the cellular level than that of homogenized models such as the bidomain or monodomain models; see, e.g., [36]. In the particular case of cardiac tissue, the use of the EMI model can help us to study cardiac conditions originating at the cellular level, especially in the case of diseases or conditions that homogenized models are not able to simulate [35]. LQT1 syndrome is another example of such a condition because its pathophysiology starts on the membrane of cardiac cells. Accordingly, we use the EMI model to study LQT1 syndrome to explicitly describe action potentials and currents on the cell membrane.

Full simulations of the heart or its subsystems have high computational requirements; see, e.g., [26] and references therein. For example, the number of cardiac cells in a full human heart is approximately two or three billion; see, e.g., [34]. In particular, this means that the computational cost of implementing the EMI model is high. Arguably, the computational requirements needed to simulate such a system may be beyond today's readily available computing power. In the meantime, the main goal of this study is to suggest a computational framework that can help professionals in telemedicine provide diagnoses or treatments in a timely manner without the need for specialized computing equipment. In particular for this study, we are interested in

Fig. 1 Depiction of the simulation domain

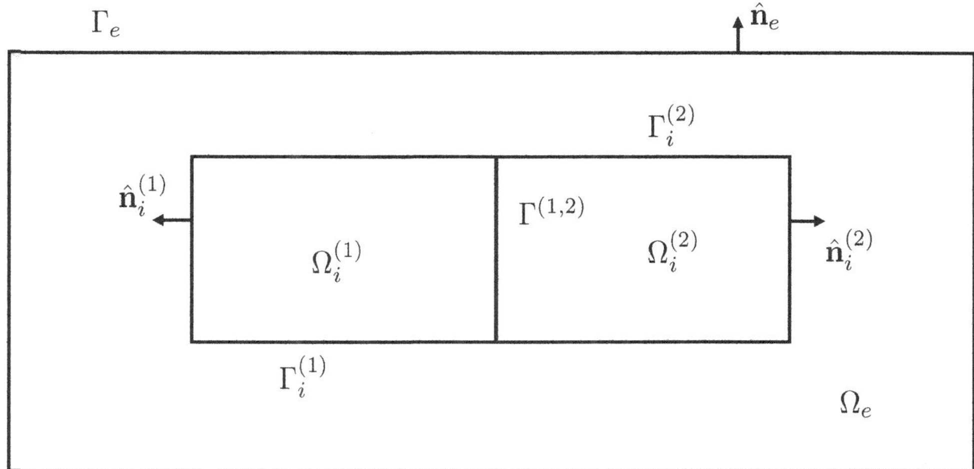

comparing the behavior of myocardial cells of patients with LQT1 syndrome to healthy myocardial cells. In doing this, we demonstrate that it is possible to capture the main effects of a condition like LQT1 in a telemedicine setting using simulations on simplistic geometries representing the basic structure of cardiac tissue and potentially explore treatment options. To achieve this, we set our simulation domain Ω to be a rectangle that contains two cardiac cells represented by two smaller rectangles of the same size that are completely inside Ω. These cells are connected to each other along one of their sides to allow them to interact during the simulations in the same way that gap junctions electrically couple neighboring cardiac cells *in vivo*.

We take Ω to have dimension $400\,\mu$m (in the x direction) by $100\,\mu$m (in the y direction), representing a two-dimensional slice of cardiac tissue. Within this rectangle, we place two smaller rectangles $\Omega_i^{(1)}$ and $\Omega_i^{(2)}$; these domains represent two cells connected along one of their sides. Both domains are of dimensions $140\,\mu$m (in the x direction) by $20\,\mu$m (in the y direction), in accordance with experimental data from [14]. The space outside the cells $\Omega_i^{(k)}$, $k = 1, 2$, and inside Ω represents the extracellular tissue and is denoted by Ω_e.

The interface between these two heart cells is denoted by $\Gamma^{(1,2)}$, and the interfaces between the cells $\Omega_i^{(k)}$ and Ω_e are denoted by $\Gamma_i^{(k)}$, $k = 1, 2$. The outer boundary of Ω_e is denoted by Γ_e. On the outer boundary Γ_e, the unit normal vector is denoted by $\hat{\mathbf{n}}_e$. On the boundaries of the cells $\Omega_i^{(k)}$, $k = 1, 2$, the unit normal vectors $\hat{\mathbf{n}}_i^{(k)}$ are chosen to point outwards from each cell. In particular, we see that $\hat{\mathbf{n}}_i^{(1)} = -\hat{\mathbf{n}}_i^{(2)}$ on the interface $\Gamma^{(1,2)}$. See Fig. 1 for a depiction of the simulation domain.

2.2   The EMI Model

We now introduce the EMI model used to simulate the interaction of cells represented by the domains described in the previous section.

With the notation as described before, we seek an extracellular potential u_e over the extracellular sub-domain Ω_e, intracellular potentials $u_i^{(k)}$ over the intracellular sub-domains $\Omega_i^{(k)}$, $k = 1, 2$, and current densities $I_m^{(k)}$ and $I^{(1,2)}$ over the interfaces $\Gamma_i^{(k)}$, $k = 1, 2$, and $\Gamma^{(1,2)}$, respectively, that satisfy the following equations:

$$-\nabla \cdot (\sigma_e \nabla u_e) = S_e, \qquad \text{in } \Omega_e, \tag{1a}$$

$$-\nabla \cdot (\sigma_i^{(k)} \nabla u_i^{(k)}) = S_i^{(k)}, \qquad \text{in } \Omega_i^{(k)}, \quad k = 1, 2, \tag{1b}$$

$$\frac{\partial v^{(k)}}{\partial t} = \frac{1}{C_m^{(k)}}(I_m^{(k)} - I_{\text{ion}}^{(k)}), \qquad \text{on } \Gamma_i^{(k)}, \quad k = 1, 2, \tag{1c}$$

$$\frac{\partial w}{\partial t} = \frac{1}{C^{(1,2)}}(I^{(1,2)} - I_{\text{gap}}), \qquad \text{on } \Gamma^{(1,2)}. \tag{1d}$$

The parameters σ_e and $\sigma_i^{(k)}$, $k = 1, 2$, are conductivities given in mS/cm, and the constants $C_m^{(k)}$, $k = 1, 2$, and $C^{(1,2)}$ represent capacitances given in μF/cm^2. The quantities S_e and $S_i^{(k)}$, $k = 1, 2$, are known source terms defined on Ω_e and $\Omega_i^{(k)}$, respectively, and $I_{\text{ion}}^{(k)}$ and I_{gap} are current densities that may depend on the transmembrane potentials $v^{(k)}$, $k = 1, 2$, and w. These potentials are defined by

$$v^{(k)} = u_i^{(k)} - u_e, \qquad \text{on } \Gamma_i^{(k)}, \quad k = 1, 2, \tag{2a}$$

$$w = u_i^{(1)} - u_i^{(2)}, \qquad \text{on } \Gamma^{(1,2)}, \tag{2b}$$

respectively. The equations in (1) are subject to the following boundary and flux conditions:

$$u_e = 0, \qquad \text{on} \quad \Gamma_e, \tag{3a}$$

$$(\sigma_e \nabla u_e) \cdot \hat{\mathbf{n}}_e = -(\sigma_i^{(k)} \nabla u_i^{(k)}) \cdot \hat{\mathbf{n}}_i^{(k)}, \qquad \text{on} \quad \Gamma_i^{(k)},\ k = 1, 2, \tag{3b}$$

$$(\sigma_i^{(2)} \nabla u_i^{(2)}) \cdot \hat{\mathbf{n}}_i^{(2)} = -(\sigma_i^{(1)} \nabla u_i^{(1)}) \cdot \hat{\mathbf{n}}_i^{(1)}, \qquad \text{on} \quad \Gamma^{(1,2)}. \tag{3c}$$

We also have

$$I_m^{(k)} = -(\sigma_i^{(k)} \nabla u_i^{(k)}) \cdot \hat{\mathbf{n}}_i^{(k)}, \qquad \text{on} \quad \Gamma_i^{(k)},\ \quad k = 1, 2, \tag{4a}$$

$$I^{(1,2)} = -(\sigma_i^{(1)} \nabla u_i^{(1)}) \cdot \hat{\mathbf{n}}_i^{(1)}, \qquad \text{on} \quad \Gamma^{(1,2)}. \tag{4b}$$

The current density $I_{\text{ion}}^{(k)}$ on $\Gamma_i^{(k)}$, $k = 1, 2$, is represented by the action potential model introduced in [33], and for brevity we refer to it as the *ten Tusscher–Panfilov (tTP) model*. In the tTP model, the ion current density $I_{\text{ion}}^{(k)}$ not only depends on the potential $v^{(k)}$, $k = 1, 2$, but it also depends on a set of state variables, denoted by $\mathbf{s}^{(k)}$, $k = 1, 2$, satisfying an ODE system

$$\frac{\partial \mathbf{s}^{(k)}}{\partial t} = \mathbf{F}(v^{(k)}, \mathbf{s}^{(k)}), \quad \text{on } \Gamma_i^{(k)}. \tag{5}$$

More details can be found in [33].

The ion current density $I_{\text{ion}}^{(k)}$ is only defined on the membrane of the cells $\Gamma_i^{(k)}$, $k = 1, 2$, and not on the intracellular interface $\Gamma^{(1,2)}$. On this part of the interface, we use a linear (passive) membrane representation of I_{gap}, defined as

$$I_{\text{gap}}(w) = \frac{1}{R^{(1,2)}} w, \quad \text{on } \Gamma^{(1,2)}, \tag{6}$$

where the constant $R^{(1,2)}$ is the resistivity of the membrane represented by $\Gamma^{(1,2)}$.

2.3 Spatial Discretization

We follow a similar approach to that in [35] to discretize the spatial variables of the EMI model in Eq. (1). For the sake of completeness, we discuss the details of such a discrete formulation. Consider a regular triangulation $\mathcal{T}_h$ of Ω such that it conforms to the interfaces $\Gamma = \Gamma_i^{(1)} \cup \Gamma_i^{(2)}$ and $\Gamma^{(1,2)}$. Denote by h the mesh size of the triangulation, defined as the maximum diameter among all the elements in $\mathcal{T}_h$. To discretize the space variables, we first define the flux

$\mathbf{q} \in H(\nabla \cdot; \Omega)$, the potential $u \in L^2(\Omega)$, and the transmembrane potential $v \in H^{1/2}(\Gamma)$ by

$$\mathbf{q} = \begin{cases} \sigma_i^{(k)} \nabla u_i^{(k)}, & \text{in } \Omega_i^{(k)}, \quad k = 1, 2, \\ \sigma_e \nabla u_e, & \text{in } \Omega_e, \end{cases} \tag{7}$$

$$u = \begin{cases} u_i^{(k)}, & \text{in } \Omega_i^{(k)}, \quad k = 1, 2, \\ u_e, & \text{in } \Omega_e, \end{cases} \tag{8}$$

and

$$v|_{\Gamma_i^{(k)}} = v^{(k)}, \quad k = 1, 2. \tag{9}$$

Let $\mathbf{p} \in H(\nabla \cdot; \Omega)$ be a test function, and let $\hat{\mathbf{n}}$ be the normal vector on $\Gamma \cup \Gamma^{(1,2)}$, chosen to point out from the intracellular domains $\Omega_i^{(k)}$, $k = 1, 2$, to the extracellular domain Ω_e, and from $\Omega_i^{(1)}$ to $\Omega_i^{(2)}$. Also, denote by σ a non-zero parameter defined by $\sigma|_{\Omega_i^{(k)}} = \sigma_i^{(k)}, k = 1, 2$, and $\sigma|_{\Omega_e} = \sigma_e$. By (3a), (9), (2b), and (7) and integrating by parts, we obtain

$$\int_\Omega \frac{1}{\sigma} \mathbf{q} \cdot \mathbf{p} = \int_{\Omega_i^{(1)}} \nabla u_i^{(1)} \cdot \mathbf{p} + \int_{\Omega_i^{(2)}} \nabla u_i^{(2)} \cdot \mathbf{p} + \int_{\Omega_e} \nabla u_e \cdot \mathbf{p}$$

$$= -\int_{\Omega_i^{(1)}} u_i^{(1)} \nabla \cdot \mathbf{p} - \int_{\Omega_i^{(2)}} u_i^{(2)} \nabla \cdot \mathbf{p} - \int_{\Omega_e} u_e \nabla \cdot \mathbf{p}$$

$$+ \int_{\partial \Omega_i^{(1)}} u_i^{(1)} \mathbf{p} \cdot \hat{\mathbf{n}}_i^{(1)} + \int_{\partial \Omega_i^{(2)}} u_i^{(2)} \mathbf{p} \cdot \hat{\mathbf{n}}_i^{(2)} + \int_{\partial \Omega_e} u_e \mathbf{p} \cdot \hat{\mathbf{n}}_e$$

$$= -\int_\Omega u \nabla \cdot \mathbf{p} + \int_{\Gamma_i^{(1)}} (u_i^{(1)} - u_e) \mathbf{p} \cdot \hat{\mathbf{n}}_i^{(1)}$$

$$+ \int_{\Gamma_i^{(2)}} (u_i^{(2)} - u_e) \mathbf{p} \cdot \hat{\mathbf{n}}_i^{(2)} + \int_{\Gamma^{(1,2)}} (u_i^{(1)} - u_i^{(2)}) \mathbf{p} \cdot \hat{\mathbf{n}}_i^{(1)},$$

$$= -\int_\Omega u \nabla \cdot \mathbf{p} + \int_\Gamma v \mathbf{p} \cdot \hat{\mathbf{n}} + \int_{\Gamma^{(1,2)}} w \mathbf{p} \cdot \hat{\mathbf{n}}.$$

Moreover, let the source term $S \in L^2(\Omega)$ be defined as $S|_{\Omega_i^{(k)}} = S_i^{(k)}$, $k = 1, 2$, and $S|_{\Omega_e} = S_e$. For $r \in L^2(\Omega)$, we obtain

$$\int_\Omega r \nabla \cdot \mathbf{q} = \int_{\Omega_i^{(1)}} r \nabla \cdot (\sigma_i^{(1)} \nabla u_i^{(1)}) + \int_{\Omega_i^{(2)}} r \nabla \cdot (\sigma_i^{(2)} \nabla u_i^{(2)}) + \int_{\Omega_e} r \nabla \cdot (\sigma_e \nabla u_e)$$

$$= -\int_{\Omega_i^{(1)}} S_i^{(1)} r - \int_{\Omega_i^{(2)}} S_i^{(2)} r - \int_{\Omega_e} S_e r$$

$$= -\int_\Omega S r.$$

Denote $\mathbf{s}|_{\Gamma_i^{(k)}} = \mathbf{s}^{(k)}$, $I|_{\Gamma_i^{(k)}} = I_{\text{ion}}^{(k)}$ and $C|_{\Gamma_i^{(k)}} = C_m^{(k)}$, $k = 1, 2$. By (3b), (3c), (4a), (4b), (7), and (9), we write (1c), (5) and (1d) in the following form:

$$\frac{dv}{dt} = \frac{1}{C}(-\mathbf{q} \cdot \hat{\mathbf{n}} - I(v, \mathbf{s})), \qquad \text{on } \Gamma,$$

$$\frac{d\mathbf{s}}{dt} = \mathbf{F}(v, \mathbf{s}), \qquad \text{on } \Gamma,$$

$$\frac{dw}{dt} = \frac{1}{C^{(1,2)}}(-\mathbf{q} \cdot \hat{\mathbf{n}} - I_{\text{gap}}(w)), \qquad \text{on } \Gamma^{(1,2)}.$$

Thus, the EMI model described by (1), (2), and (3) is reduced to a differential-algebraic equation (DAE) problem as follows: given a source term $S \in L^2(\Omega)$, we are to find the flux $\mathbf{q} \in H(\nabla\cdot\,; \Omega)$, the potential $u \in L^2(\Omega)$ and transmembrane potentials $v \in H^{1/2}(\Gamma)$ and $w \in H^{1/2}(\Gamma^{(1,2)})$, and the state variables $\mathbf{s} \in H^{1/2}(\Gamma)$ satisfying

$$\int_\Omega \frac{1}{\sigma} \mathbf{q} \cdot \mathbf{p} + \int_\Omega u \nabla \cdot \mathbf{p} - \int_\Gamma v \mathbf{p} \cdot \hat{\mathbf{n}} - \int_{\Gamma^{(1,2)}} w \mathbf{p} \cdot \hat{\mathbf{n}} = 0, \quad (11a)$$

$$\int_\Omega r \nabla \cdot \mathbf{q} = -\int_\Omega S r, \tag{11b}$$

$$\frac{dv}{dt} = \frac{1}{C}(-\mathbf{q} \cdot \hat{\mathbf{n}} - I(v, \mathbf{s})), \quad \text{on } \Gamma, \tag{11c}$$

$$\frac{d\mathbf{s}}{dt} = \mathbf{F}(v, \mathbf{s}), \quad \text{on } \Gamma, \tag{11d}$$

$$\frac{dw}{dt} = \frac{1}{C^{(1,2)}}(-\mathbf{q} \cdot \hat{\mathbf{n}} - I_{\text{gap}}(w)), \quad \text{on } \Gamma^{(1,2)}, \tag{11e}$$

for all $\mathbf{p} \in H(\nabla\cdot\,; \Omega)$ and $r \in L^2(\Omega)$.

2.4   Time Evolution via Operator Splitting

The time evolution of the DAE system Eq. (11) is performed using *operator splitting*; e.g., see [6,36] and references therein. Operator splitting is a common divide-and-conquer approach to solving DAEs. The idea is that a given problem can be divided into sub-problems that are easier to handle than the entire problem. For example, specialized solution techniques may exist for some or all of the sub-problems. The desired end result is an algorithm that is either more tractable or efficient than one applied to the problem as a whole.

To this end, we first gather all of the unknowns into the vector $\mathbf{y} = (\mathbf{q}, u, v, \mathbf{s}, w)^T$ and rewrite Eq. (11) as a single DAE system

$$\frac{d}{dt}\mathbf{A}\mathbf{y} = \mathbf{f}^{\{I\}}(\mathbf{y}) + \mathbf{f}^{\{E\}}(\mathbf{y}), \quad \mathbf{y}(0) = \mathbf{y}_0, \tag{12}$$

where $\mathbf{y}_0$ is given, the matrix $\mathbf{A}$ is defined such that the matrix-vector multiplication $\mathbf{A}\mathbf{y}$ results in the following vector:

$$\mathbf{A}\mathbf{y} = \begin{pmatrix} 0 \\ 0 \\ v \\ \mathbf{s} \\ w \end{pmatrix}, \tag{13}$$

and the functions $\mathbf{f}^{\{I\}}$ and $\mathbf{f}^{\{E\}}$ define the splitting. We take

$$\mathbf{f}^{\{I\}}(\mathbf{y}) = \begin{pmatrix} \int_\Omega \frac{1}{\sigma} \mathbf{q} \cdot \mathbf{p} + \int_\Omega u \nabla \cdot \mathbf{p} - \int_\Gamma v \mathbf{p} \cdot \hat{\mathbf{n}} - \int_{\Gamma^{(1,2)}} w \mathbf{p} \cdot \hat{\mathbf{n}} \\ \int_\Omega r \nabla \cdot \mathbf{q} + \int_\Omega S r \\ \frac{1}{C}(-\mathbf{q} \cdot \hat{\mathbf{n}}) \\ 0 \\ \frac{1}{C^{(1,2)}}(-\mathbf{q} \cdot \hat{\mathbf{n}} - I_{\text{gap}}(w)) \end{pmatrix} \tag{14}$$

and

$$\mathbf{f}^{\{E\}}(\mathbf{y}) = \begin{pmatrix} 0 \\ 0 \\ -\frac{1}{C}I(v, \mathbf{s}) \\ \mathbf{F}(v, \mathbf{s}) \\ 0 \end{pmatrix}. \tag{15}$$

Splitting in this way isolates the (nonlinear) cell membrane model, evaluated on the cellular membrane, from the rest of the problem, which is linear. This allows us to apply explicit methods to update the cell variables on Γ and requires only linear solves for applying implicit methods to the rest of the problem.

We apply the first-order Godunov operator splitting to advance the state of the system from t_n to $t_{n+1} = t_n + \Delta t$:

1. Solve $\frac{d}{dt}\mathbf{A}\tilde{\mathbf{y}} = \mathbf{f}^{\{E\}}(\tilde{\mathbf{y}})$ with $\tilde{\mathbf{y}}(t_n) = \mathbf{y}_n$ to find $\tilde{\mathbf{y}}(t_{n+1})$.
2. Solve $\frac{d}{dt}\mathbf{A}\hat{\mathbf{y}} = \mathbf{f}^{\{I\}}(\hat{\mathbf{y}})$ with $\hat{\mathbf{y}}(t_n) = \tilde{\mathbf{y}}(t_{n+1})$ to find $\hat{\mathbf{y}}(t_{n+1})$.
3. Assign $\mathbf{y}_{n+1} = \hat{\mathbf{y}}(t_{n+1})$.

For steps 1 and 2, any time-integration method can be applied in principle, but because the Godunov method introduces a first-order splitting error, there is no advantage in using methods of order higher than one from this perspective. Furthermore, because the cell model equations are nonlinear and not too stiff, there may be advantages to using an explicit method.

For step 1, we use the forward Euler method for N substeps,

$$\mathbf{A}\tilde{\mathbf{y}}_{n,j+1} = \mathbf{A}\tilde{\mathbf{y}}_{n,j} + \frac{\Delta t}{N}\mathbf{f}^{\{E\}}(\tilde{\mathbf{y}}_{n,j}), \quad j = 0, 1, \ldots, N-1, \quad \tilde{\mathbf{y}}_{n,0} = \mathbf{y}_n, \tag{16}$$

to obtain $\tilde{\mathbf{y}}_{n+1} = \tilde{\mathbf{y}}_{n,N}$ as an approximation for $\tilde{\mathbf{y}}(t_{n+1})$. Then, we employ the backward Euler method for step 2. That is, we solve the system

$$\mathbf{A}\hat{\mathbf{y}}_{n+1} - \Delta t \mathbf{f}^{\{I\}}(\hat{\mathbf{y}}_{n+1}) = \mathbf{A}\tilde{\mathbf{y}}_{n+1}, \qquad (17)$$

for $\hat{\mathbf{y}}_{n+1}$ as an approximation for $\hat{\mathbf{y}}(t_{n+1})$. With these two methods, we think of the discrete time solution to Eq. (11) having fixed timesteps of size Δt, where we must update the cell model using smaller timesteps of size $\Delta t/N$ with $N > 1$ to maintain stability of the cell model ODE solutions.

Overall Algorithm

Inputs: v and w at $t_0 = 0$, time step size Δt, and final time t_f
$n = 0$
while ($t_n < t_f$)
     Compute $\tilde{\mathbf{y}}_{n+1}$ by (16)
     Solve (17) for $\hat{\mathbf{y}}_{n+1}$
     $\mathbf{y}_{n+1} = \hat{\mathbf{y}}_{n+1}$
     $t_{n+1} = t_n + \Delta t$
     $n \leftarrow n + 1$
end while

The finite element method was used to solve the linear system in (17). We employ an RT1-P1d-P1c-P1c scheme, where RT1 denotes the Raviart–Thomas finite element of order one, P1d is the piecewise linear finite element, and P1c is the continuous linear finite element on both interfaces Γ and $\Gamma^{(1,2)}$. The flux $\mathbf{q}$ is discretized with RT1 elements, the potential u is discretized with P1d elements, and the transmembrane potentials v and w are discretized with P1c elements defined on the interfaces.

Algorithm 2.4 outlines the general procedure of the operator splitting method applied to perform the simulations reported. This algorithm was fully implemented in the FreeFem++ library [15]. The tTP model was obtained from the CellML repository [9] and converted to the correct format with the OpenCOR environment [12] to be able to incorporate the cell model in the FreeFem++ library.

3   Results

We now present simulations of the EMI model with the use of the methods discussed in the previous section. In the first simulation, we consider the parameters and measurements corresponding to healthy heart cells. In the second simulation, we modify certain parameters to simulate cells that exhibit LQT1 syndrome. We compare the action potential duration up to 90% repolarization (APD90) and I_{Ks} activity of both under baseline conditions as well as in the presence of sympathetic activation through β-adrenergic receptors of the heart to mimic the effects of exercise on individuals with LQT1, a common trigger for arrhythmia. We then conduct a final simu-

Table 1 Parameters for the EMI model common to all simulations

Parameter	Value
$C_m^{(1)}$	$1\,\mu\mathrm{F/cm}^2$
$C_m^{(2)}$	$1\,\mu\mathrm{F/cm}^2$
$C^{(1,2)}$	$1\,\mu\mathrm{F/cm}^2$
$\sigma_i^{(1)}$	$5\,\mathrm{mS/cm}$
$\sigma_i^{(2)}$	$5\,\mathrm{mS/cm}$
σ_e	$20\,\mathrm{mS/cm}$
$R^{(1,2)}$	$0.0015\,\mathrm{kVcm}^2/\mathrm{A}$

Table 2 Parameters used in simulations as percentages of values from ten Tusscher and Panfilov [33]

Simulation	G_{Ks} (%)	G_{CaL} (%)
Control baseline	100	100
Control + Sympathetic activation	100	300
LQT1 baseline	13	100
LQT1 + Sympathetic activation	13	300
LQT1 + β-blocker	13	50

lation in which we observe the theoretical effects of β-blocker therapy on an individual presenting with LQT1.

The EMI model and the tTP model require parameter values such as conductances and resistivities. The parameters for the EMI model that are common to all the simulations are presented in Table 1. The parameters needed in the tTP model can be found in [33]. Changes made to the tTP parameter values for the various simulations are found in Table 2. The parameters G_{Ks} and G_{CaL} are expressed as percentages used to modify the conductance parameters in the I_{Ks} and L-type I_{Ca} currents.

A stimulus current with a magnitude of $52\,\mu\mathrm{A}/\mu\mathrm{F}$ is applied in 1 ms pulses to the tTP model on the left side of cell 1. All measurements are taken from the center of the right side of cell 2 so that an action potential is only observed when the applied stimulus initiates one that propagates through the cells.

3.1   Baseline LQT1 Activity

Parameters for LQT1 syndrome were generated by adjusting I_{Ks} conductance (G_{Ks}) at a point in the membrane domain to match experimentally determined APD90 and I_{Ks} current density curves from [20]. Experimental data were acquired from human-induced pluripotent stem cell cardiomyocytes from an LQT1 patient with a mutation (heterozygous deletion of exon 7) in the pore region of the KCNQ1 channel. A

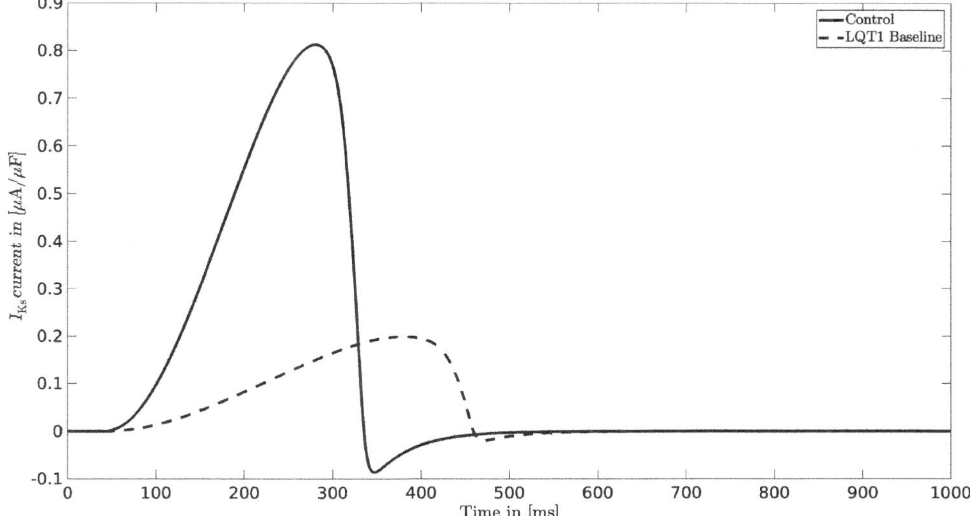

Fig. 2 Current density I_{Ks} of healthy tissue (solid line) and tissue with LQT1 (dashed line)

current density plot of I_{Ks} acquired from our simulations can be seen in Fig. 2. It shows an approximately 75.6% reduction in I_{Ks} current density in a cell with LQT1 compared with the control; this reduction is well within the range of reported experimental data [3,7,20,22].

3.2 LQT1 Activity with Activation of Sympathetic Nervous System

It is known that β-adrenergic stimulation, often coupled with exercise, is arrhythmogenic in individuals with LQT1 syndrome [29,31]. In order to observe these effects, sympathetic activity was simulated by adjusting the conductance (G_{CaL}) of the L-type calcium current (I_{Ca}) until I_{Ca}-voltage curves in the range of pharmacologically induced sympathetic activity was achieved [13]. Calcium current peaks approximately doubled upon a threefold increase of G_{CaL} relative to baseline values. Pacing frequencies of 1.0 Hz, 2.0 Hz, and 2.5 Hz were applied to observe effects of sympathetic activity coupled with both resting and active heart rates.

An action potential of healthy and LQT1 cells is shown in Fig. 3, both in the presence and absence of sympathetic activation. There was an approximately 23% increase in APD90 between the baseline control and the control with sympathetic activation; such an increase is in the range of experimentally determined data [11,19]. APD90 of LQT1 cells was increased by approximately 37% compared with control, also in accordance with the same experimental data cited in the previous section [20]. APD90 of LQT1 cells with sympathetic activation was prolonged further by approximately 47%, slightly

lower than but still within the range of the 52% reported in [19].

Our results demonstrate that a noticeable difference in APD can be both simulated and observed in a healthy individual compared to an individual with LQT1 syndrome. Our simulation also shows that LQT1 symptoms are more pronounced when coupled with sympathetic tone, in agreement with experimentally determined data [17,19,30]. Traces can be found in Fig. 4, showing the shape of the action potentials of healthy cells with sympathetic tone (top) versus the action potentials of LQT1 cells with sympathetic tone (middle), both paced at a slightly active heart rate 2 Hz. Early afterdepolarizations (EADs) are seen in the LQT1 traces, a hallmark feature of LQT syndromes [19]. These indicate that the cell did not have enough time to repolarize before the next stimulus, thus increasing the risk for an arrhythmia to occur. Similar results not shown here were observed at a pacing frequency of 2.5 Hz.

The first line of action for prophylactic management of LQT Syndrome is the use of β-blockers [24]. However, β-blockers have proven to be more effective for LQT1 compared with other LQT syndromes [25]. It has also been shown that β-blockers are more effective for certain genetic variants of LQT1 compared with others [18]. We show here that the action of β-blockers, i.e., attenuated sympathetic activity, can be represented using a cardiac model. In order to do this, we partially restrict L-type I_{Ca} activity by reducing G_{CaL} by 50%. After doing that, the APD90 was reduced to close to the control value: from an approximately 37% prolongation to only approximately 1% (Fig. 5). We observe these rectifying effects also in the presence of a higher pacing frequency, simulating a slightly elevated heart rate (see bottom trace of Fig. 4).

Fig. 3 Action potential of a healthy cell (solid line), a healthy cell in the presence of sympathetic activation (dashed-dotted line), a cell with LQT1 (dashed line), and a cell with LQT1 in the presence of sympathetic activation (dotted line)

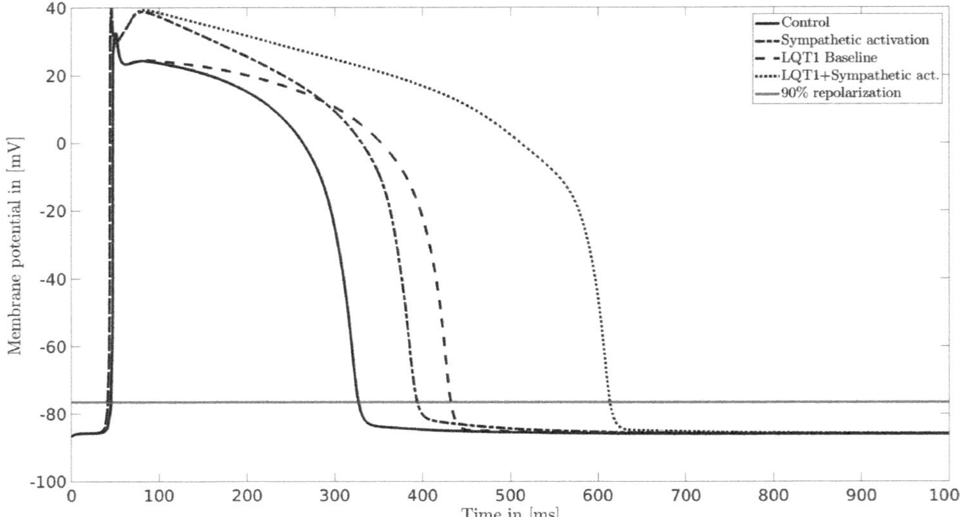

Fig. 4 Action potential traces of healthy cells with sympathetic activation (top, solid line), LQT1 cells with sympathetic activation (middle, dashed line), and LQT1 cells in the presence of simulated β-blockers (bottom, dotted line)

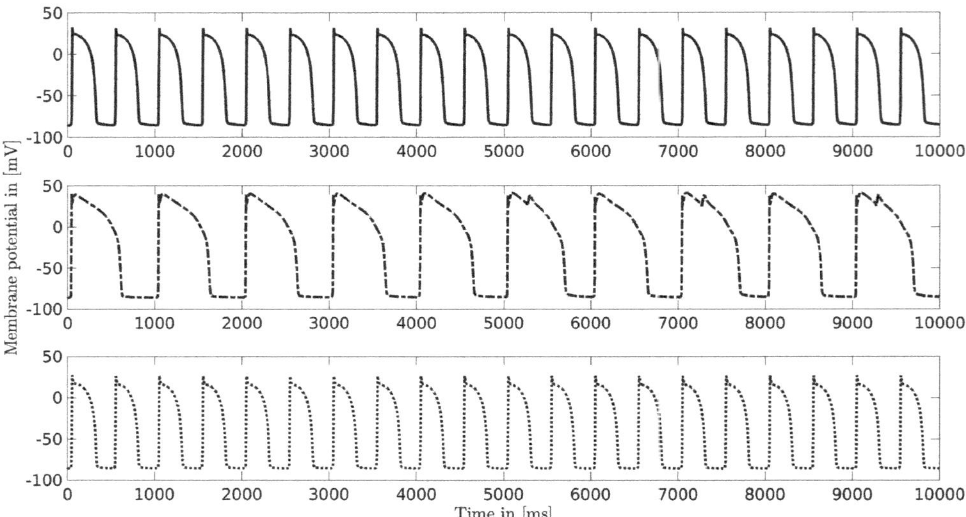

Fig. 5 Action potential of control (solid line), LQT1 (dashed line), and LQT1 in the presence of β-blockers (dotted line)

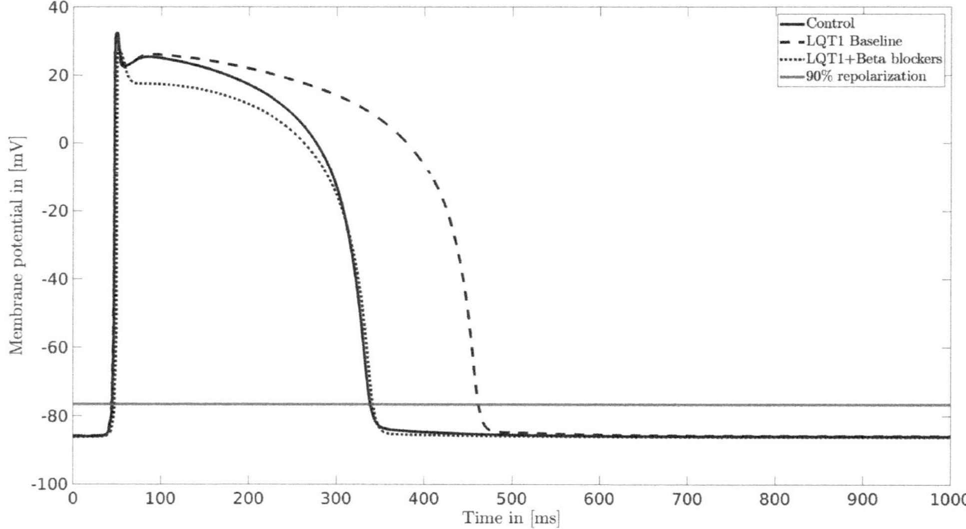

4   Discussion

Through the use of the EMI model, cardiac simulations can assist in the observation, diagnosis, and treatment of LQT1 syndrome in both clinical and telemedicine settings. Cardiac simulation models have recently drawn attention for their potential in advancing precision medicine [8]. The quality of diagnosis and treatment delivery in the field of cardiovascular medicine can be greatly improved by the use of personalized cardiac models. In a context where personalized models are becoming an integral part of the vision of health care, cardiac models have a directly beneficial role to play in telemedicine. In the case of a patient suspected to have LQT Syndrome, they could submit a genetic sample by mail, and a cardiac model resolved at the cellular level could be constructed for them on the basis of their unique genetic code. A physician could then conduct a remote analysis using the simulation to observe whether there is a prolongation of the action potential duration. Furthermore, if the physician found no differences initially, they could simulate exercise using the model, thus inducing sympathetic tone, and this may reveal arrhythmogenic mechanisms that were missed previously, potentially leading to a diagnosis. A benefit of this even in an in-person setting is that it would allow for diagnoses to be made without needing to induce arrhythmia in real time—something that is both difficult to do remotely and risky whether in-person or not.

We have also shown that this technology can aid in a more accurate determination of treatment for LQT1 syndrome. Although LQT1 syndrome always affects the I_{Ks} current, it is caused by different mutations that alter the KCNQ1/KCNE1 channel in various ways [18,25]. This may cause patients to react to treatments differently. The ability to identify exactly which parameter is affected by a specific mutation allows for greater specificity when determining a treatment. Currently, the standard method of treatment for LQTS is β-blockers [24]. Using the cardiac model such as the one we have presented, the effects of β-blockers could be realistically emulated, and a physician would be able to see whether the effects it would have on their patient's heart would be beneficial or not.

In addition, although we did not explore other LQT syndromes in this paper, the unique parameters of each one may be programmed into the model to allow a physician to distinguish between LQT syndromes. There are different arrhythmogenic triggers for each one [16], and the effects of these triggers could also be simulated in the same way that exercise was simulated for LQT1 in this study. A promising treatment could then be selected for the patient based on their particular form of LQTS. Such a procedure could of course be extended to many other cardiac conditions.

5   Conclusions

Whether it is due to transportation challenges, long wait times, or a public health risk such as COVID-19, it is not always possible for a patient to receive prompt in-person medical attention. In the case of LQT syndrome, these challenges may result in serious consequences for patient health, including arrhythmia and cardiac arrest. In this study, we obtained the parameters needed for both healthy cardiac tissue and cardiac tissue known to have LQT1 syndrome and demonstrated that this disease can be accurately represented at the cellular level using the EMI model. We also showed that triggers and therapies can be explored for this syndrome remotely, without ever putting the patient at risk. Using the EMI model, we have outlined how heart simulations can offer a solution to the challenges of cardiac telemedicine by being both accurate and customizable. Along those lines, we described how heart simulations may contribute to the field of personalized medicine, whether in-person or remotely.

References

[1] Abrams, D.J., Macrae, C.A.: Long QT syndrome. Circulation **129**(14), 1524–1529 (2014). https://doi.org/10.1161/CIRCULATIONAHA.113.003985

[2] Agudelo-Toro, A., Neef, A.: Computationally efficient simulation of electrical activity at cell membranes interacting with self-generated and externally imposed electric fields. Journal of neural engineering **10**(2), 026019 (2013)

[3] Aidery, P., Kisselbach, J., Schweizer, P.A., Becker, R., Katus, H.A., Thomas, D.: Biophysical properties of mutant KCNQ1 S277L channels linked to hereditary long QT syndrome with phenotypic variability. Biochimica et Biophysica Acta - Molecular Basis of Disease **1812**(4), 488–494 (2011). https://doi.org/10.1016/j.bbadis.2011.01.008

[4] Barnett, M.L., Ray, K.N., Souza, J., Mehrotra, A.: Trends in Telemedicine Use in a Large Commercially Insured Population, 2005-2017. JAMA **320**(20), 2147–2149 (2018). https://doi.org/10.1001/jama.2018.12354

[5] Bestsennyy, O., Gilbert, G., Harris, A., Rost, J.M..C.: Telehealth: A post-COVID-19 reality? (2020). https://www.mckinsey.com/industries/healthcare-systems-and-services/our-insights/telehealth-a-quarter-trillion-dollar-post-covid-19-reality

[6] Cervi, J., Spiteri, R.J.: High-order operator splitting for the bidomain and monodomain models. SIAM J. Sci. Comput. **40**(2), A769–A786 (2018). https://doi.org/10.1137/17M1137061

[7] Chen, J., Weber, M., Yon Um, S., Walsh, C.A., Tang, Y., McDonald, T.V.: A dual mechanism for I Ks current reduction by the pathogenic mutation KCNQ1-S277L. PACE - Pacing and Clinical Electrophysiology **34**(12), 1652–1664 (2011). https://doi.org/10.1111/j.1540-8159.2011.03190.x

[8] Corral-Acero, J., Margara, F., Marciniak, M., Rodero, C., Loncaric, F., Feng, Y., Gilbert, A., Fernandes, J.F., Bukhari, H.A., Wajdan, A., Martinez, M.V., Santos, M.S., Shamohammdi, M., Luo, H., Westphal, P., Leeson, P., DiAchille, P., Gurev, V., Mayr, M., Geris, L., Pathmanathan, P., Morrison, T., Cornelussen, R., Prinzen, F., Delhaas, T., Doltra, A., Sitges, M., Vigmond, E.J., Zacur, E., Grau, V., Rodriguez, B., Remme, E.W., Niederer, S., Mortier, P., McLeod, K., Potse, M., Pueyo, E., Bueno-Orovio, A., Lamata, P.: The 'Digital Twin' to enable the vision of precision cardiology. European Heart Journal (2020). https://doi.org/10.1093/eurheartj/ehaa159. Ehaa159

[9] Cuellar, A.A., Lloyd, C.M., Nielsen, P.F., Bullivant, D.P., Nickerson, D.P., Hunter, P.J.: An overview of cellml 1.1, a biological model description language. SIMULATION 79(12), 740–747 (2003). https://doi.org/10.1177/0037549703040939

[10] Dorsey, E.R., Topol, E.J.: State of telehealth. New England Journal of Medicine 375(2), 154–161 (2016). https://doi.org/10.1056/NEJMra1601705. PMID: 27410924

[11] Eckel, L., Gristwood, R.W., Nawrath, H., Owen, D.A., Satter, P.: Inotropic and electrophysiological effects of histamine on human ventricular heart muscle. The Journal of Physiology 330(1), 111–123 (1982). https://doi.org/10.1113/jphysiol.1982.sp014332

[12] Garny, A., Hunter, P.J.: OpenCOR: a modular and interoperable approach to computational biology. Frontiers in Physiology 6, 26 (2015). https://www.frontiersin.org/article/10.3389/fphys.2015.00026

[13] Gaur, N., Rudy, Y., Hool, L.: Contributions of ion channel currents to ventricular action potential changes and induction of early afterdepolarizations during acute hypoxia. Circulation Research 105(12), 1196–1203 (2009). https://doi.org/10.1161/CIRCRESAHA.109.202267

[14] Gerdes, A.M., Kellerman, S.E., Moore, J.A., Muffly, K.E., Clark, L.C., Reaves, P.Y., Malec, K.B., Mckeown, P.P., Schocken, D.D.: Structural remodeling of cardiac myocytes in patients with ischemic cardiomyopathy. Circulation 86(2), 426–430 (1992). https://doi.org/10.1161/01.CIR.86.2.426

[15] Hecht, F.: New development in freefem++. J. Numer. Math. 20(3-4), 251–265 (2012). https://freefem.org/

[16] Hintsa, T., Puttonen, S., Toivonen, L., Kontula, K., Swan, H., Keltikangas-Järvinen, L.: A history of stressful life events, prolonged mental stress and arrhythmic events in inherited long QT syndrome. Heart 96(16), 1281–1286 (2010). https://doi.org/10.1136/hrt.2009.190868

[17] Jost, N., Virág, L., Bitay, M., Takács, J., Lengyel, C., Biliczki, P., Nagy, Z., Bogáts, G., Lathrop, D.A., Papp, J.G., Varró, A.: Restricting Excessive Cardiac Action Potential and QT Prolongation. Circulation 112(10), 1392–1399 (2005). https://doi.org/10.1161/CIRCULATIONAHA.105.550111

[18] Kobori, A., Sarai, N., Shimizu, W., Nakamura, Y., Murakami, Y., Makiyama, T., Ohno, S., Takenaka, K., Ninomiya, T., Fujiwara, Y., Matsuoka, S., Takano, M., Noma, A., Kita, T., Horie, M.: Additional gene variants reduce effectiveness of beta-blockers in the LQT1 form of long QT syndrome. Journal of Cardiovascular Electrophysiology 15(2), 190–199 (2004). https://doi.org/10.1046/j.1540-8167.2004.03212.x

[19] Liu, G., Choi, B., Ziv, O., Li, W., De Lange, E., Qu, Z., Koren, G.: Differential conditions for early after-depolarizations and triggered activity in cardiomyocytes derived from transgenic LQT1 and LQT2 rabbits. Journal of Physiology 590(5), 1171–1180 (2012)

[20] Ma, D., Wei, H., Lu, J., Huang, D., Liu, Z., Loh, L.J., Islam, O., Liew, R., Shim, W., Cook, S.A.: Characterization of a novel KCNQ1 mutation for type 1 long QT syndrome and assessment of the therapeutic potential of a novel IKs activator using patient-specific induced pluripotent stem cell-derived cardiomyocytes. Stem Cell Research & Therapy 6(1), 39 (2015). https://doi.org/10.1186/s13287-015-0027-z

[21] Matsa, E., Burridge, P.W., Wu, J.C.: Human stem cells for modeling heart disease and for drug discovery (2014). www.ScienceTranslationalMedicine.org

[22] Moretti, A., Bellin, M., Welling, A., Jung, C.B., Lam, J.T., Bott-Flügel, L., Dorn, T., Goedel, A., Höhnke, C., Hofmann, F., Seyfarth, M., Sinnecker, D., Schömig, A., Laugwitz, K.L.: Patient-specific induced pluripotent stem-cell models for long-qt syndrome. New England Journal of Medicine 363(15), 1397–1409 (2010). https://doi.org/10.1056/NEJMoa0908679. PMID: 20660394

[23] Morini, E., Sangiuolo, F., Caporossi, D., Novelli, G., Amati, F.: Application of Next Generation Sequencing for personalized medicine for sudden cardiac death (SCD). Frontiers in Genetics 5(FEB) (2015). https://www-ncbi-nlm-nih-gov.cyber.usask.ca/pmc/articles/PMC4345839/

[24] Moss, A.J.: Management of patients with the hereditary long qt syndrome. Journal of Cardiovascular Electrophysiology 9(6), 668–674 (1998)

[25] Moss, A.J., Zareba, W., Hall, W.J., Schwartz, P.J., Crampton, R.S., Benhorin, J., Vincent, G.M., Locati, E.H., Priori, S.G., Napolitano, C., Medina, A., Zhang, L., Robinson, J.L., Timothy, K., Towbin, J.A., Andrews, M.L.: Effectiveness and Limitations of Beta-Blocker Therapy in Congenital Long-QT Syndrome. Circulation 101(6), 616–623 (2000). https://doi.org/10.1161/01.CIR.101.6.616

[26] Potse, M., Saillard, E., Barthou, D., Coudière, Y.: Feasibility of Whole-Heart Electrophysiological Models With Near-Cellular Resolution. In: CinC 2020 - Computing in Cardiology. Rimini / Virtual, Italy (2020). https://hal.inria.fr/hal-02943513

[27] Reumann, M., Gurev, V., Rice, J.J.: Computational modeling of cardiac disease: Potential for personalized medicine. Personalized Medicine 6(1), 45–66 (2009). https://doi.org/10.2217/17410541.6.1.45

[28] Robbins, J.: KCNQ potassium channels: Physiology, pathophysiology, and pharmacology. Pharmacology and Therapeutics 90(1), 1–19 (2001). https://doi.org/10.1016/S0163-7258(01)00116-4

[29] Sakaguchi, T., Shimizu, W., Itoh, H., Noda, T., Miyamoto, Y., Nagaoka, I., Oka, Y., Ashihara, T., Ito, M., Tsuji, K., Ohno, S., Makiyama, T., Kamakura, S., Horie, M.: Age- and genotype-specific triggers for life-threatening arrhythmia in the genotyped long QT syndrome. Journal of Cardiovascular Electrophysiology 19(8), 794–799 (2008). https://doi.org/10.1111/j.1540-8167.2008.01138.x

[30] Schreieck, J., Wang, Y., Gjini, V., Korth, M., Zrenner, B., Schömig, A., Schmitt, C.: Differential effect of beta-adrenergic stimulation on the frequency-dependent electrophysiologic actions of the new class iii antiarrhythmics dofetilide, ambasilide, and chromanol 293. Journal of Cardiovascular Electrophysiology 8(12), 1420–1430 (1997)

[31] Schwartz, P., Priori, S., Spazzolini, C., Moss, A.: Genotype-phenotype correlation in the long-QT syndrome: Gene-specific triggers for life-threatening arrhythmias. Circulation 103(1), 89–95 (2001). http://search.proquest.com/docview/212672014/

[32] Stinstra, J., Henriquez, C., MacLeod, R.: Comparison of microscopic and bidomain models of anisotropic conduction. In: 2009 36th Annual Computers in Cardiology Conference (CinC), pp. 657–660 (2009)

[33] Ten Tusscher, K.H.W.J., Panfilov, A.V.: Cell model for efficient simulation of wave propagation in human ventricular tissue under normal and pathological conditions. Physics in Medicine and Biology 51(23), 6141–6156 (2006)

[34] Tirziu, D., Giordano, F.J., Simons, M.: Cell communications in the heart. Circulation 122(9), 928–937 (2010). https://www.ahajournals.org/doi/abs/10.1161/CIRCULATIONAHA.108.847731

[35] Tveito, A., Jæger, K.H., Kuchta, M., Mardal, K.A., Rognes, M.E.: A cell-based framework for numerical modeling of electrical conduction in cardiac tissue. Frontiers in Physics **5**(OCT), 1–18 (2017). https://doi.org/10.3389/fphy.2017.00048

[36] Tveito, A., Mardal, K., Rognes, M.: Modeling Excitable Tissue. Simula SpringerBriefs on Computing. Springer International Publishing (2020). https://www.springer.com/gp/book/9783030611569

[37] Wade, V.A., Karnon, J., Elshaug, A.G., Hiller, J.E.: A systematic review of economic analyses of telehealth services using real time video communication (2010). https://bmchealthservres.biomedcentral.com/articles/10.1186/1472-6963-10-233